Introduction to Epidemiology

FOURTH EDITION

RAY M. MERRILL, PhD, MPH

Brigham Young University
Provo, Utah

THOMAS C. TIMMRECK, PhD

California State University
San Bernardino, California

JONES AND BARTLETT PUBLISHERS
Sudbury, Massachusetts
BOSTON TORONTO LONDON SINGAPORE

World Headquarters
Jones and Bartlett Publishers
40 Tall Pine Drive
Sudbury, MA 01776
978-443-5000
info@jbpub.com
www.jbpub.com

Jones and Bartlett Publishers Canada
6339 Ormindale Way
Mississauga, Ontario
L5V 1J2
CANADA

Jones and Bartlett Publishers International
Barb House, Barb Mews
London W6 7PA
UK

Jones and Bartlett's books and products are available through most bookstores and online booksellers. To contact Jones and Bartlett Publishers directly, call 800-832-0034, fax 978-443-8000, or visit our website, www.jbpub.com.

Substantial discounts on bulk quantities of Jones and Bartlett's publications are available to corporations, pro fessional associations, and other qualified organizations. For details and specific discount information, contact the special sales department at Jones and Bartlett via the above contact information, or send an email to specialsales@jbpub.com.

ISBN-13: 978-0-7637-3582-1
ISBN-10: 0-7637-3582-5

Library of Congress Cataloging-in-Publication Data
Merrill, Ray M.
Introduction to epidemiology.—4th ed. / by Ray M. Merrill, Thomas C. Timmreck.
p. ; cm.
Rev. ed. of: An introduction to epidemiology / Thomas C. Timmreck. 3rd ed. c2002.
Includes bibliographical references and index.
ISBN 0-7637-3582-5
1. Epidemiology. I. Timmreck, Thomas C. II. Timmreck, Thomas C. Introduction to epidemiology. III. Title.
[DNLM: 1. Epidemiologic Methods. 2. Epidemiology.
WA 950
M571t 2005]
RA651.T56 2006
614.4--dc22
6048
200502684

Production Credits
Publisher: Mike Brown
Production Director: Amy Rose
Associate Editor: Kylah Goodfellow McNeill
Production Assistant: Rachel Rossi
Marketing Manager: Marissa Hederson
Manufacturing Buyer: Therese Connell
Composition: Auburn Associates, Inc.
Cover Design: Kristin E. Ohlin
Cover Image: ©James Dawson/Image Farm Inc./Alamy Images
Printing and Binding: Malloy, Inc.
Cover Printing: Malloy, Inc.

Printed in the United States of America
10 09 08 07 06 10 9 8 7 6 5 4 3 2

Dedication

To the memory of my gracious and loving mother
Barbara H. Merrill
(1939–2005)

Contents

About the Authors

Ray M. Merrill, Ph.D., M.P.H. has been actively involved in epidemiology since his professional career began in 1995. As a Cancer Prevention Fellow at the National Cancer Institute, he worked with leading researchers in the area of cancer epidemiology. In 1998 he joined the faculty in the Department of Health Science at Brigham Young University, Provo, Utah, where he continued his research in epidemiology. Since 1999, he has also held an adjunct faculty position in the Department of Family and Preventive Medicine at the University of Utah. In 2001, he spent a sabbatical working in the Unit of Epidemiology for Cancer Prevention at the International Agency for Research on Cancer Administration, Lyon, France. He has won various awards for his research in cancer epidemiology. He currently teaches introductory and advanced level classes in epidemiology and biostatistics. He has more than 100 professional publications in epidemiology and public health journals. Dr. Merrill is currently a full professor of epidemiology and biostatistics at Brigham Young University.

Thomas C. Timmreck, Ph.D. began his professional career in the field of public health, health science, and health services in 1971. His work brought him to public health departments, community health services, hospitals, nursing homes, environmental health services, and both public and private social and health agencies. Dr.Timmreck served on the full-time faculty at Texas Tech University, Idaho State University, Northern Arizona University, and was formerly a Professor of Public Health and Health Care Administration, Department of Health Science and Human Ecology at California State University San Bernardino.

With a Ph.D. in health science from the University of Utah, and two master's degrees, one in community health and community health education from Oregon State University, and one in counseling psychology and human relations and behavior from Northern Arizona University, Dr. Timmreck, a Registered Sanitarian, taught public health and epidemiology courses for more than 23 years.

The author of more than 50 professional publications, and four nationally published books, Dr. Timmreck has added greatly to the fields of public health, health services, long-term care and gerontology, health education and health promotion, and behavioral health. Dr. Timmreck authored the first three editions of *Introduction to Epidemiology,* and asked Dr. Merrill to participate as lead author of this fourth edition.

Preface

The field of epidemiology has come a long way since the days of infectious disease investigations by such scientists as Louis Pasteur, Robert Koch, and John Snow. Historically, the main causes of death were due to a single pathogen, a single cause of disease. Epidemiologists had the challenge of isolating a single bacteria, virus, or parasite. In modern times, advances in nutrition, housing conditions, sanitation, water supply, antibiotics, and immunization programs has resulted in a decrease in various infectious diseases but an increase in many noninfectious diseases and conditions. Consequently, the scope of epidemiology has expanded to include the study of acute and chronic noninfectious diseases and conditions. Advances in biology, medicine, statistics, and social and behavioral sciences have greatly aided epidemiologic study.

This book was written as an introductory epidemiology text for the student who has minimal training in the biomedical sciences and statistics. *Introduction to Epidemiology* is based on the premise that the advanced analysis of empirical research studies, using advanced statistical methods, are more akin to biostatistics than epidemiology and, therefore, are not included in this book. Many recent books bearing the title of epidemiology are in fact biostatistics books, with limited information on the basics of epidemiological investigations or the study of epidemics. Epidemiology is unique from biostatistics in that emphasis is placed on completing the causal picture. Identifying causal factors and modes of transmission, with the assistance of statistical tools and biomedical information, reflects the primary aim of epidemiology. This book maintains that focus.

Chapter 1 presents the foundations of epidemiology, including definitions, concepts, and applications of the field. Chapter 2 covers historical developments in epidemiology. Chapter 3 looks at several important disease concepts in epidemiology. Chapters 4–6 focus on descriptive epidemiology: several design strategies and statistical measures are presented in these chapters. Chapter 7 presents design strategies and statistical methods used in analytic epidemiology. Chapter 8 covers design strategies and ethical issues associated with experimental studies. Chapter 9 considers the basics of statistical associations versus causal associations. Chapter 10 focuses on basic concepts and approaches used field epidemiology. Finally, Chapter 11 presents chronic disease epidemiology.

Preface to the Fourth Edition

Epidemiology is the foundation upon which public health is built. What we know about causes of disease and health-related events, we have learned through epidemiologic study. As the leading causes of disease and death have moved from infectious to noninfectious disease and conditions, epidemiology has advanced accordingly. This fourth edition captures the evolution of the discipline, with a greater emphasis on acute and chronic noninfectious disease than previous editions. This fourth edition also better aligns selected epidemiologic measures with descriptive and analytic epidemiologic studies. Descriptive and analytic research designs used in epidemiology, along with conditions associated with their use, and their strengths and weaknesses, are more fully developed in this edition.

This fourth edition offers an easy and effective approach to learning epidemiology, which includes case reports and news files. The case reports and news files represent applications of commonly used research designs in epidemiology. The chapter topics were selected to represent the fundamentals of epidemiology. Learning objectives are presented at the beginning of each chapter. The chapters are divided into concise sections with several examples. Tables and figures are used to summarize and clarify important concepts and information. Key words are bolded in the text and defined. Study questions with descriptive answers are provided at the end of each chapter.

Foreword

Epidemiology is a fun and challenging subject to study, as well as an interesting field to pursue as a career. Most undergraduate degree programs and graduate programs in public health, environmental health, occupational health and industrial hygiene, health education and health promotion, health services administration, and other health-related degree programs require a basic introductory course in epidemiology. *Introduction to Epidemiology* can also be a valuable guide for practicing epidemiologists. Thus, it is hoped that this book will be a useful and practical source for introductory epidemiology courses, as well as for epidemiologists working in the field. Readers of this book may be specialists in international projects in developing countries, industrial hygienists within major industrial plants, infectious disease nurses in hospitals and medical centers, chronic disease epidemiologists in government agencies, behavioral scientists conducting behavioral health epidemiological investigations, or staff epidemiologists in local public health departments.

CHAPTER

1

Foundations of Epidemiology

OBJECTIVES

After completing this chapter you will be able to

- Define epidemiology.
- Define descriptive epidemiology.
- Define analytic epidemiology.
- Identify some activities performed in epidemiology.
- Explain the role of epidemiology in public health practice and individual decision making.
- Define epidemic, endemic, and pandemic.
- Describe common source, propagated, and mixed epidemics.
- Define the concepts and principles of case as used in epidemiology.
- Describe the epidemiology triangle for infectious disease.
- Describe the advanced epidemiology triangle for chronic diseases and behavioral disorders.
- Define the 3 levels of prevention used in public health and epidemiology.
- Understand the basic vocabulary used in epidemiology.

INTRODUCTION

Epidemiology is the study of the distribution and determinants of health-related states or events in human populations and the application of this study to the prevention and control of health problems.[1] Epidemiology is commonly referred to as the basic science or foundation of public health. The word *epidemiology* is based on the Greek words *epi,* a prefix meaning "on, upon, or befall"; *demos,* a root meaning "the people"; and *logos,* a suffix meaning "the study of." In accordance with medical terminology the suffix is read first, then the prefix and the root. Thus the word epidemiology, taken literally, refers to the study of that which befalls people. An example of a disease that has had widespread consequences on human populations throughout the world is acquired immunodeficiency syndrome (AIDS), caused by the human immunodeficiency virus (HIV). The estimated number of people living with HIV in 2004 was 39.4 million, and the estimated number of AIDS deaths in that same year was 3.1 million.[2]

Epidemiology involves sound methods of scientific investigation. Epidemiologic investigations involve descriptive and analytic methods, which draw on statistical techniques for describing data, and evaluation of hypotheses, biological principles, and causal theory. Both descriptive and analytic epidemiology will be considered at length in later chapters. Briefly, descriptive epidemiology involves characterization of the distribution of health-related states or events. Analytic epidemiology involves finding and quantifying associations, testing hypotheses, and identifying causes of health-related states or events.[3]

Evaluating the distribution of disease means to identify the frequency and pattern of health-related states or events among people in the population. Frequency refers to the number of cases or deaths and the relationship between the number of cases or deaths and the size of the population. Typically the number of cases or deaths is more meaningful when considered in reference to the size of the population, especially when comparing risks of disease among groups. For example, despite differences in population sizes across time or among regions, meaningful comparisons can be made of the burden of HIV/AIDS by using proportions or percentages. In 2004, the estimated percentage of adults 15–49 years of age with HIV/AIDS was 7.4% in sub-Saharan Africa, 2.3% in the Caribbean, 0.8% in Eastern Europe and Central Asia, and 0.6% in North America.[2]

Pattern refers to describing health-related states or events by who is experiencing the health-related state or event (person), where the occurrence of the state or event is highest or lowest (place), and when the state or event occurs most or least (time). In other words, epidemiologists are interested in identifying the people involved and why these people are affected and not others, where the people are affected and why in this place and not others, and when the state or event occurred and why at this time and not others.

For example, in 1981 the Centers for Disease Control and Prevention (CDC) reported that 5 young men went to 3 different hospitals in Los Angeles, California, with confirmed *Pneumocystis carinii* pneumonia. These men were all identified as homosexuals.[4] On July 27, 1982, this illness was called AIDS, and in 1983, the Institut Pasteur in France found the human immunodeficiency virus, which causes AIDS.[5]

Identifying the determinants or determining factors of health-related states or events is a primary function of epidemiology. However, identifying causal associations is complex and typically requires making a judgment about several conditions. A step toward understanding causation is identifying risk factors for disease. A risk factor has been defined as a behavior, environmental exposure, or inherent human characteristic that is associated with an important health condition.[6] In other words, a risk factor is a condition that is associated with the increased probability of a health-related state or event. For example, smoking is a risk factor for chronic diseases such as heart disease, stroke, and several cancers (including cancers of the oral cavity and pharynx, esophagus, pancreas, larynx, lung and bronchus, urinary bladder, kidney and renal pelvis, and cervix).[7–10]

"Health-related states or events" is used in the definition of epidemiology to capture the fact that epidemiology involves more than just the study of disease states (eg, cholera, influenza, pneumonia); it also includes the study of events (eg, injury, drug abuse, and suicide) and of behaviors and conditions associated with health (eg, physical activity, nutrition, seat belt use, and provision and use of health services).

Epidemiology not only involves the study of the distribution and determinants of health-related states or events in human populations, but it also involves the application of this study to the prevention and control of health problems. Results of epidemiologic investigations can provide public health officials with information related to who is at greatest risk for disease, where the disease is most common, when the disease occurs most frequently, and what public health programs might be most effective. Such information may lead to more efficient resource allocation and to more appropriate application of health programs designed to educate, prevent, and control disease. Epidemiologic information can also assist individuals in making informed decisions about their health behavior.

ACTIVITIES IN EPIDEMIOLOGY

An **epidemiologist** studies the occurrence of disease or other health-related events in specified populations, practices epidemiology, and controls disease.[1] Epidemiologists may be involved in a range of activities, which include

- Identifying risk factors for disease, injury, and death
- Describing the natural history of disease
- Identifying individuals and populations at greatest risk for disease
- Identifying where the public health problem is greatest
- Monitoring diseases and other health-related events over time
- Evaluating the efficacy and effectiveness of prevention and treatment programs
- Providing information useful in health planning and decision making for establishing health programs with appropriate priorities
- Assisting in carrying out public health programs
- Being a resource person
- Communicating public health information

The interdependence of these activities is evident. For example, carrying out an intervention program requires clearance from an institutional review board and, often, other organizations and agencies. As is also the case for funding agencies, these groups require quantifiable justification of needs and of the likelihood of success. This presupposes that the risk factors are known, that there is an understanding of the natural history of the disease, and that there are answers to the person, place, and time questions as well as some evidence of the probable success of the intervention. Being a resource person in this process implies that you have a good understanding of the health problem as it relates to the individual and community; the rationale and justification for intervention, along with corresponding goals and objectives; and an ability to communicate in a clear and concise manner.[11] All of this implies a good understanding of epidemiologic methods.

In their professional work, epidemiologists may focus on specific areas, such as epidemiologic methods, infectious disease, chronic disease, oral and dental health epidemiology, pharmacoepidemiology, psychiatric epidemiology, social epidemiology, reproductive epidemiology, and more. Training for these various focus areas is broad, yet the training required in each of the areas typically includes statistics and medicine.

Epidemiologists are employed by the appropriate health agencies at all levels of local, state, and federal government. They find careers in health care organizations, private and voluntary health organizations, hospitals, the military, and private industry. Epidemiologists are also employed by universities and medical schools to teach and/or conduct research.

ROLE OF EPIDEMIOLOGY IN PUBLIC HEALTH PRACTICE

Epidemiologic information plays an important role in meeting public health objectives aimed at promoting physical, mental, and social well-being in the population. Epidemiologic findings contribute to preventing and controlling disease, injury, disability, and death by providing information that leads to informed public health policy and planning as well as individual health decision making. Some useful information provided to health policy officials and individuals through epidemiology is listed in Table 1.1.

Public health assessment identifies if, where, and when health problems occur and serves as a guide to public health planning, policy making, and resource allocation. The state of health of the population should be compared to the availability, effectiveness, and efficiency of current health services. Most areas of the United States have surveillance systems that monitor the morbidity and mortality of the community by person, place, and time. Public health surveillance has been defined as the ongoing systematic collection, analysis, interpretation, and dissemination of health data.[12] Surveillance information about disease epidemics, breakdowns in vaccination or prevention programs, and health disparities among special populations is important for initiating and guiding action.

Accurate assessment requires standard case definitions and adequate levels of reporting. A standard set of criteria, or **case definition**, ensures that cases are consistently diagnosed, regardless of where or when they were identified and who diagnosed the case. Higher levels of reporting ensure accurate representation of the health problem. However, even low levels of reporting can provide important information as to the existence and potential problems of a given health state or event.

When evaluating a prevention or control program, both the efficacy and the effectiveness of the program should be considered. Although these terms are related, they have distinct meanings. **Efficacy** refers to the ability of a program to produce a desired effect among those who participate in the program compared with those who do not.[3,13] **Effectiveness**, on the other hand, refers to the ability of a program to produce benefits among those who are offered the program.[3,13] For example, suppose a strict dietary intervention program is designed to aid in the recovery process of heart attack patients. If those who comply with the program have much better recoveries than those who do not adhere to the program, the program is efficacious. However, if complience is low because of, for example, the amount, cost, and types of foods involved in the program, the program is not effective.

TABLE 1.1 Types of epidemiologic information useful for influencing public health policy and planning and individual health decisions

1. Public health assessment
   - Surveillance
     - Identifying individuals and populations at greatest risk for disease
     - Identifying where the public health problem is greatest
     - Monitoring diseases and other health-related events over time
2. Finding causes of disease
   - Identifying the primary agents associated with disease, disorders, or conditions
   - Identifying the mode of transmission
   - Combining laboratory evidence with epidemiologic findings
3. Completing the clinical picture
   - Identifying who is susceptible to disease
   - Identifying the types of exposures capable of causing disease
   - Describing the pathologic changes that occur, the stage of subclinical disease, and the expected length of this subclinical phase of the disease
   - Identifying the types of symptoms that characterize the disease
   - Identifying probable outcomes (recovery, disability, or death) associated with different levels of the disease
4. Evaluating the program
   - Identifying the efficacy of the public health program
   - Measuring the effectiveness of the public health program

Similarly, suppose a physical activity program involving skiing was shown to be efficacious, but the cost of skiing and the technical skills associated with it made it ineffective in the general public. Finally, it must be taken into account that the administration of some interventions might require the presence of individuals with advanced medical training and technically advanced equipment. In certain communities, lack of available health resources may limit the availability of such programs, making them ineffective although they may be efficacious.

EPIDEMICS, ENDEMICS, AND PANDEMICS

Historically epidemiology was developed in order to investigate epidemics of infectious disease. An **epidemic** is the occurrence in a community or region of cases of an illness, specific health-related behavior, or other health-related events clearly in excess of normal expectancy.[1] Public health officials often use the term *outbreak,* which is used synonymously with epidemic but actually refers to an epidemic confined to a localized area.[6] An epidemic may result from exposure to a common source at a point in time or through intermittent or continuous exposure over days, weeks, or years. An epidemic may also result from exposure propagated through gradual spread from host to host. It is possible for an epidemic to originate from a common source and then, by secondary spread, be communicated from person to person.

The word **"endemic"** refers to the ongoing, usual, or constant presence of a disease in a community or among a group of people; a disease is said to be endemic when it continually prevails in a region.[1] For example, influenza, although it follows a seasonal trend with the highest number of cases in the winter months, is considered endemic if the pattern is consistent from year to year. A **pandemic** is an epidemic affecting or attacking the population of an extensive region, country, or continent.[1]

Several epidemics of cholera have been reported since the early 1800s. In 1816, an epidemic of cholera occurred in Bengal, India, and then became pandemic as it spread across India, extending as far as China and the Caspian Sea before receding in 1826.[14] Other cholera epidemics that also became pandemic involved Europe and North America (1829–1851), Russia (1852–1860), Europe and Africa (1863–1875), Europe and Russia (1899–1923), and Indonesia, El Tor, Bangladesh (India), and the Union of Soviet Socialist Republics (USSR) (1961–1966).[14] Examples of case reports of cholera, provided by John Snow along with descriptions of two cholera epidemics investigated by Snow, are presented in Case Study I: Snow on Cholera (Appendix I).

In the United States, cholera is now classified as an endemic disease. Between 1992 and 1999, the annual numbers of cases reported have been 103, 25, 39, 23, 4, 6, 17, and 6, respectively.[15] Other examples of diseases classified now as endemic in the United States include botulism, brucellosis, and plague.

Epidemics are often described by how they spread through the population. Two primary types of infectious-disease epidemics are common-source and propagated epidemics. **Common-source epidemics** arise from a specific source, whereas **propagated epidemics** arise from infections transmitted from one infected person to another. Transmission can be through direct or indirect routes. Common-source epidemics tend to result in more cases occurring more rapidly and sooner than is seen in host-to-host epidemics. Identifying the common source of exposure and removing it typically causes the epidemic to rapidly abate. On the other hand, host-to-host epidemics rise and fall more slowly. Some examples of common-source epidemic diseases are anthrax, traced to milk or meat from infected animals; botulism, traced to soil-contaminated food; and cholera, traced to fecal contamination of food and water. Some examples of propagated epidemic diseases are tuberculosis, whooping cough, influenza, and measles.

In some diseases, natural immunity or death can decrease the susceptible population. Resistance to the disease can also occur with treatment or immunization, all of which reduce susceptibility. Disease transmission is usually a result of direct person-to-person contact or of contact with fomites, vehicles, or vectors. Syphilis and other sexually transmitted diseases (STDs) are examples of direct transmission. Hepatitis B and HIV/AIDS in needle-sharing drug users are examples of **vehicleborne transmission**. Malaria spread by mosquitoes is an example of **vectorborne transmission**.

Some disease outbreaks may have both common-source and propagated epidemic features. A **mixed epidemic** occurs when victims of a common-source epidemic have person-to-person contact with others and spread the disease, resulting in a propagated outbreak. In some cases it is difficult to determine which came first. During the mid-1980s, at the beginning of the AIDS epidemic in San Francisco, HIV spread rapidly in bathhouses. Homosexual men had sexual contact before entering the bathhouses, yet the bathhouses would be considered the common source aspect of the epidemic, and the person-to-person spread through sexual intercourse would be the source of direct transmission. Direct disease transmission from person-to-person contact occurred in some individuals before and after entering a bathhouse. The bathhouses (the common source) were clearly a point for public health intervention and control, so the bathhouses were closed in an attempt to slow the epidemic.

CASE CONCEPTS IN EPIDEMIOLOGY

When an epidemic is confirmed and the epidemiology investigation begins, one activity of the epidemiologist is to look for and examine cases of the disease. A **case** is a person who has been diagnosed with a disease. Any individual in a population group identified as having a particular disease, disorder, injury, or condition is also considered a case. A clinical record of an individual, someone identified in a screening process, or a person identified from a survey of the population or general data registry can also be an epidemiologic case. Thus the epidemiologic definition of a case is broader than the clinical definition because a variety of criteria can be used to identify cases in epidemiology.

In an epidemic, the first disease case in the population is the **primary case**. The first disease case brought to the attention of the epidemiologist is the **index case**. The index case is not always the primary case. Those persons who become infected and ill once a disease has been introduced into a population and who became infected from contact with the primary case are **secondary cases**. A **suspect case** is an individual (or a group of individuals) who has all of the signs and symptoms of a disease or condition yet has not been diagnosed as having the disease or had the cause of the symptoms connected to a suspected **pathogen** (ie, any virus, microorganism, or other substance that causes disease).[1] For example, a cholera outbreak could be in progress and a person could have vomiting and diarrhea, symptoms consistent with cholera. This is a suspect case; the presence of cholera bacteria in the person's body has not been confirmed, and the disease has not been definitely identified as cholera because it could be one of the other gastrointestinal diseases, such as salmonella food poisoning.

As indicated previously, as epidemics occur across time and in different places, each case must be described in exactly the same way each time in order to standardize disease investigations. As cases occur in each separate epidemic, they must be described and diagnosed consistently—and with the same diagnostic criteria—from case to case. When standard disease diagnosis criteria are used by all the people assisting in outbreak investigations, the epidemiologist can compare the numbers of cases of a disease that occur in one outbreak (numbers of new cases in a certain place and time) with those in different outbreaks of the same disease (cases from different epidemics in different places and times). Computerized laboratory analysis that is now available, even in remote communities, has enhanced the ability of those involved to arrive at a case-specific definition. With advanced computer-assisted support directly and quickly available from the CDC, case definition of almost all diseases has become extremely accurate and specific.

Different levels of diagnosis (suspect, probable, or confirmed) are generally used by the physician who is assisting in epidemic investigations. As more information (such as laboratory results) becomes available to the physician, the physician generally upgrades the diagnosis. When all criteria are met for the case definition, the case is classified as a confirmed case. If the case definition is not matched, then the exposed person is labeled "not a case," and other possible diseases are considered until the case definition fits. Elaborate diagnoses are not always needed in those epidemics in which obvious symptoms can be quickly seen, such as measles and chicken pox.[3]

If people become ill enough to require hospitalization, the severity of the illness is of concern. **Case severity** is found by looking at several variables that are effective measures of it. One such measure is the average length of stay in a hospital. The longer the hospital stay, the greater the severity of the illness. Subjectively, severity is also measured by how disabling or debilitating the illness is, the chances of recovery, how long the person is ill, and how much care the person (case) needs.[16–19]

THE EPIDEMIOLOGY TRIANGLE

When the colonists settled America, they introduced smallpox to the Native Americans. Epidemics became rampant, and entire tribes died as a result. In the 1500s, the entire native population of the island of Jamaica died when smallpox was introduced. Poor sanitation and basic knowledge of disease; the low levels of immunity; the various modes of transmission; and the environmental conditions all allowed such epidemics to run wild and wipe out entire populations. A multitude of epidemiologic circumstances allowed such epidemics to happen. The interrelatedness of 4 epidemiologic factors often contributed to an outbreak of a disease: (1) the role of the host, (2) the agent or disease-causing organism, (3) the environmental circumstances needed for a disease to thrive, survive, and spread, and (4) time-related issues.

The traditional triangle of epidemiology is shown in Figure 1.1. This triangle is based on the communicable disease model and is useful in showing the interaction and interdependence of agent, host, environment, and time as used in the investigation of diseases and epidemics. The **agent** is the cause of the disease; the **host** is an organism, usually a human or an animal, that harbors the disease; the **environment** is those surroundings and conditions external to the human or animal that cause or allow disease transmission; and **time** accounts for incubation periods, life expectancy of the host or the pathogen, and duration of the course of the illness or condition.

Agents of infectious diseases include bacteria, viruses, parasites, fungi, and molds. With regard to noninfectious disease, disability, injury, or death, agents can include chemicals from dietary foods, tobacco smoke, solvents, radiation or heat, nutritional deficiencies, or other substances, such as rattlesnake poison. One or several agents may contribute to an illness.

A host offers subsistence and lodging for a pathogen and may or may not develop the disease. The level of immunity, genetic makeup, level of exposure, state of health, and over-

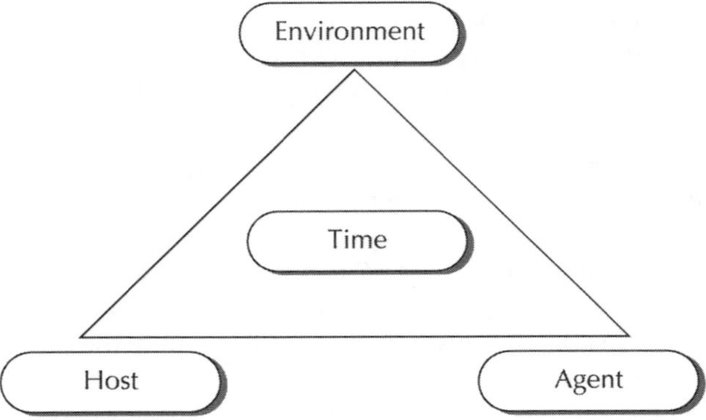

FIGURE 1.1 The Triangle of Epidemiology.

all fitness of the host can determine the effect a disease organism will have on it. The makeup of the host and the ability of the pathogen to accept the new environment can also be a determining factor because some pathogens thrive only under limited ideal conditions. For example, many infectious disease agents can exist only in a limited temperature range.

Environmental factors can include the biological aspects as well as the social, cultural, and physical aspects of the environment. The surroundings in which a pathogen lives and the effect the surroundings have on it are a part of the environment. Environment can be within a host or external to it in the community. Finally, time includes severity of illness in relation to how long a person is infected or until the condition causes death or passes the threshold of danger toward recovery. Delays in time from infection to when symptoms develop, duration of illness, and threshold of an epidemic in a population are time elements with which the epidemiologist is concerned.

The primary mission of epidemiology is to provide information that results in breaking one of the legs of the triangle, thereby disrupting the connection among environment, host, and agent, and stopping the outbreak. On the basis of epidemiologic information, public health efforts are able to prevent and control health-related states and events (Figure 1.2). An epidemic can be stopped when one of the elements of the triangle is interfered with, altered, changed, or removed from existence so that the disease no longer continues along its mode of transmission.

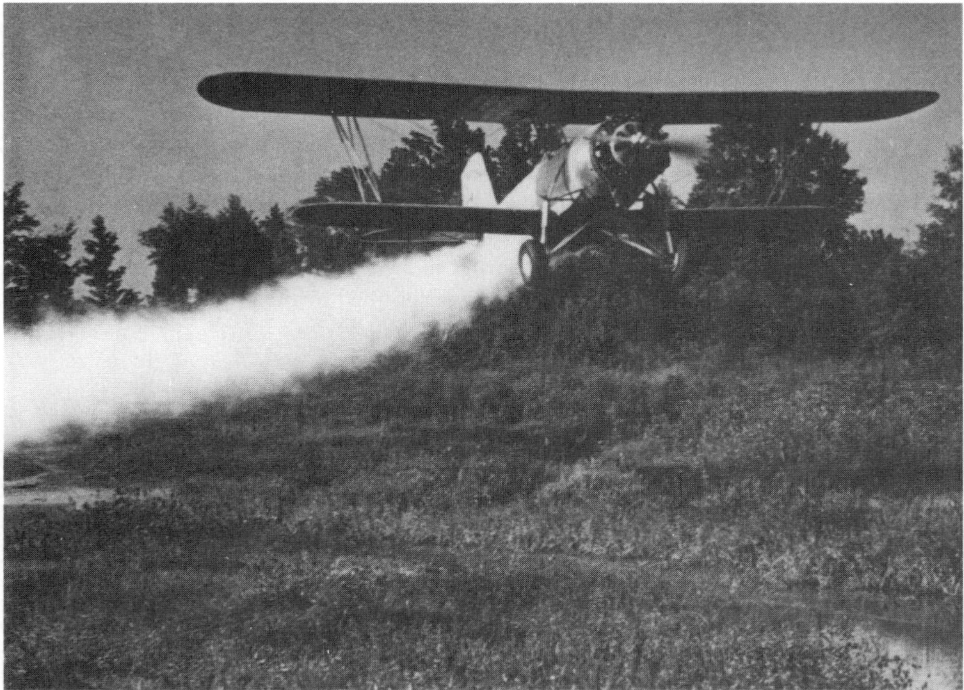

FIGURE 1.2 Airplanes are often used to spray the watery breeding places (environment) of mosquitoes in an effort to kill this *vector* of malaria, St. Louis encephalitis, and yellow fever. (Picture courtesy of Centers for Disease Control and Prevention, Atlanta, Georgia)

SOME DISEASE TRANSMISSION CONCEPTS

Several disease transmission concepts that relate to or influence the epidemiology triangle are fomites, vectors, reservoirs, and carriers.

Fomites (fomes = singular) are objects such as clothing, towels, and utensils that can harbor a disease agent and are capable of transmitting it.[1] An example of transmission of cutaneous anthrax from drums to a woman is shown in Figure 1.3.

A **vector** is an invertebrate animal (eg, tick, mite, mosquito, bloodsucking fly) capable of transmitting an infectious agent among vertebrates.[1] A vector can spread an infectious agent from an infected animal or human to other susceptible animals or humans through its waste products, bite, body fluids, or indirectly through food contamination.

A **reservoir** is the habitat (living or nonliving) in or on which an infectious agent lives, grows, and multiplies and on which it depends for its survival in nature.[1,3] As infectious organisms reproduce in the reservoir, they do so in a manner that allows disease to be transmitted to a susceptible host. Humans often serve as both reservoir and host. A disease transmitted to a human from an animal is referred to as a **zoonosis**. The World Health Organization states that zoonoses are those diseases and infections that are transmitted between vertebrate animals and man.[20]

A **carrier** contains, spreads, or harbors an infectious organism (Figure 1.4). The infected person (or animal) harboring the disease-producing organism often lacks discernible clinical manifestation of the disease, yet the person or animal serves as a potential source of infection and disease transmission to other humans (or animals). The carrier condition can exist throughout the entire course of a disease if it is not treated, and its presence can be unapparent because the carrier may not be sick (healthy carriers). Some people can even be carriers for their entire lives. An example of this was Typhoid Mary (see Chapter 2, "Historic Developments in Epidemiology"). Some carriers can be cured of this condition. Typhoid Mary may have been cured by surgery (removal of the gallbladder provides a cure in 60% of all typhoid carriers). If she had lived in modern times, antibiotics would have been effective.[16–18] Tuberculosis is another example of a disease commonly known to have carriers.

Carriers have been found to have several different conditions or states. Traditionally, five types of carriers have been identified by the public health and medical fields.

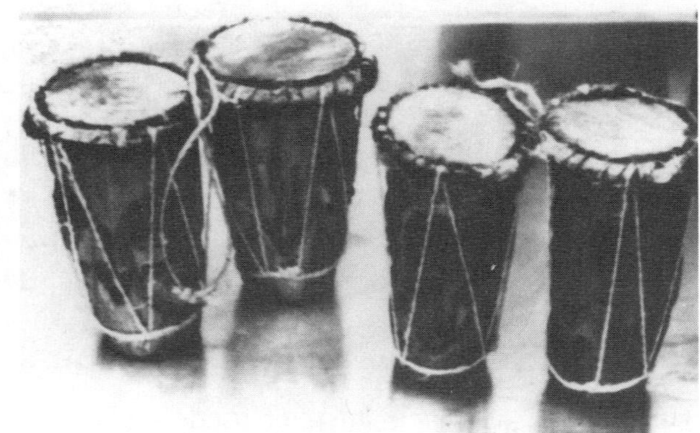

FIGURE 1.3 These drums, purchased in Haiti, served as a *fomite* and were responsible for transmitting cutaneous anthrax to the 22-year-old female who purchased them. (Picture courtesy of Centers for Disease Control and Prevention, Atlanta, Georgia)

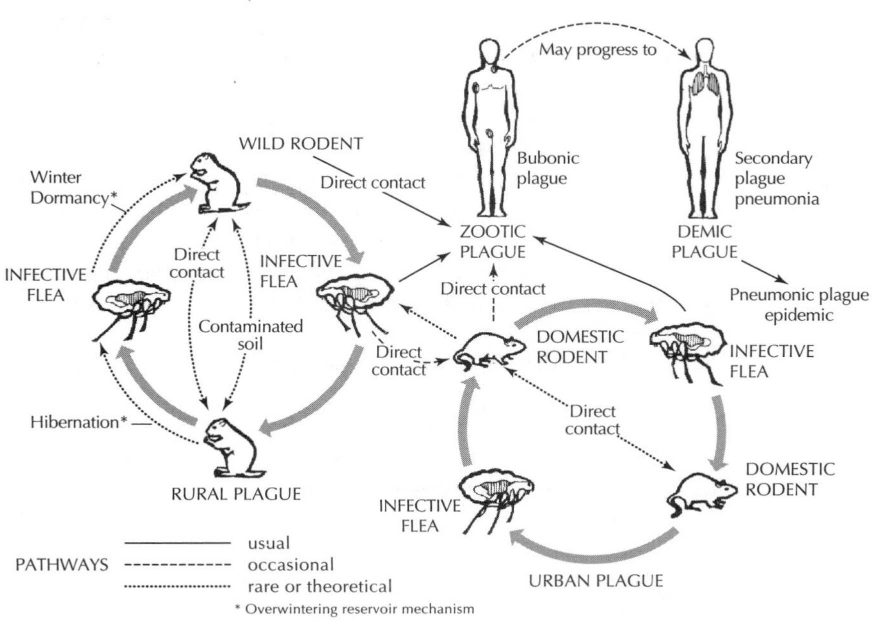

FIGURE 1.4 Rodents and coyotes are often *carriers* of bubonic plague. Fleas serve as *vectors* in transmitting this disease to humans as shown in these epidemiological cycles of the bubonic plague. (Courtesy of Centers for Disease Control and Prevention, Atlanta, Georgia)

1. **Active carriers.** Individuals who have been exposed to and harbor a disease-causing organism (pathogen) and who have done so for some time, even though they may have recovered from the disease.
2. **Convalescent carriers.** Individuals who harbor a pathogen and who, although in the recovery phase of the course of the disease, are still infectious.
3. **Healthy carriers (also called passive carriers).** Individuals who have been exposed to and harbor a pathogen but have not become ill or shown any of the symptoms of the disease. This could be referred to as a subclinical case.
4. **Incubatory carriers.** Individuals who have been exposed to and harbor a pathogen, are in the beginning stages of the disease, are showing symptoms, and have the ability to transmit the disease.
5. **Intermittent carriers**. Individuals who have been exposed to and harbor a pathogen and who can spread the disease at different places or intervals.[21,22]

MODES OF DISEASE TRANSMISSION

There are 2 general **modes of disease transmission**, direct transmission and indirect transmission.

Direct transmission is the direct and immediate transfer of the pathogen from a host/reservoir to a susceptible host. Direct transmission can occur through direct physical contact or direct person-to-person contact (see News File p 13), such as touching with contaminated hands, skin-to-skin contact, kissing, or sexual intercourse.

Indirect transmission occurs when pathogens or agents are transferred or carried by some intermediate item, organism, means, or process to a susceptible host, resulting in disease. Fomites, vectors, air currents, dust particles, water droplets, water, food, oral–fecal contact, and other mechanisms that effectively transfer disease-causing organisms are means of indirect disease transmission. **Airborne transmission** occurs when droplets or dust particles carry the pathogen to the host and cause infection. This may result when a person sneezes, coughs, or talks, spraying microscopic pathogen-carrying droplets into the air that can be breathed in by nearby susceptible hosts. It also occurs when droplets are carried through a building's heating or air conditioning ducts or are spread by fans throughout a building or complex of buildings. Waterborne transmission occurs when a pathogen such as cholera or shigellosis is carried in drinking water, swimming pools, streams, or lakes used for swimming. **Vehicleborne transmission** is related to fomites, such as eating utensils, clothing, washing items, combs, shared drinking bottles, and so on.

Some epidemiologists classify droplet spread as direct transmission because it usually takes place within a few feet of the susceptible host and because it is direct. Logically, however, the droplets from a sneeze or cough use the intermediary mechanism of the droplet to carry the pathogen; thus it is an indirect transmission. This is also a form of person-to-person transmission, and influenza and the common cold are commonly spread this way. Droplets can also be spread by air-moving equipment and air-circulation processes (heating and air conditioning) within buildings, which carry droplet-borne disease great distances, often to remote locations, causing illness. Such equipment has been implicated in cases of tuberculosis and Legionnaire's disease.

Some vectorborne disease transmission processes are simple mechanical processes, such as when the pathogen, in order to spread, uses a host (eg, a fly, flea, louse, or rat) as a mechanism for a ride, for nourishment, or as part of a physical transfer process. This is called **mechanical transmission**. When the pathogen undergoes changes as part of its life cycle while within the host/vector and before being transmitted to the new host, it is called **biological transmission**. Biological transmission is easily seen in malaria, in which the female *Anopheles* mosquito's blood meal is required for the *Plasmodium* protozoan parasite to complete its sexual development cycle. This can occur only with the ingested blood nutrients found in the intestine of the *Anopheles* mosquito.

CHAIN OF INFECTION

There is a close association between the triangle of epidemiology and the **chain of infection** (Figure 1.5). Disease transmission occurs when the pathogen leaves the reservoir through a

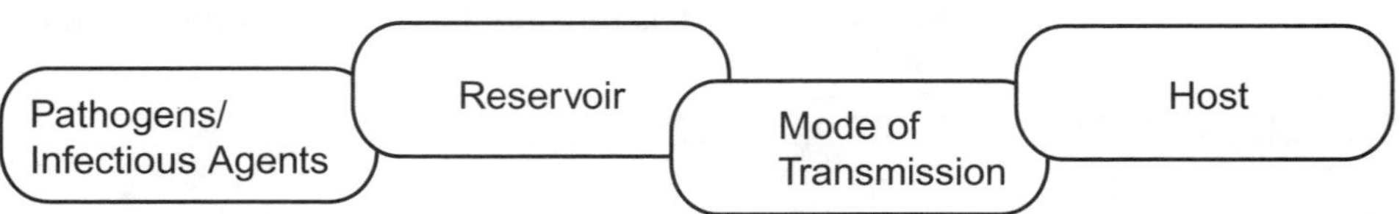

FIGURE 1.5 The chain of infection.

portal of exit and is spread by one of several modes of transmission. The pathogen or disease-causing agent enters the body through a **portal of entry** and infects the host if the host is susceptible.

Pathogens can include bacteria, viruses, worms, chemicals, or any other plant or animal substance or factor that can cause disease, disability, illness, syndrome, or death. The reservoir is the medium or habitat in which pathogens or infectious agents thrive, propagate, and multiply. Reservoirs are humans, animals, or certain environmental conditions or

NEWS FILE

Pediculosis (Person-to-Person Transmission)

Head Lice: The Epidemic Continues

Some people think of head lice as a nuisance that bothers only the lower class and those with bad personal hygiene. Yet a nationwide epidemic of pediculosis continues to run rampant in both public and private schools.

The bloodsucking lice (*Anoplura* order) prefer mammal hosts and rarely infest even closely related species, including pets. Head lice limit themselves to the hair of the head near the nape of the neck and the ears. The life cycle of head lice is spent on the host, usually on the same person. The 3-stage growth cycle of egg, nymph, and adult takes about 3 weeks. When head lice are not on the host, they die in a day or two. The head louse is very small, about 2 to 3 mm, and can be found grasping the hair shaft near the scalp with its special claws. The adult female louse lives about a month, laying 150 or more eggs called nits, about 10 a day. Nits are not to be confused with solidified globules of hair spray or dandruff. The yellowish-white, oval-shaped nit found glued to the bottom of the hair shaft takes about a week to hatch.

Little disease is transmitted through lice, but they themselves are a problem. They suck blood and inject saliva during the infestation, causing itching and secondary infections from excreta, bites, and scratching.

The louse cannot jump or fly, so transmission occurs either directly, from contact with an infested person, or indirectly, through fomites such as shared scarves, hats, coats, brushes, combs, sweaters, and bedding. Schools are particularly vulnerable because children may try on and wear each other's clothing. Because lice like a frequent blood meal and a warm and fuzzy environment, person-to-person transmission is most common. Control comes largely from not sharing combs, brushes, and head clothing or sleeping with infested persons.

The only way to get rid of nits and lice is to use pesticide treatment, which comes in the form of special shampoos, cream rinses, and topical lotions, with shampoos containing permethrin being most common and effective if used according to directions. Clothing and bedding must be washed in hot soapy water and dried in a hot dryer to destroy lice and nits. Nits must also be removed from the hair with fine-toothed combs. Children should be kept out of school until treatment is complete and successful.

(Source: California Morbidity. Division of Communicable Disease Control, California Department of Health Services; 1996.)

substances, such as food, feces, or decaying organic matter, that are conducive to the growth of pathogens. Two types of human or animal reservoirs are generally recognized: symptomatic (ill) persons who have a disease and carriers who are asymptomatic and can still transmit the disease.

Once a pathogen leaves its reservoir, it follows its mode of transmission to a susceptible host, either by direct transmission (person-to-person contact) or by indirect transmission (airborne droplets or dust particles, vectors, fomites, food). The final link in the chain of infection is thus the susceptible individual or host, usually a human or an animal. The host is generally protected from invasion of pathogens by the skin, mucous membranes, and the body's physiological responses (weeping of mucous membranes to cleanse themselves, acidity in the stomach, cilia in the respiratory tract, coughing, and the natural response of the immune system). If the pathogen is able to enter the host, the result will most likely be illness if the host has no immunity to the pathogen.

Susceptibility is based on level of immunity. Natural immunity can come from genetic makeup; that is, some people seem better able to resist disease than others. Active immunity occurs when the body develops antibodies and antigens in response to a pathogen invading the body. Passive immunity comes from antibodies entering a baby through the placenta or from antitoxin or immune globulin injections.[3]

ADVANCED TRIANGLE OF EPIDEMIOLOGY

The epidemiology triangle as used in a discussion of communicable disease is basic and foundational to all epidemiology. However, infectious diseases are no longer the leading cause of death in industrialized nations, so a more advanced model of the triangle of epidemiology is needed. This new model includes all facets of the communicable disease model, and to make it more relevant and useful with regard to today's diseases, conditions, disorders, defects, injuries, and deaths, it also reflects the causes of current illnesses and conditions. Behavior, lifestyle factors, environmental causes, ecologic elements, physical factors, and chronic diseases must be taken into account. Figure 1.6 presents an adapted and advanced model of the triangle of epidemiology, better reflecting the behavior, lifestyle, and chronic disease issues found in modern times.

The advanced model of the triangle of epidemiology, like the traditional epidemiology triangle, is not comprehensive or complete. However, the advanced model recognizes that disease states and conditions affecting a population are complex and that there are many causative factors. The term *agents* is replaced with *causative factors,* which implies the need to identify multiple causes or etiologic factors of disease, disability, injury, and death. In Chapter 9, "Statistical and Causal Associations," the web of causation is presented as an effective method of investigation into chronic disease and behaviorally founded causes of disease, disability, injury, and death. The web of causation shows the importance of looking for many causes or an array of contributing factors to various maladies.

LEVELS OF PREVENTION

Three types of prevention have been established in public health: primary prevention, secondary prevention, and tertiary prevention.

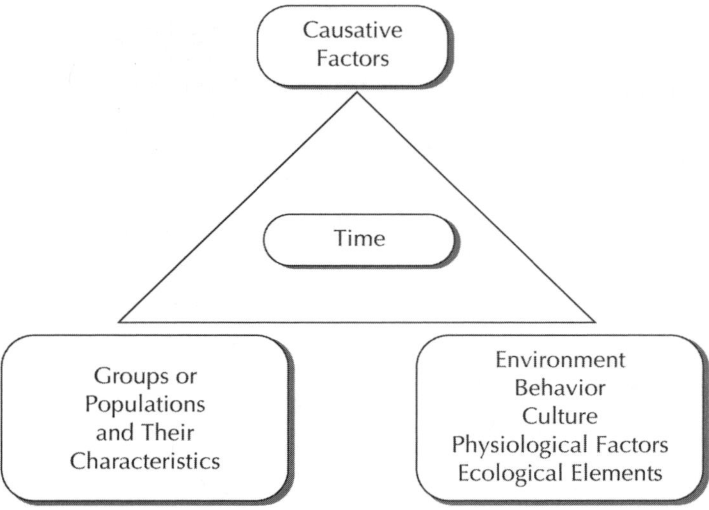

FIGURE 1.6 Advanced model of the triangle of epidemiology.

Primary Prevention

Primary prevention is preventing a disease or disorder before it happens. Health promotion, health education, and health protection are 3 main facets of primary prevention. Lifestyle changes, community health education, school health education, good prenatal care, good behavioral choices, proper nutrition, and ensuring safe and healthy conditions at home, school, and the workplace are all primary prevention activities. Fundamental public health measures and activities such as sanitation; infection control; immunizations; protection of food, milk, and water supplies; environmental protection; and protection against occupational hazards and accidents are all basic to primary prevention. Basic personal hygiene and public health measures have had a major impact on halting communicable disease epidemics. Immunizations, infection control (eg, hand washing), refrigeration of foods, garbage collection, solid and liquid waste management, water supply protection and treatment, and general sanitation have reduced infectious disease threats to populations.

Because of successes in primary prevention efforts directed at infectious diseases, noninfectious diseases are now the main causes of death in the United States and industrialized nations (Table 1.2).[23,24] The leading factors contributing to the causes of death (Figure 1.7) are smoking and tobacco use, alcohol and substance abuse, accidents, inadequate diet, lack of physical fitness, emotional and mental health problems, and environmental health concerns. Prevention at its basic levels now has to be behaviorally directed and lifestyle oriented. Efforts at the primary prevention level have to focus on influencing individual behavior and protecting the environment. In the future the focus on treatment and health care by physicians should be lessened and replaced with a major effort in the area of primary prevention, including adequate economic support for prevention programs and activities.[16–19]

TABLE 1.2 Leading causes of death in the United States in 1900[23] and in 2000[24]

1900		*2000*	
Pneumonia and influenza	11.8%	Heart diseases	29.6%
Tuberculosis	11.3%	Cancer	23.0%
Diarrhea, enteritis, ulcerations of the intestines	8.3%	Cerebrovascular diseases	7.0%
Heart diseases	8.0%	Chronic obstructive pulmonary diseases	5.1%
Intracranial lesions of vascular origin	6.2%	Accidents	4.1%
Nephritis	5.2%	Diabetes mellitus	2.9%
Accidents	4.2%	Pneumonia and influenza	2.7%
Cancer	3.7%	Alzheimer's diseases	2.1%
Senility	2.9%	Nephritis	1.5%
Diphtheria	2.3%	Septicemia	1.3%
All other	36.1%	All other	20.7%
	100.0%		100.0%

Two related terms are **active primary prevention** and **passive primary prevention.** Active primary prevention requires behavior change on the part of the individual (eg, begin exercising, stop smoking, reduce dietary fat intake). Passive primary prevention does not require behavior change on the part of the individual (eg, eating vitamin-enriched foods, drinking fluoridated water).

Secondary Prevention

Secondary prevention is aimed at the health screening and detection activities used to identify disease. If pathogenicity (the ability to cause disease) is discovered early, diagnosis and early treatment can prevent conditions from progressing and from spreading within the population and can stop or at least slow the progress of disease, disability, disorders, or death.[1] Secondary prevention aims to block the progression of disease or prevent an injury from developing into an impairment or disability.[16,17,20]

Tertiary Prevention

The aim of the third level of prevention is to retard or block the progression of a disability, condition, or disorder in order to keep it from advancing and requiring excessive care. **Tertiary prevention** consists of limiting any disability by providing rehabilitation where disease, injury, or a disorder has already occurred and has caused damage. At this level the goal is to help those diseased, disabled, or injured individuals to avoid wasteful use of health care services and avoid becoming dependent on health care practitioners and health care institutions. Prompt diagnosis and treatment, followed by proper rehabilitation and posttreatment recovery, proper patient education, behavior changes, and lifestyle changes, are all necessary so that diseases or disorders will not recur. At the very minimum, the progression of the disease or disorder or injury needs to be slowed and checked.[25,26]

Rehabilitation is any attempt to restore an afflicted person to a useful, productive, and satisfying lifestyle and to provide the highest quality of life possible, given the extent of the disease and disability. Rehabilitation is one component of tertiary prevention. Patient education, aftercare, health counseling, and some aspects of health promotion can be important components of tertiary prevention.

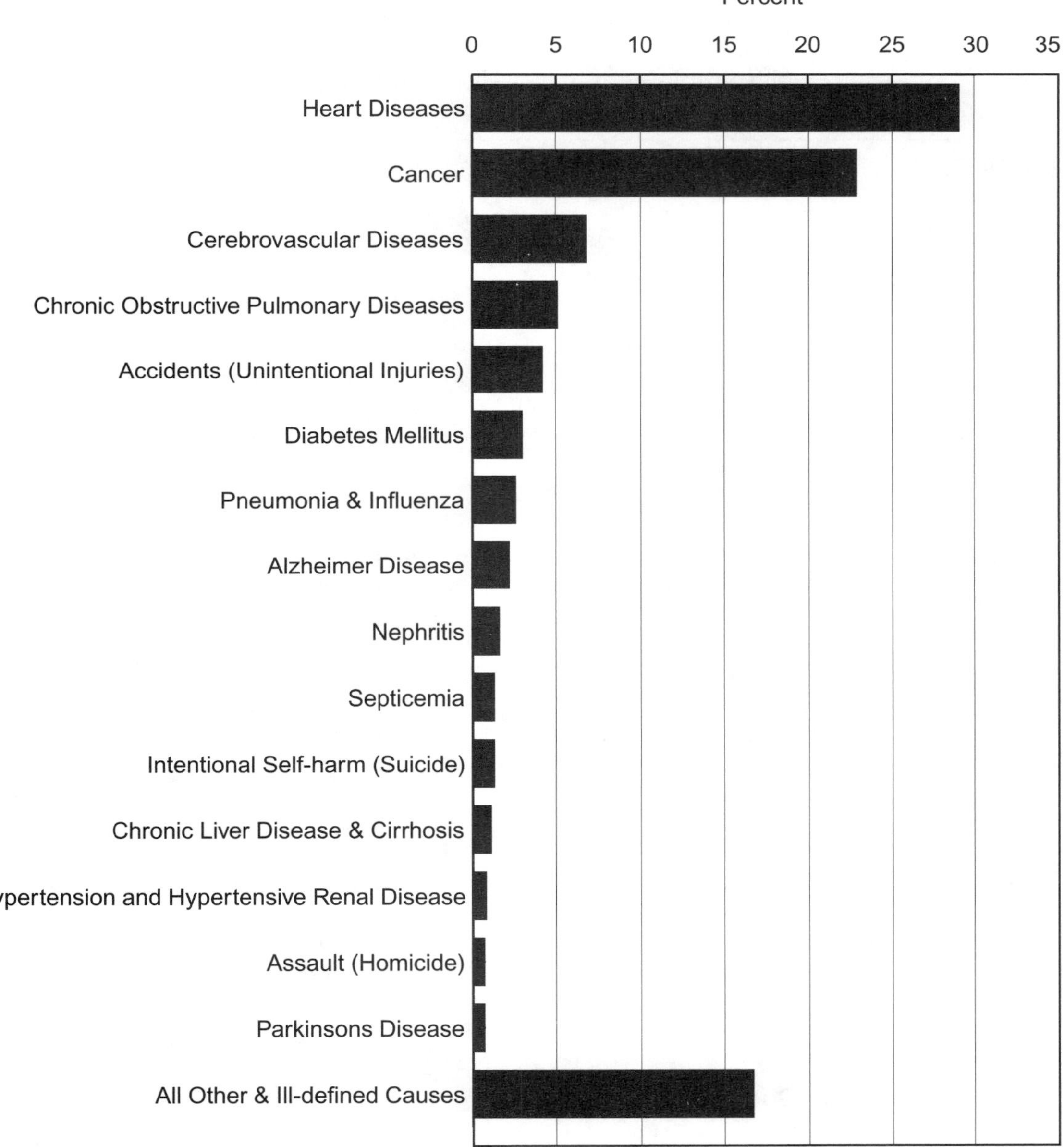

FIGURE 1.7 Leading causes of disease in the United States, 2000. *Source:* Centers for Disease Control and Prevention. US Mortality Public Use Data Tape, 2000. National Center for Health Statistics, 2002.

SUMMARY

Epidemiology is the process of describing and understanding public health problems and the application of this knowledge to the promotion of physical, mental, and social well-being in the population. Epidemiology involves applying scientific models to the description of the frequency and pattern of health-related states or events, the identification of the causes of health-related states or events and modes of transmission, and the guidance of public health planning and decision making. Epidemiologic information is intended to guide health officials and assist individuals in making informed health behavior changes.

EXERCISES

Key Terms

Define the following terms.

Active carrier
Active primary prevention
Agent
Airborne transmission
Analytic epidemiology
Biological transmission
Carrier
Case
Case definition
Case severity
Chain of infection
Common-source epidemic
Convalescent carrier
Direct transmission
Effectiveness
Efficacy
Endemic
Environment
Epidemic
Epidemiologist
Epidemiology
Fomite
Healthy carrier
Host
Incubatory carrier
Index case
Indirect transmission
Intermittent carrier
Mechanical transmission
Mixed epidemic
Modes of disease transmission
Pandemic
Passive carrier
Passive primary prevention
Pathogen
Portal of entry
Portal of exit
Primary case
Propagated epidemic
Rehabilitation
Reservoir
Secondary case
Secondary prevention
Suspect case
Tertiary prevention
Time
Vector
Vectorborne transmission
Vehicleborne transmission
Zoonosis

Study Questions

1.1 The definition of epidemiology includes the terms "distribution" and "determinants." Describe the meaning of these terms.

1.2 Epidemiology involves the study of more than just infectious diseases. Explain.

1.3 Describe the chain of infection.

1.4 List 4 types of epidemiologic information useful for influencing public health policy and planning and individual health decisions.

1.5 Define efficacy and effectiveness and provide examples of both.

Use the following information to answer questions 1.6 and 1.7.

Emergency Medical Services (EMS) responses were made to 1,551 nonindustrial injuries resulting from falls. Of total falls, 869 (56%) occurred at home, and 682 (44%) occurred elsewhere. The very young (<4 years old) and the very old (80+ years) were the most vulnerable to falls. Persons over age 60 accounted for 44% of the total emergency calls for nonindustrial falls. On weekends most injuries from falls occurred in the home. Time pattern analysis revealed that the greatest number of injuries from falls at home occurred in the late afternoon and evening, between 3:00 PM and midnight. Callers from three socioeconomic strata were identified from census tract information. Age and sex were tabulated for the 3 strata areas based on falls in the home. The greatest use of EMS was by those over 60 years of age in all 3 strata levels. Those aged 40–59 years in the low socioeconomic group and infants through 9 years of age in the low socioeconomic group were next highest users. The highest socioeconomic group had the lowest rates for each age group.[26] The percentages given are out of total emergency EMS responses. Table 1.3 represents percentages of falls per total population based on the rates per 100,000 people. In Table 1.3

- population for the high socioeconomic group was 143,798
- population for the medium socioeconomic group was 249,381
- population for the low socioeconomic group was 138,413

1.6 With what you have learned from the scenario just described, what can you say about the role age plays in falls? Present statistics and provide a discussion of reasons for the age-related statistics and differences.

TABLE 1.3 Home falls and emergency medical service response in the state of Washington

Age Group	*High Socio-economic Rate/100,000*	*% Total Population*	*Medium Socio-economic Rate/100,000*	*% Total Population*	*Low Socio-economic Rate/100,000*	*% Total Population*
0–9	87.95	3.8	199.88	6.4	260.24	2.9
10–19	35.94	4.8	87.43	6.7	104.81	2.9
20–39	29.69	8.2	60.77	14.9	104.76	9.1
40–59	60.66	6.8	168.42	9.7	288.89	5.1
60+	444.05	3.4	355.18	9.3	420.66	5.9
TOTAL	—	27.05	—	46.91	—	26.04

1.7 Explain the effect of socioeconomic status on falls as responded to by EMS as shown in Table 1.3.

1.8 Explain the epidemiology triangle and compare and contrast it with the advanced epidemiology triangle.

1.9 Review Figure 1.7 and explain the implications of the 15 leading causes of death for public health. Include the 3 levels of prevention.

1.10 HIV/AIDS can be transmitted from an infected person to another person through blood, semen, vaginal fluids, and breast milk. High-risk behaviors include homosexual practices; unprotected oral, vaginal, or anal sexual intercourse; and needle sharing. Discuss how this information can be used in public health action and individual decision making.

REFERENCES

1. *Stedman's Medical Dictionary for the Health Professions and Nursing*. 5th ed. New York, NY: Lippincott, Williams & Wilkins; 2005.
2. Joint United Nations Programme on HIV/AIDS and World Health Organization. Global summary of the AIDS epidemic December 2004. Available at: http://www.unaids.org/wad2004/EPI_1204_pdf_en/EpiUpdate04_en.pdf. Accessed May 3, 2005.
3. Page RM, Cole GE, Timmreck TC. *Basic Epidemiologic Methods and Biostatistics. A Practical Guidebook*. Boston, MA: Jones and Bartlett; 1995.
4. Centers for Disease Control and Prevention (CDC). Pneumocystis pneumonia—Los Angeles. *MMWR*. 1981;30:250–252.
5. CDC. Possible transfusion-associated acquired immune deficiency syndrome (AIDS)—California. *MMWR*. 1982;31:652–654.
6. Last JM, ed. *A Dictionary of Epidemiology*. 3rd ed. New York, NY: Oxford University Press; 1995.
7. Rigotti NA, Pasternak RC. Cigarette smoking and coronary heart disease: Risks and management. *Cardiol Clin*. 1996;14:51–68.
8. Shinton R. Lifelong exposures and the potential for stroke prevention: The contribution of cigarette smoking, exercise, and body fat. *J Epidemiol Community Health*. 1997;51:138–143.
9. US Department of Health and Human Services (DHHS). The health benefits of smoking cessation: A Report of the Surgeon General, 1990. Rockville, MD: Centers for Disease Control, Center for Chronic Disease Prevention and Health Promotion, Office on Smoking and Health, 1990. (DHHS Publication No. (CDC) 90-8416).
10. US DHHS. Reducing the Health Consequences of Smoking: 25 Years of Progress. A Report of the Surgeon General, 1989. Rockville, MD: Centers for Disease Control, Office on Smoking and Health, 1989. (DHHS Publication No. (CDC) 89-8411).
11. Merrill RM, White GL Jr. Why health educators need epidemiology. *Educ Health*. 2002; 15:215–221.
12. Thacker SB, Berkelman RL. Public health surveillance in the United States. *Epidemiol Rev*. 1988;10:164–190.
13. Oleckno WA. *Essential Epidemiology: Principles and Application*. Long Grove, IL: Waveland Press; 2002.
14. Pandemics. Pandemics through history. Available at: http://www.absoluteastronomy.com/encyclopedia/p/pa/pandemic.htm. Accessed May 3, 2005.
15. Chang M, Glynn MK, Groseclose SL. Endemic, notifiable bioterrorism-related diseases, United States, 1992–1999. *Emerg Infect Dis*. 2003;9:5. Available at: http://www.cdc.gov/ncidod/eid/vol9no5/02-0477.htm. Accessed May 4, 2005.

16. Timmreck TC. *Health Services Cyclopedic Dictionary*. 3rd ed. Sudbury, MA: Jones and Bartlett; 1997.
17. Mausner J, Bahn AK. *Epidemiology: An Introductory Text*. Philadelphia, PA: WB Saunders; 1974.
18. Shindell S, Salloway JC, Oberembi CM. *A Coursebook in Health Care Delivery*. New York, NY: Appleton-Century-Crofts; 1976.
19. Lilienfeld AM, Lilienfeld DE. *Foundations of Epidemiology*. 2nd ed. New York, NY: Oxford University Press; 1980.
20. World Health Organization. Zoonoses: Second report of the Joint WHO/FAO Expert Committee; 1959.
21. Thomas CL, ed. *Taber's Cyclopedic Medical Dictionary*. 14th ed. Philadelphia, PA: FA Davis; 1981.
22. Nester EW, McCarthy BJ, Roberts CE, Pearsall NN. *Microbiology*. New York, NY: Holt, Rinehart & Winston; 1973.
23. CDC. Leading causes of disease, 1900–1998. Available at: http://www.cdc.gov/nchs/data/statab/lead1900_98.pdf. Accessed May 10, 2005.
24. CDC. *US Mortality Public Use Data Tape, 2000*. National Center for Health Statistics; 2000. Available at: http://webapp.cdc.gov/sasweb/ncipc/leadcaus10.html. Accessed September 12, 2005.
25. Picket G, Hanlon JJ. *Public Health: Administration and Practice*. St. Louis, MO: Times Mirror/Mosby; 1990.
26. MacMahon B, Pugh TF. *Epidemiology Principles and Methods*. Boston, MA: Little, Brown and Company; 1970.

CHAPTER

2

Historic Developments in Epidemiology

OBJECTIVES

After completing this chapter you will be able to

- Describe important historic events in the field of epidemiology.
- List several individuals who contributed to and helped shape the field of epidemiology.
- Recognize the application of certain epidemiologic concepts, principles, and study design methods.

INTRODUCTION

The history of epidemiology has involved many key players who sought to understand and explain illness, injury, and death from an observational scientific perspective. These individuals also sought to provide information for the prevention and control of health-related states and events in the population. They advanced the study of disease from a supernatural viewpoint to a viewpoint based on a scientific foundation; from no approach for assessment to systematic methods for summarizing and describing public health problems; from no clear understanding of the natural course of disease to a knowledge of the probable causes, modes of transmission, and health outcomes; and from no means for preventing and controlling disease to effective approaches for solving public health problems.

Initially, epidemiologic knowledge advanced slowly, with large segments in time where little or no advancement in the field occurred. The time from Hippocrates (460–377 BC), who attempted to explain disease occurrence from a rational viewpoint, to John Graunt (AD 1620–1674), who described disease occurrence and death with the use of systematic methods and who developed and calculated life tables and life expectancy, and Thomas Sydenham (1624–1689), who approached the study of disease from an observational angle rather than a theoretical one, was 2,000 years. Approximately 200 years later, William Farr (1807–1883) advanced John Graunt's work in order to better describe epidemiologic problems. In the 19th century, John Snow, Ignaz Semmelweis, Louis Pasteur, Robert Koch, and others also made important contributions to the field of epidemiology. Since then, the science of epidemiology has rapidly progressed. Although it is impossible to identify all of the contributors to the field of epidemiology in this chapter, several of these individuals and their contributions are considered here.

HIPPOCRATES, THE FIRST EPIDEMIOLOGIST

Hippocrates was a physician who became known as the father of medicine and the first epidemiologist. His three books; *Epidemic I*, *Epidemic III*, and *On Airs, Waters and Places*, attempted to describe disease from a rational rather than a supernatural basis. He observed that different diseases occurred in different locations. He noted that malaria and yellow fever most commonly occurred in swampy areas. He also introduced terms like *epidemic* and *endemic*.[1–4]

Hippocrates gave advice to persons wishing to pursue the science of medicine and provided insights on the effects of the seasons of the year and of hot and cold winds. He believed the properties of water should be examined and advised that the source of water should be considered.[1–4] Is the water from a marshy soft-ground source, or is the water from the rocky heights? Is the water brackish and harsh? Hippocrates also made some noteworthy observations on the behavior of the populace. He believed the effective physician should be observant of peoples' behavior, such as eating, drinking, and other activity. Did they eat lunch, eat too much, or drink too little? Were they industrious?

For traveling physicians, Hippocrates suggested they become familiar with local diseases and with the nature of those prevailing diseases. He believed that as time passed the physician should be able to tell what epidemic diseases might attack and in what season and that this could be determined by the settings of the stars. Sources of water, how water sets or flows, and smells were always considered in his study of disease states.[1–4]

Hippocrates identified **hot** and **cold diseases** and, consequently, hot and cold treatments. Hot diseases were treated with cold treatments, and cold diseases required hot treatments. The process of deciding whether a disease was hot or cold was complex. An example is diarrhea, which was considered a hot disease and was believed to be cured with a cold treatment such as eating fruit.[1–4]

Hippocrates also ascribed to and incorporated into his theory what is now considered the **atomic theory**; that is, the belief that everything is made of tiny particles. He theorized that there were four types of atoms: earth atoms (solid and cold), air atoms (dry), fire atoms (hot), and water atoms (wet). Additionally, Hippocrates believed that the body was composed of four humors: phlegm (earth and water atoms), yellow bile (fire and air atoms), blood (fire and water atoms), and black bile (earth and air atoms). Sickness was thought to be caused by an imbalance of these humors, and fever was thought to be caused by too much blood. The treatment for fever was to reduce the amount of blood in the body through bloodletting or the application of bloodsuckers (leeches). Imbalances were ascribed to a change in the body's "constitution." Climate, moisture, stars, meteorites, winds, vapors, and diet were thought to cause imbalances and contribute to disease. Diet was both a cause and cure of disease. Cures for illness and protection from disease came from maintaining a balance and avoiding imbalance in the constitution.

The essentials of epidemiology noted by Hippocrates included observations on how diseases affected populations and how disease spread. He further addressed issues of diseases in relation to time and seasons, place, environmental conditions, and disease control, especially as it related to water and the seasons. The broader contribution to epidemiology made by Hippocrates was that of epidemiologic observation. His teachings about how to observe any and all contributing or causal factors of a disease are still sound epidemiologic concepts.[1–4]

DISEASE OBSERVATIONS OF SYDENHAM

Thomas Sydenham (1624–1689), although a graduate of Oxford Medical School, did not at first practice medicine but served in the military and as a college administrator. While at All Souls College, Oxford, he became acquainted with Robert Boyle, a colleague who sparked Sydenham's interest in diseases and epidemics. Sydenham went on to get his medical license, and he spoke out for strong empirical approaches to medicine and close observations of disease. Sydenham wrote the details of what he observed about diseases without letting various traditional theories of disease and medical treatment influence his work and observations. From this close observation process, he was able to identify and recognize different diseases. Sydenham published his observations in a book in 1676 titled *Observationes Medicae*.[4]

One of the major works of Sydenham was the classification of fevers plaguing London in the 1660s and 1670s. Sydenham came up with three levels or classes of fevers: continued fevers, intermittent fevers, and smallpox. Some of Sydenham's theories were embraced while others were criticized, mostly because his ideas and observations went against the usual Hippocratic approaches. He treated smallpox with bed rest and normal bed covers. The treatment of the time, based on the Hippocratic theory, was to use heat and extensive bed coverings. He was met with good results but was erroneous in identifying the cause of the disease.[4]

Sydenham was persecuted by his colleagues, who at one time threatened to take away his medical license for irregular practice that did not follow the theories of the time. However, he gained a good reputation with the public, and some young open-minded physicians agreed with his empirical principles. Sydenham described and distinguished different diseases, including some psychological maladies. He also advanced useful treatments and remedies including exercise, fresh air, and a healthy diet, which other physicians rejected at the time.[4]

THE EPIDEMIOLOGY OF SCURVY

In the 1700s, it was observed that armies lost more men to disease than to the sword. James Lind (1716–1794), a Scottish naval surgeon, focused on illnesses in these populations. He observed the effect of time, place, weather, and diet on the spread of disease. His 1754 book *A Treatise on Scurvy* identified the symptoms of scurvy and the fact that the disease became common in sailors after as little as a month at sea.[3,4]

Lind noticed that while on long ocean voyages, sailors would become sick from **scurvy**, a disease marked by spongy and bleeding gums, bleeding under the skin, and extreme weakness. He saw that scurvy began to occur after 4–6 weeks at sea. Lind noted that even though the water was good and the provisions were not tainted, the sailors still fell sick. Lind pointed out that the months most common to scurvy were April, May, and June. He also observed that cold, rainy, foggy, and thick weather were often present. Influenced by the Hippocratic theory of medicine, Lind kept looking to the air as the source of disease. Dampness of the air, damp living arrangements, and life at sea were the main focus of his observations as he searched for an explanation of the cause of disease and, most of all, the cause of scurvy.[5] Although not correct about the link with weather and climate at sea, Lind looked at all sides of the issue and considered what was happening to the sick. He then compared their experience with the experiences of those who were healthy.

When Lind began to look at the diet of the mariners, he observed that the sea diet was extremely gross and hard on digestion. Concerned with the extent of sickness in large numbers of sailors, Lind set up some experiments with mariners. In 1747, while serving on the HMS *Salisbury,* he conducted an experimental study on scurvy. He took 12 ill patients who had all the classic symptoms of scurvy. He put the sailors in 6 groups of 2 and varied the diet of each group. Two men received a quart of cider a day, and 2 others were given an unspecified elixir 3 times a day. One pair was treated with seawater, and another was fed with a combination of garlic, mustard, and horseradish. Two men were given spoonfuls of vinegar, and the last 2 were given 2 oranges and a lemon every day. The most sudden and visible good effects were seen in those eating oranges and lemons. In 6 days, the 2 eating citrus were fit for duty. All the others had putrid gums, spots, lassitude, and weakness of the knees. Free of symptoms, the two citrus-eating sailors were asked to nurse the others who were still sick. Thus Lind observed that oranges and lemons were the most effective remedies for scurvy at sea.[5]

The epidemiologic contributions of Lind were many. He was concerned with the occurrence of disease in large groups of people. Lind not only participated in the identification of the effect of diet on disease, but he made clinical observations, used experimental design, asked classic epidemiologic questions, observed population changes and their effect on disease, and considered sources of disease, including place, time, and season.

COWPOX AND ITS EPIDEMIOLOGIC CONNECTION TO SMALLPOX

In England, Benjamin Jesty, a farmer/dairyman in the mid-1700s, noticed his milkmaids never got **smallpox**, a disease characterized by chills, fever, headache, and backache, with eruption of pimples that blister and form pockmarks. However, the milkmaids did develop cowpox from the cows. Jesty believed there was a link between acquiring cowpox and not getting smallpox. In 1774, Jesty exposed his wife and children to cowpox to protect them from smallpox. It worked: the exposed family members developed immunity to smallpox. Unfortunately, little was publicized about Jesty's experiment and observations.[4]

The experiment of Jesty and similar reported experiences in Turkey, the Orient, America, and Hungary were known to Edward Jenner (1749–1823), an English rural physician. He personally observed that dairymen's servants and milkmaids got cowpox and did not get smallpox. For many centuries the Chinese had made observations about weaker and stronger strains of smallpox. They learned that it was wise to catch a weaker strain of the disease. If one had a weak strain of the disease, one would not get the full disease later on. This was termed **variolation**.[3,4]

In the late 1700s, servants were often the ones who milked the cows. Servants were also required to tend to the sores on the heels of horses affected with cowpox. The pus and infectious fluids from these sores were referred to as "the grease" of the disease. Left unwashed because of a lack of concern about sanitation and cleanliness, the servants' grease-covered hands would then spread the disease to the cows during milking. The cowpox in turn was transmitted to the dairymaids. Jenner observed that when a person had cowpox, this same person would not get smallpox if exposed to it. Jenner attempted to give a dairymaid, exposed to a mild case of cowpox in her youth, a case of cowpox by cutting her arm and rubbing some of the infectious "grease" into the wound. She did not get ill. Cowpox was thus found to shield against smallpox.[3,4] Jenner invented a vaccination for smallpox with this knowledge. The vaccine was used to protect populations from this disease.[3,4,6]

On October 26, 1977, World Health Organization workers supposedly tracked down the world's last case of naturally occurring smallpox. The patient was 23-year-old Ali Maow Maalin, a hospital cook in Merka, Somalia. (Two cases of smallpox occurred in 1978 as a result of a laboratory accident.) Because it is believed that smallpox has been eradicated from the earth, vaccinations have been halted. However, some public-health and health care professionals are skeptical and fear that such acts may set the stage for an unexpected future epidemic of smallpox because the pathogen still exists in military and government labs. As unvaccinated persons proliferate, so does the risk of future smallpox epidemics.

EPIDEMIOLOGY OF CHILDBED FEVER IN A LYING-IN HOSPITAL

Historically, epidemiology was centered on the study of the great epidemics: cholera, bubonic plague, smallpox, and typhus. As the diseases were identified and differentiated, the focus of epidemiology changed. Such a change in focus came through the work of another physician–epidemiologist, Ignaz Semmelweis, in the early to mid-1800s.[7]

In the 1840s, one of the greatest fears a pregnant mother had was dying of **childbed fever** (a uterine infection, usually of the placental site, after childbirth). Babies were born to mothers with the usual risks that warranted obstetric assistance, and this often resulted in an uneventful birth. However, after the birth of the child, the mother would get an infection and die of childbed fever, a streptococcal disease. Many times the child would become infected and die as well. After many years of observing the course of the disease and the symptoms associated with childbed fever, Semmelweis began a series of investigations.[7]

The Viennese Maternity Hospital (called a lying-in hospital), of which Semmelweis was clinical director, was divided into 2 clinics. The first clinic consistently had greater numbers of maternal deaths than the second clinic. In 1846, the maternal mortality rate of this clinic was 5 times greater than that of the second clinic, and over a 6-year period, it was 3 times as great. Semmelweis observed that the mothers became ill either immediately during birth or within 24–36 hours after delivery. The mothers died quickly of rapidly developing childbed fever. Often the children would soon die as well. This was not the case in the second clinic.[7]

Semmelweis observed it was not the actual labor that was the problem but the examination of the patients seemed to be connected to the onset of the disease. Through clinical observation, retrospective study, collection and analysis of data on maternal deaths and infant deaths, and clinically controlled experimentation, he was able to ascertain that the communication of childbed fever was through germs passed from patient to patient by the physician in the process of doing pelvic examinations. Semmelweis discovered that, unlike in the second clinic, the medical students would come directly from the death house after working at autopsy of infected and decaying dead bodies and then would conduct pelvic exams on the mothers ready to give birth. Hand washing or any form of infection control was not a common practice. Unclean hands with putrefied cadaver material on student doctors' hands were used to conduct the routine daily pelvic exams, and the practice was never questioned. There was no reason to be concerned about clean hands because the theory of medicine that was accepted at the time relied on the Hippocratic theory of medicine and the idea that disease developed spontaneously. Semmelweis observed that a whole row of patients became ill while patients in the adjacent row stayed healthy.[7]

Semmelweis discovered that any infected or putrefied tissue, whether from a living patient or a cadaver, could cause disease to spread. In order to destroy the cadaverous or putrefied matter on the hands, it was necessary that every person, physician or midwife, performing an examination wash their hands in chlorinated lime on entering the labor ward in clinic 1. At first, Semmelweis said it was only necessary to wash during entry to the labor ward, but a cancerous womb was discovered to also cause the spread of the disease, and thus Semmelweis required washing with chlorinated lime between each examination. When strict adherence to hand washing was required of all medical personnel who examined patients in the maternity hospital, mortality rates fell at unbelievable rates. In 1842 the percentage of deaths was 12.1% (730 of 6,024) compared with 1.3% (91 of 7,095) in 1848.[7]

At this time in the history of public health the causes of disease were unknown, yet suspected. It was known that hand washing with chlorinated lime between each examination reduced the illness and deaths from childbed fever, but even with the evidence of this success Semmelweis's discovery was discounted by most of his colleagues.[7] Today, it is known that hand washing is still one of the best sanitation practices for medical and laypeople alike. What Ignaz Semmelweis discovered is still one of the easiest disease- and infection-control methods known.

JOHN SNOW'S INVESTIGATION OF CHOLERA IN LONDON

In the 1850s, John Snow (1813–1858) was a respected physician and the anesthesiologist to Queen Victoria of England. He is noted for his medical work with the royal family, including the administration of chloroform to the queen at the birth of her children. However, Snow is most famous for his pioneering work in epidemiology. Among epidemiologists Snow is considered one of the most important contributors to the field. Many of the tactics, approaches, concepts, and methodologies used by Snow in his epidemiologic work are still useful and valuable in epidemiologic work today.[8–10]

Throughout his medical career Snow studied cholera. **Cholera** is a disease characterized by watery diarrhea, loss of fluid and electrolytes, dehydration, and collapse. From his studies he established sound and useful epidemiologic methods. He observed and recorded important factors related to the course of disease. In the later part of his career, Snow conducted 2 major investigative studies of cholera. The first involved a descriptive epidemiologic investigation of a cholera outbreak in the Soho district of London in the Broad Street area. The second involved an analytic epidemiologic investigation of a cholera epidemic in which he compared death rates from the disease according to where sufferers got their water, either the Lambeth Water Company or the Southwark and Vauxhall Water Company.[8–10]

In the mid-1840s, in the Soho and Golden Square districts of London, a major outbreak of cholera occurred. Within 250 yards of the intersection of Cambridge Street and Broad Street, about 500 fatal attacks of cholera occurred in 10 days. Many more deaths were averted because of the flight of most of the population. Snow was able to identify incubation times, length of time from infection until death, modes of transmission of the disease, and the importance of the flight of the population from the dangerous areas. He also plotted statistics based on dates and mortality rates. He studied sources of contamination of the water, causation and infection, and the flow of the water in the underground aquifer by assessing water from wells and pumps. He found that nearly all deaths had taken place within a short distance of the Broad Street pump.

Snow observed that in the Soho district there were two separate populations of persons not so heavily affected by the cholera epidemic, nor were death rates equal to those of the surrounding populations. A brewery with its own wells and a workhouse, also with its own water source, were the protected populations. Snow used a spot map (sometimes called a dot map) to identify the locations of all deaths. He plotted data on the progress of the course of the epidemic, the occurrence of new cases, and when the epidemic started, peaked, and subsided. Snow examined the water, movement of people, sources of exposure, transmission of the disease between and among close and distant people, and possible causation. Toward the end of the epidemic, as a control measure, as protection from any reoccurrence, and as a political statement to the community, Snow removed the handle from the Broad Street pump.[8–10]

In his early days as a practicing physician before the Broad Street outbreak, Snow recorded detailed scenarios of several cases of cholera, many of which he witnessed first-hand. Many of the details he chose to record were epidemiologic in nature, such as various modes of transmission of cholera, incubation times, cause-effect association, clinical observations and clinical manifestations of the disease, scientific observations on water and the different sources (including observations made with a microscope), temperature, climate, diet, what the differences were between those who got the disease and those who did not, and immigration and emigration differences.[8–10]

In 1853, a larger cholera outbreak occurred in London. London had not had a cholera outbreak for about 5 years. During this period, the Lambeth Water Company moved their intake source of water upriver on the Thames, from opposite Hungerford Market to a source above the city, Thames Ditton. By moving the source of water upriver to a place above the sewage outlets, Lambeth was able to draw water free from London's sewage, contamination, and pollution. The Southwark and Vauxhall Water Company, however, did not relocate its source of water. Throughout the south district of the city both water companies had pipes down every street. The citizens were free to pick and choose which water company they wanted for their household water. Thus, by mere coincidence, Snow encountered a populace using water randomly selected throughout the south district. Snow could not have arranged better sampling techniques than those which had occurred by chance.[8–10]

The registrar general in London published a "Weekly Return of Births and Deaths." On November 26, 1853, the Registrar General observed from a table of mortality that mortality rates were fairly consistent across the districts supplied with the water from the Hungerford market area. The old supply system of Lambeth and the regular supply of the Southwark and Vauxhall Company were separate systems but drew water from the same area in the river. The registrar general also published a mortality list from cholera. Snow developed comparison tables on death by source of water by subdistricts. Snow was able to conclude that the water drawn upriver solely by Lambeth Water Company caused no deaths. The water drawn downstream, in areas that were below the sewage inlets, mostly by Southwark and Vauxhall Water Company, was associated with very high death rates.[8–10]

Gaining cooperation and permission from the registrar general, Snow was supplied with addresses of persons who had died from cholera. He went into the subdistrict of Kennington One and Kennington Two and found that 38 of 44 deaths in this subdistrict received their water from Southwark and Vauxhall Company. Each house had randomly selected different water companies, and many households did not know from which one they received water. Snow developed a test that used chloride of silver to identify which water source each household had by sampling water from within the houses of those he contacted. Snow was eventually able to tell the source of water by appearance and smell.[8–10]

Vital statistics data, death rates, and location, when compared with water supply sources, presented conclusive evidence as to the source of contamination. A report to Parliament showed that in the 30,046 households that were supplied water by the Southwark and Vauxhall Company, 286 persons died of cholera. Of the 26,107 houses supplied by Lambeth, only 14 died of cholera. The death rate was 71 per 10,000 in Southwark and Vauxhall households and 5 per 10,000 for Lambeth households. The mortality at the height of the epidemic in households supplied with water by Southwark and Vauxhall was 8 to 9 times greater than in those supplied by Lambeth. Snow was finally able to prove his hypothesis that contaminated water passing down the sewers into the river, then being drawn from the rive and distributed through miles of pipes into peoples' homes produced cholera throughout the community. Snow showed that cholera was a **waterborne** disease that traveled in both surface and groundwater supplies[8–10] (see News File p 31).

Snow laid the groundwork for descriptive and analytic epidemiologic approaches found useful in epidemiology today. He identified various modes of transmission and incubation times and, in his second study, employed a comparison group to more definitively establish a cause-effect association. It was not until Koch's work in 1883 in Egypt, when he isolated and cultivated *Vibrio cholerae,* that the accuracy and correctness of Snow's work was proved and accepted.[3,4,8–10]

CONTRIBUTION OF PASTEUR AND KOCH TO EPIDEMIOLOGY

In the 1870s, on journeys into the countryside of Europe, it was not uncommon to see dead sheep lying in the fields. These sheep had died from **anthrax**, which most commonly occurs in animals but can also occur in humans. Anthrax was a major epidemic that plagued the farmers and destroyed them economically.[3,4]

By this time, Louis Pasteur (1822–1895), a French chemist, had been accepted into France's Academy of Medicine for his work in microbiology. Pasteur had distinguished himself as a scientist and a respected contributor to the field of medicine and public health (even though it was not recognized as a separate field at the time). Pasteur had already iden-

NEWS FILE

Preventing Cholera

A Simple Filtration Procedure Produces a 48% Reduction in Cholera

Cholera continues to plague developing countries and surfaces sporadically throughout the world. In 2001, an estimated 184,311 cases and 2,728 deaths were reported by the World Health Organization. Yet the number of cases and deaths may be much higher because illness and death associated with *Vibrio cholerae* tends to be underreported as a result of surveillance difficulties and threat of economic and social consequences.

Researchers developed a simple filtration procedure involving both nylon filtration and sari cloth (folded four to eight times) filtration for rural villagers in Bangladesh to remove *Vibrio cholerae* attached to plankton in environmental water. The research hypothesis was that removing the copepods (with which *Vibrio cholerae* is associated) from water used for household purposes, including drinking, would significantly reduce the prevalence of cholera. The study was conducted over a 3-year period.

Both the nylon filtration group and the sari filtration group experienced significantly lower cholera rates than the control group. Both filters were comparable in removing copepods as well as particulate matter from the water. The study estimated that the sari cloth filtration reduced the occurrence of cholera by about 48%. Given the low cost of sari cloth filtration, this prevention method has considerable potential in lowering the occurrence of cholera in developing countries.

(Source: Colwell RR, Huq A, Islam MS, et al. Reduction of cholera in Bangladeshi villages by simple filtration. Proc Natl Acad Sci. *2003;100(3):1051–1055.)*

tified the cause of rabies and many other devastating diseases. Because of his many past successes in microbiology, Pasteur had confidence in his ability to take on the challenge of conquering anthrax.[3,4]

Pasteur was convinced that it was the bacteria identified as anthrax that caused the disease. The anthrax bacteria were always present on **necropsy** (autopsy) of sheep that died from anthrax. It was unclear, however, why the course of the disease occurred the way it did. The cause-effect association seemed to have some loopholes in it. How did the sheep get anthrax? How were the sheep disposed of? Why did the anthrax occur in some areas and not in others? How was the disease transmitted? How did the disease survive? All were questions that Louis Pasteur sought to answer.

Pasteur observed that the dead sheep were buried. The key and insightful discovery was that anthrax spores and/or bacteria were brought back to the surface by earthworms. Koch had previously shown that the anthrax bacteria existed in silkworms and that anthrax was an intestinal disease. Pasteur made the earthworm connection.

Pasteur and his assistants had worked on a vaccine for anthrax for months, and in 1881 an anthrax vaccine was discovered. After a presentation at the Academy of Sciences in Paris, Pasteur was challenged to prove that his vaccine was effective. Pasteur put his career and reputation at stake to prove that his vaccine would work, that disease was caused by microorganisms, and that a cause-effect association exists between a particular microbe and a certain disease.

Pasteur agreed to the challenge with a public demonstration to prove his vaccination process could prevent sheep from getting anthrax. He went to a farm in rural France where 60 sheep were provided for the experiment. He was to vaccinate 25 of the sheep with his new vaccine. After the proper waiting time, Pasteur was then to inoculate 50 of the sheep with a virulent injection of anthrax. Ten sheep were to receive no treatment and were used to compare to the survivors of the experiment (a control group). Pasteur was successful. The inoculated sheep lived, the unvaccinated sheep died, and the control group had no changes. Pasteur successfully demonstrated that his methodology was sound, that vaccinations were sound approaches in disease control, and that bacteria were indeed causes of disease.

Historically many scientists have contributed to the methodology used in epidemiology. Robert Koch (1843–1910) lived in Wollstein, a small town near Breslau, in rural Germany (Prussia). Koch was a private practice physician and district medical officer. Because of his compelling desire to study disease experimentally, he set up a laboratory in his home and purchased equipment, including photography equipment, out of his meager earnings. Robert Koch became a key medical research scientist in Germany in the period of the explosion of knowledge in medicine and public health, and he used photography to take the first pictures of microbes in order to show the world that microorganisms do in fact exist and that they are what cause disease.[3,4,11]

In the 1870s, Koch showed that anthrax was transmissible and reproducible in experimental animals (mice). He identified the spore stage of the growth cycle of microorganisms. The epidemiologic significance that Koch demonstrated was that the anthrax bacillus was the *only* organism that caused anthrax in a susceptible animal.

In 1882, Koch discovered the tubercle bacillus with the use of special culturing and staining methods. Koch and his assistant also perfected the concept of steam sterilization. In Egypt and India, he and assistants discovered the cholera bacterium and proved that it was transmitted by drinking water, food, and clothing. Incidental to the cholera investigations, Koch also found the microorganisms that cause infectious conjunctivitis. One of his major contributions to epidemiology was a paper on waterborne epidemics and how they can be largely prevented by proper water filtration.[3,4,11]

Koch, who began as a country family physician, pioneered the identification of microorganisms and many different bacteria that caused different diseases as well as pure culturing techniques for growing microorganisms in laboratory conditions. Some of the major public health contributions that Koch made were the identification of the tuberculosis and cholera microorganisms and the establishment of the importance of water purification in disease prevention. He was the recipient of many honors throughout his life, including the Nobel Prize in 1905 for his work in microbiology.[3,4,11,12]

Both Pasteur and Koch were successful in putting to rest a major misguided notion of medicine at the time: that the diseases were a result of "spontaneous generation;" that is, organisms would simply appear out of other organisms, a fly would spontaneously appear out of garbage, etc.[8]

THE MICROSCOPE AND ITS CONTRIBUTION TO EPIDEMIOLOGY

The important findings of Koch, Pasteur, Snow, and many others in this era of sanitation and microbe discovery would have been impossible without the use of the microscope.

Koch's camera would not have been invented if the microscope had not been developed and its lenses adapted to picture taking.

The microscope first found scientific use in the 1600s through the work of Cornelius Drebbel (1572–1633), the Janssen brothers of the Netherlands (1590s), and Antoni Van Leeuwenhoek (1632–1723). The microscope was used for medical and scientific purposes by Athanasius Kircher of Fulda (1602–1680). In 1658 in Rome he wrote his publication *Scrutinium Pestis.* He conducted experiments on the nature of putrefaction and showed how microscopic living organisms and maggots develop in decaying matter. He also discovered that the blood of plague patients was filled with countless "worms" not visible to the human eye.

Most of the credit goes to Leeuwenhoek for the advancement, development, and perfection of the use of the microscope. He was the first to effectively apply the microscope in the study of disease and medicine, even though he was not a physician. Because of a driving interest in the microscope, Leeuwenhoek was able to devote much time to microscopy, owning over 247 microscopes and over 400 lenses (many of which he ground himself). He was the first to describe the structure of the crystalline lens.

Leeuwenhoek made contributions to epidemiology. He did a morphologic study of red corpuscles in the blood. He saw the connection of arterial circulation to venous circulation in the human body through the microscopic study of capillary networks. With his microscope, Leeuwenhoek contributed indirectly to epidemiology through microbiology by discovering "animalcules" (microscopic organisms, later called microbes, bacteria, and microorganisms).

In addition to epidemiology and microbiology, chemistry and histology were also developed because of the advent of the microscope, which influenced advances in the study and control of diseases.[4,13]

JOHN GRAUNT AND VITAL STATISTICS

Another major contributor to epidemiology, but in a different manner, was John Graunt (1620–1674). In 1603 in London, a systematic recording of deaths was commenced and was called the "bills of mortality." It is summarized in Figure 2.1. This was the first major contribution to record keeping on a population and was the beginning of the vital statistics aspect of epidemiology. Graunt, when he took over the work, systematically recorded ages, sex, who died, what killed them, where the deaths occurred, and when. Graunt also recorded how many persons per year died of what kind of event or disease (Figure 2.1).[4,11]

Through the analysis of the bills of mortality already developed for London, Graunt summarized mortality data and developed a better understanding of diseases as well as sources and causes of death. Using the data and information he collected, Graunt wrote a book, *Natural and Political Observations Made Upon the Bills of Mortality.* From the bills of mortality, Graunt identified variations in death according to sex, residence, season, and age. Graunt was the first to develop and calculate life tables and life expectancy. He divided deaths into two types of causes: acute (struck suddenly) and chronic (lasted over a long period of time).[4,11]

When Graunt died, little was done to continue his good work until 200 years later, when William Farr (1807–1883) was appointed registrar general in England. Farr built on the ideas of Graunt. The concept of "political arithmetic" was replaced by a new term, "statistics." Farr extended the use of vital statistics and organized and developed a modern vital statistics system, much of which is still in use today. Another important contribution of Farr was to promote the idea that some diseases, especially chronic diseases, can have a **multifactorial etiology**.[14]

The Diseases And Casualties This Year Being 1632

Disease	Number	Disease	Number
Abortive and Stillborn	445	Jaundies	43
Afrighted	1	Jawfaln	8
Aged	628	Impostume	74
Ague	43	Kil'd by Several Accident	46
Apoplex, and Meagrom	17	King's Evil	38
Bit with a mad dog	1	Lethargie	2
Bloody flux, Scowring, and Flux	348	Lunatique	5
Brused, Issues, Sores, and Ulcers	28	Made away themselves	15
Burnt and Scalded	5	Measles	80
Burst, and Rupture	9	Murthered	7
Cancer, and Wolf	10	Over-laid/starved at nurse	7
Canker	1	Palsie	25
Childbed	171	Piles	8
Chrisomes, and Infants	2,268	Plague	8
Cold and Cough	55	Planet	13
Colick, Stone, and Strangury	56	Pleurisie, and Spleen	36
Consumption	1,797	Purples, and Spotted Fever	38
Convulsion	241	Quinsie	7
Cut of the Stone	5	Rising of the Lights	98
Dead in the street and starved	6	Sciatica	1
Dropsie and Swelling	267	Scurvey, and Itch	9
Drowned	34	Suddenly	62
Executed and Prest to death	18	Surfet	86
Falling Sickness	7	Swine Pox	6
Fever	1,108	Teeth	470
Fistula	13	Thrush, Sore Mouth	40
Flox and Small Pox	531	Tympany	13
French Pox	12	Tissick	34
Gangrene	5	Vomiting	1
Gowt	4	Worms	27
Grief	11		

Christened	Buried
Males 4,994	Males 4,932
Females 4,590	Females 4,603
In All 9,584	In All 9,535

Increased in the Burials in the 122 Parishes, and at the Pesthouse this year - 993

Decreased of the Plagues in the 122 Parishes, and at the Pesthouses this year - 266

FIGURE 2.1 Selections from *Natural and Political Observations Made Upon the Bills of Mortality* by John Graunt (First Edition 1662). (*Source:* Johns Hopkins Press: Baltimore, 1937)

RAMAZZINI: OCCUPATIONAL HEALTH AND INDUSTRIAL HYGIENE

Bernardino Ramazzini (1633–1714) was born in Carpi near Modena, Italy. He received his medical training at the University of Parma and did postgraduate studies in Rome. Ramazzini eventually returned to the town of Modena where he became a professor of medicine at the local university. He was interested in the practical problems of medicine and not in the study of ancient theories of medicine, a fact not well received by his colleagues. Through Ramazzini's continuous curiosity and his unwillingness to confine himself to the study of ancient medical theories, he became recognized for his innovative approaches to medical and public health problems. For example, in 1692, at the age of 60, Ramazzini was climbing down into 80-foot wells, taking temperature and barometric readings, trying to discover the origin and rapid flow of Modena's spring water. He tried to associate barometric readings with the cause of disease by taking daily readings during a **typhus** (infectious disease characterized by high fever, a transient rash, and severe illness) epidemic.[3,4,11,13]

Ramazzini came upon a worker in a cesspool. In his conversation with the worker, Ramazzini was told that continued work in this environment would cause the worker to go blind. Ramazzini examined the worker's eyes after he came out of the cesspit and found them bloodshot and dim. After inquiring about other effects of working in cesspools and privies, he was informed that only the eyes were affected.[3,4,11,13]

The event with the cesspool worker turned his mind to a general interest in the relation of work to health. He began work on a book that would become influential in the area of occupational medicine and provided related epidemiologic implications. The book, titled *The Diseases of Workers,* was completed in 1690 but not published until 1703. It was not acceptable to pity the poor or simple laborers in this period of time, which caused Ramazzini to delay the publication because he thought it would not be accepted.[3,4,11,13]

Ramazzini observed that disease among workers arose from two causes. The first, he believed, was from the harmful character of the materials that workers handled because the materials often emitted noxious vapors and very fine particles that could be inhaled. The second cause of disease was ascribed to certain violent and irregular motions and unnatural postures imposed on the body while working.[3,4,11,13]

Ramazzini described the dangers of poisoning from lead used by potters in their glaze. He also identified the danger posed by the use of mercury as used by mirror makers, goldsmiths, and others. He observed that very few of these workers reached old age. If they did not die young, their health was so undermined that they prayed for death. He observed that many had palsy of the neck and hands, loss of teeth, vertigo, asthma, and paralysis. Ramazzini also studied those who used or processed organic materials such as mill workers, bakers, starch makers, tobacco workers, and those who processed wool, flax, hemp, cotton, and silk—all of whom suffered from inhaling the fine dust particles in the processing of the materials.[3,4,11,13]

Ramazzini further examined the harmful effects of the physical and mechanical aspects of work, such as varicose veins from standing, sciatica caused by turning the potter's wheel, and ophthalmia found in glassworkers and blacksmiths. Kidney damage was seen to be suffered by couriers and those who rode for long periods, and hernias appeared among bearers of heavy loads.[3,4,11,13]

Major epidemiologic contributions made by Ramazzini were not only his investigation into and description of work-related maladies but his great concern for prevention. Ramazzini suggested that the cesspool workers fasten transparent bladders over their eyes to protect them, take long rest periods, or if their eyes were weak, get into a different line of work. In discussing the various trades, he suggested changing posture, exercising, providing adequate ventilation in workplaces, and avoiding extreme temperatures in the workplace.

Ramazzini was an observant epidemiologist. He described the outbreak of lathyrism in Modena in 1690. He also described the malaria epidemics of the region and the Paduan cattle plague in 1712.[3,4,11,13]

TYPHOID MARY

In the early 1900s, 350,000 cases of typhoid occurred each year in the United States. **Typhoid fever** is an infectious disease characterized by a continued fever, physical and mental depression, rose-colored spots on the chest and abdomen, diarrhea, and sometimes intestinal hemorrhage or perforation of the bowel. An Irish cook, Mary Mallon, referred to as Typhoid Mary, was believed to be responsible for 53 cases of typhoid fever in a 15-year period.[12]

George Soper, a sanitary engineer studying several outbreaks of typhoid fever in New York City in the 1900s, found the food and water supply no longer suspect as the primary means of transmission of typhoid. Soper continued to search for other means of communication of the disease. He began to look to people instead of fomites, food, and water.

He discovered that Mary Mallon had served as a cook in many homes that were stricken with typhoid. The disease always seemed to follow, but never preceded, her employment. Bacteriologic examination of Mary Mallon's feces showed that she was a chronic carrier of typhoid. Mary seemed to sense that she was giving people sickness, because when typhoid appeared, she would leave with no forwarding address. Mary Mallon illustrated the importance of concern over the chronic typhoid carrier causing and spreading typhoid fever. Like 20% of all typhoid carriers, Mary suffered no illness from the disease. Epidemiologic investigations have shown that carriers might be overlooked if epidemiologic searches are limited to the water, food, and those with a history of the disease.[12,15]

From 1907 to 1910, Mary was confined by health officials. The New York Supreme Court upheld the community's right to keep her in custody and isolation. Typhoid Mary was released in 1910, through legal action she took, and she disappeared almost immediately. Two years later typhoid fever occurred in a hospital in New Jersey and a hospital in New York. More than 200 people were affected. It was discovered that Typhoid Mary had worked at both hospitals as a cook but under a different name. This incident taught public health officials and epidemiologists the importance of keeping track of carriers. It also showed that typhoid carriers should never be allowed to handle food or drink intended for public consumption. In later years Typhoid Mary voluntarily accepted isolation. Typhoid Mary died at age 70.[12,15]

The investigating, tracking, and controlling of certain types of diseases that can affect large populations were epidemiologic insights gained from the Typhoid Mary experience. The importance of protecting public food supplies and the importance of the investigative aspects of disease control were again reinforced and further justified as public health measures.

VITAMINS AND THE CURE OF NUTRITIONAL DISEASES

In the middle to late 1800s, bacteria were being identified as the major causes of disease. However, the discovery of microorganisms and their connection to disease clouded the discovery of the causes of other life-threatening diseases. Beriberi, rickets, and pellagra were still devastating the populations around the world. It was believed in 1870 that up to one third of the poor children in the inner city areas of major cities in the world suffered from serious rickets. Biochemistry was being advanced, and new lines of investigation were opening up. In the 1880s, it was observed that when young mice were fed purified diets, they died quickly. When fed milk, they flourished. In 1887, a naval surgeon, T. K. Takaki, eradicated beriberi from the Japanese navy by adding vegetables, meat, and fish to their diet, which up until then was mostly rice. In 1889, at the London Zoo, it was demonstrated that rickets in lion cubs could be cured by feeding them crushed bone, milk, and cod liver oil.[11,16,17]

The first major epidemiologic implications of deficiency illnesses came in 1886 when the Dutch commissioned the firm of C. A. Pekelharing and Winkler who sent Christian

Eijkman (1858–1930), an army doctor, to the East Indies to investigate the cause of beriberi. Eijkman observed that chickens fed on polished rice developed symptoms of beriberi and recovered promptly when the food was changed to whole rice, but he mistakenly attributed the cause of the disease to a neurotoxin. Eijkman and G. Grijns (1865–1944), a physiologist, suggested that beriberi was a result of the lack of some essential substance in the outer layer of the rice grain. In 1905, Pekelharing conducted a series of experiments based on Eijkman's observations, was more thorough in his work, and came to the same conclusions.

In 1906 Frederick Gowland Hopkins (1861–1947), a British biochemist, did similar studies with a concern for the pathogenesis of rickets and scurvy. Hopkins suggested that other nutritional factors exist beyond the known ones of protein, carbohydrates, fat, and minerals, and these must be present for good health.

In 1911 Casimir Funk (1884–1967), a Polish chemist, isolated a chemical substance that he believed belonged to a class of chemical compounds called amines. Funk added the Latin term for life, *vita*, and invented the term "vitamine." He authored the book *Vitamines.* In 1916, E. V. McCollum showed that two factors were required for the normal growth of rats, a fat-soluble "A" factor found in butter and fats and a water-soluble "B" factor found in nonfatty foods like whole grain rice. These discoveries set the stage for labeling **vitamins** by letters of the alphabet. McCollum in the United States and E. Mellanby in Great Britain showed that the "A" factor was effective in curing rickets. It was also demonstrated that the "A" factor contained two separate factors. A heat-stable factor was identified and found to be the one responsible for curing rickets. A heat-labile factor that was capable of healing xerophthalmia (dryness of the conjunctiva leading to a diseased state of the mucous membrane of the eye resulting from vitamin A deficiency) was also discovered. The heat-stable factor was named vitamin D, and the heat-labile factor was termed vitamin A.[11,16–18]

The discovery of vitamin D connected observations about rickets and cod liver oil. Cod liver oil cured rickets because it contains vitamin D. It was observed that children exposed to sunshine were less likely to get rickets. In Germany in 1919, Kurt Huldschinsky (1883–1940) showed that exposing children to artificial sunshine also cured rickets. It was shown that vitamin D was produced in the body when sunshine acted on its fats. It was later discovered that the anti-beriberi substance vitamin B was also effective against pellagra.[11,16,17]

In this era, the role of social and economic factors was observed to contribute much to the causation of disease, especially poverty conditions, which clearly contributed to nutritional deficiencies.[11]

BEGINNING OF EPIDEMIOLOGY IN THE UNITED STATES

In 1850, Lemuel Shattuck published the first report on sanitation and public health problems in the Commonwealth of Massachusetts. Shattuck was a teacher, sociologist, and statistician, and he served in the state legislature. He was chair of a legislative committee to study sanitation and public health. The report set forth many public health programs and needs for the next century. Of the many needs and programs suggested, several of them were epidemiologic in nature. One of the things needed to ensure that epidemiology, its investigations, and the all-important control and prevention aspects of its work be achieved is an organized and structured effort. The organized effort has to come through an organization sponsored by the government.

Shattuck's report set forth the importance of establishing state and local boards of health. It recommended that an organized effort to collect and analyze vital statistics be established. Shattuck also recommended the exchange of health information, sanitary inspections, research on tuberculosis, and the teaching of sanitation and prevention in medical schools. The health of school children was also of major concern. As a result of the report, boards of health were established, with state departments of health and local public health departments soon to follow, organizations through which epidemiologic activities took place.[19,20]

Quarantine conventions were held in the 1850s. The first in the United States was in Philadelphia in 1857. The prevention of typhus, cholera, and yellow fever was discussed. Port quarantine and the hygiene of immigrants were also of concern. Public health educational activities began at this time. In 1879 the first major book on public health, which included epidemiologic topics, was published by A. H. Buck. The book was titled *Hygiene and Public Health*.[19,20]

The infectious nature of yellow fever was established in 1900 (Figure 2.2). In 1902 the United States Public Health Service was founded, and in 1906 the Pure Food and Drug Act was passed. Standard methods of water analysis were also adopted in 1906. The pasteurization of milk was shown to be effective in controlling the spread of disease in 1913, and in this same year the first school of public health, the Harvard School of Public Health, was established.[19,20]

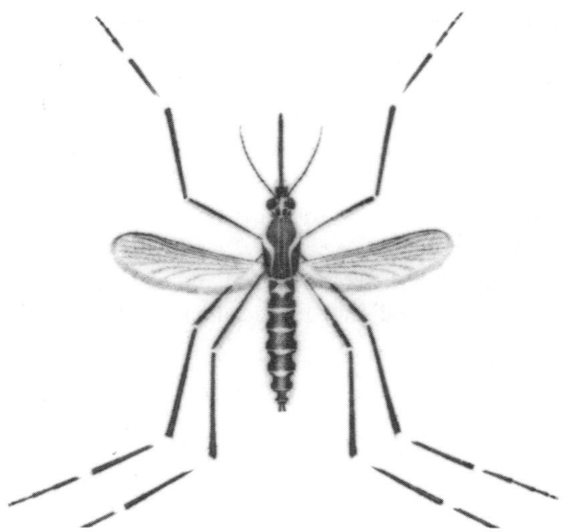

FIGURE 2.2 It has been said "that of all the people who ever died, half of them died from the bite of the mosquito." For thousands of years it was not known that the mosquito was responsible for diseases such as yellow fever and malaria. These two diseases are still not fully contained in many parts of the world. In 1900, Walter Reed, M.D., a U.S. Army physician working in the tropics, made the epidemiological connection between the mosquito (*Aedes aegypti* species) and yellow fever. (Pictures courtesy of Centers for Disease Control and Prevention, Atlanta, Georgia)

HISTORICAL DEVELOPMENT OF MORBIDITY IN EPIDEMIOLOGY

An epidemiology professional of the early 1900s who helped advance the study of disease statistics (morbidity) was Edgar Sydenstricker. The development of a morbidity statistics system in the United States was quite slow. One problem was that morbidity statistics cannot be assessed and analyzed in the same manner that death (mortality) statistics are. Sydenstricker struggled with the mere definition of sickness and recognized that to all persons, disease is an undeniable and frequent experience. Birth and death come to a person only once but illness comes often. This was especially true in Sydenstricker's era when sanitation, public health, microbiology, and disease control and prevention measures were still being developed.[21]

In the early 1900s morbidity statistics of any given kind were not regularly collected on a large scale. Interest in disease statistics came only when the demand for them arose from special populations and when the statistics would prove useful socially and economically. Additionally, Sydenstricker noted that there were barriers to collecting homogeneous morbidity data in large amounts: differences in data collection methods and definitions; time elements; and the existence of peculiar factors that affect the accuracy of all records.[21]

Sydenstricker suggested that morbidity statistics be classified into five general groups in order to be of value.

1. Reports of communicable disease. Notification of those diseases for which reasonably effective administrative controls have been devised.
2. Hospital and clinical records. These records were viewed as being of little value in identifying incidence or prevalence of illness in populations. (At this time most people were treated at home unless they were poor and in need of assistance.) Such records are only of value for clinical studies.
3. Insurance and industrial establishment and school illness records. The absence of records of illnesses in workers in large industries in the United States was of concern because it added to the difficulty of defining and explaining work-related illness. Criteria for determining disability from illness or injury at work and when sick benefits should be allowed were not well developed. Malingering was also considered, as was its effect on the illness rates of workers. It was suggested that if illness records showing absence from school were kept with a degree of specificity, they could be of value to the understanding of the effect of disease on these populations.
4. Illness surveys. Illness surveys have been used by major insurance companies to determine the prevalence of illness in a specific population. House-to-house canvass approaches have been used. Incidence of diseases within a given period is not revealed by such methods, whereas chronic-type diseases are found to be of higher incidence (which should be expected and predicted).
5. Records of the incidence of illness in a population continuously or frequently observed. To benefit epidemiologic studies, 2 study methods were employed: (1) determination of the annual illness rate in a representative population, and (2) development of an epidemiologic method whereby human populations could be observed in order to determine the existence of an incidence of various diseases as they were manifested under normal conditions within the community.[21]

A morbidity study by Sydenstricker and his colleagues under the direction of the United States Public Health Service in Hagerstown, Maryland, 1921–1924, was conducted. The study involved 16,517 person-years of observation or an equivalent population of 1,079 individuals who were observed for 28 months beginning in 1921. Illnesses discovered in field investigations, when family members reported being sick or when researchers observed a sick person, were recorded during each family visit. A fairly accurate record of actual illness was obtained by a community interview method. Two findings included were that only 5% of illnesses were of short duration of one day or less, and that 40% were not only disabling but caused bed confinement as well. An accurate data-gathering process was developed from the experience.[21]

In the study, 17,847 cases of illness were recorded in a 28-month period. An annual rate of 1,081 per 1,000 person-years was observed, about one illness per person-year. The illness rate was 100 times the annual death rate in the same population.[21]

The most interesting results of this first morbidity study were the variations of incidence of illness according to age. Incidence of frequent attacks of illness, four or more a year, was highest (45%) in children aged 2–9 years and lowest in those aged 20–24 years (11%). By age 35, the rate rose again, to 21%. When severity of illness was looked at, it was found that the greatest resistance to disease was in children between 5 and 14 years. The lowest resistance to disease was in early childhood, 0–4 years, and toward the end of life.[21,22]

FRAMINGHAM HEART STUDY

In 1948 the Framingham, Massachusetts, cardiovascular disease study was launched. The aim of the study was to determine which of the many risk factors contribute most to cardiovascular disease. At the beginning, the study involved 6,000 persons between 30 and 62 years of age. These persons were recruited to participate in a cohort study that spanned 30 years, with 5,100 residents completing the study. In each of the 30 years, medical exams and other related testing activities were conducted with the participants. The study was initially sponsored by the National Health Institute of the United States Public Health Service and the Massachusetts Department of Public Health, along with the local Framingham Health Department.[23–25]

The site for the study was determined by several factors. It was implied that Framingham was a cross-section of Americana and was a typical small American city. Framingham had a fairly stable population, one major hospital was used by most of the people in the community, an annual updated city population list was kept, and a broad range of occupations, jobs, and industries were represented. The study approach used in the Framingham study was a prospective cohort study.[23–25]

The diseases of most concern in the study were coronary heart disease, rheumatic heart disease, congestive heart failure, angina pectoris, stroke, gout, gallbladder disease, and eye conditions. Several clinical categories of heart disease were distinguished in this study: myocardial infarction, angina pectoris, coronary insufficiency, and death from coronary heart disease as shown by a specific clinical diagnosis.[23–25]

Many study design methods and approaches were advanced in the investigation, such as cohort tracking, population selection, sampling, issues related to age of the population, mustering population support, community organization, a specific chronic disease focus, and analysis of the study findings.

CIGARETTE SMOKING AND CANCER

Following World War II, vital statistics indicated a sharp increase in deaths attributed to lung cancer. The first epidemiologic reports suggesting a link between cigarette smoking and lung cancer appeared in the early 1950s.[26–30] By the time of the 1964 report by the Surgeon General of the United States, there had been 29 case-control studies and 7 prospective cohort studies published, all showing a significantly increased risk of lung cancer among tobacco smokers.[31]

The first case-control studies that assessed the association between smoking and lung cancer were conducted in the late 1940s by Wynder and Graham in the United States (1950) and Doll and Hill in Great Britain (1950).[32,33] These studies first identified cases with lung cancer and controls and then investigated whether people with lung cancer differed from others without the disease with respect to their smoking history. Both studies showed that lung cancer patients were more likely to have been smokers.

The first cohort study assessing the association between smoking and lung cancer was conducted in 1951 by Doll and Hill.[34,35] Physicians in Great Britain were sent a questionnaire to determine their smoking habits. They were then followed over a 25-year period with death certificate information collected to determine if deaths were attributed to lung cancer or some other cause. The study found that smokers were 10 times more likely to die of lung cancer than nonsmokers.

The case-control and cohort study designs used by these researchers remain commonly used in epidemiologic research today.

EXERCISES

Key Terms

Define the following terms.

Anthrax
Atomic theory
Childbed fever
Cholera
Hot and cold diseases
Multifactorial etiology
Necropsy
Scurvy
Smallpox
Typhoid fever
Typhus
Variolation
Vitamin
Waterborne

Study Questions

2.1 Match the individuals in Column A with their historical contributions in Column B.

Column A		Column B
___ Hippocrates	A.	Identified the cause of rabies
	B.	Invented a vaccination for smallpox
___ Thomas Sydenham	C.	Published the first report on sanitation and public health problems
___ James Lind		
	D.	Introduced the terms epidemic and endemic
___ Benjamin Jesty	E.	Showed an association between smoking and lung cancer using case-control and cohort study designs
___ Edward Jenner	F.	Chronic healthy (passive) carrier of typhoid fever, causing over 50 cases

___ Ignaz Semmelweis
___ John Snow
___ Louis Pasteur
___ Robert Koch
___ John Graunt
___ William Farr
___ Bernardino Ramazzini
___ Mary Mallon
___ T. K. Takaki
___ Lemuel Shattuck
___ Edgar Sydenstricker
___ Doll and Hill

G. Applied experimental methods to identify that oranges and lemons were effective remedies for scurvy at sea
H. Insisted that observation should drive the study of the course of disease
I. With Pasteur, established the germ theory of disease
J. Exposed his wife and children to cowpox
K. Eradicated beriberi in a group with certain foods
L. Associated certain occupational exposures to disease
M. Conducted descriptive and analytic epidemiologic studies investigating cholera epidemics in London
N. Developed and calculated life tables and life expectancy
O. Identified the importance of washing hands to prevent the spread of disease
P. Developed a modern vital statistics system
Q. Developed morbidity statistics

2.2 List some of the contributions of the microscope to epidemiology.

2.3 What two individuals contributed to the birth of vital statistics?

2.4 What type of epidemiologic study was used by James Lind?

2.5 What types of epidemiologic studies were used by Doll and Hill?

REFERENCES

1. Hippocrates. Airs, waters, places. In: Buck C, Llopis A, Najera E, Terris M, eds. *The Challenge of Epidemiology: Issues and Selected Readings.* Washington, DC: World Health Organization; 1988:18–19.
2. *Dorland's Illustrated Medical Dictionary.* 25th ed. Philadelphia, PA: Saunders; 1974.
3. Cumston CG. *An Introduction to the History of Medicine.* New York, NY: Alfred A. Knopf; 1926.
4. Garrison FH. *History of Medicine.* Philadelphia, PA: Saunders; 1926.
5. Lilienfeld AM, Lilienfeld DE. *Foundations of Epidemiology.* 2nd ed. New York, NY: Oxford; 1980:30–31.
6. Jenner E. An inquiry into the causes and effects of the variolae vaccine. In: Buck C, Llopis A, Najera E, Terris M, eds. *The Challenge of Epidemiology: Issues and Selected Readings.* Washington, DC: World Health Organization; 1988:31–32.
7. Semmelweis I. The etiology, concept, and prophylaxis of childbed fever. In: Buck C, Llopis A, Najera E, Terris M, eds. *The Challenge of Epidemiology: Issues and Selected Readings.* Washington, DC: World Health Organization; 1988:46–59.
8. Benenson AS, ed. *Control of Communicable Diseases in Man.* 15th ed. Washington, DC: American Public Health Association; 1990:367–373.
9. Snow J. *On the Mode of Communication of Cholera.* 2nd ed, 1855. Reprinted by Commonwealth Fund, New York, NY; 1936.
10. Snow J. On the mode of communication of cholera. In: Buck C, Llopis A, Najera E, Terris M, eds. *The Challenge of Epidemiology: Issues and Selected Readings.* Washington, DC: World Health Organization; 1988:42–45.
11. Rosen G. *A History of Public Health.* New York, NY: MD Publications; 1958.

12. Nester EW, McCarthy BJ, Roberts CE, Pearsall NN. *Microbiology: Molecules, Microbes and Man*. New York, NY: Holt, Rinehart and Winston; 1973.
13. Seelig MG. *Medicine: An Historical Outline*. Baltimore: Williams and Wilkins; 1925.
14. Fox JP, Hall CE, Elveback LR. *Epidemiology: Man and Disease*. New York, NY: Macmillan Company; 1970.
15. Health News. *Medical Milestone: Mary Mallon, Typhoid Mary*. November 1968. New York, NY: New York Department of Health; 1968.
16. Krause MV, Hunscher MA. *Food, Nutrition and Diet Therapy*. 5th ed. Philadelphia, PA: Saunders; 1972.
17. Guthrie HA. *Introductory Nutrition*. St. Louis, MO: Mosby; 1975.
18. Clayton T, ed. *Taber's Medical Dictionary*. 14th ed. Philadelphia, PA: Davis; 1981:762.
19. Green L, Anderson C. *Community Health*. 5th ed. St. Louis, MO: Times Mirror/Mosby; 1986.
20. Picket G, Hanlon J. *Public Health: Administration and Practice*. 9th ed. St. Louis, MO: Times Mirror/Mosby; 1990.
21. Sydenstricker E. A study of illness in a general population. *Public Health Rep*. 1926;61:12.
22. Sydenstricker E. Sex difference in the incidence of certain diseases at different ages. *Public Health Rep*. 1928;63:1269–1270.
23. Miller DF. *Dimensions of Community Health*. 3rd ed. Dubuque, IA: William C. Brown; 1992.
24. Hennekens CH, Buring JE. *Epidemiology in Medicine*. Boston, MA: Little, Brown and Company; 1987.
25. Dawber TR, Kannel WB, Lyell LP. An approach to longitudinal studies in a community: The Framingham study. *Ann NY Acad Sci.* 1963;107:539–556.
26. Doll R, Hill AB. Smoking and carcinoma of the lung: Preliminary report. *BMJ*. 1950;2:739.
27. Norr R. Cancer by the carton. *Read Dig*. December 1952:7–8.
28. Cigarettes. What CU's test showed: The industry and its advertising, and how harmful are they? *Consum Rep*. February 1953: 58–74.
29. Miller LM, Monahan J. The facts behind the cigarette controversy. *Read Dig*. July 1954:1–6.
30. Tobacco smoking and lung cancer. *Consum Rep*. February 1954:54,92.
31. United States Department of Health and Human Services. *Smoking and Health: Report of the Advisory Committee to the Surgeon General of the Public Health Service*. Washington, DC: US Government Printing Office; 1964. Publication PHS 1103.
32. Wynder EL, Graham EA. Tobacco smoking as a possible etiologic factor in bronchiogenic carcinoma. A study of six hundred and eighty-four proved cases. *J Am Med Assoc*. 1950;143: 329–336.
33. Doll R, Hill AB. Smoking and carcinoma of the lung: Preliminary Report. *BMJ*. 1950;2:739–748.
34. Doll R, Hill AB. Mortality in relation to smoking: Ten years' observations of British doctors. *BMJ*. 1964;1:1399–1410.
35. Doll R, Peto R. Mortality in relation to smoking. Twenty years' observations on male British doctors. *BMJ*. 1976;2:1525.

CHAPTER

3

Practical Disease Concepts in Epidemiology

OBJECTIVES

After completing this chapter you will be able to

- Define disease.
- Classify acute and chronic diseases according to infectivity and communicability.
- Identify various classifications of diseases and conditions and their sources and modes of transmission.
- Understand the major stages in the disease process.
- Know the five major categories of disease.
- Identify the role of zoonoses in communicable disease in humans.
- Discuss notifiable disease reporting in the United States.
- Discuss immunity and immunizations against infectious diseases.
- Identify the changing emphasis of epidemiologic study.
- Be familiar with common nutritional deficiency diseases and disorders.
- Be familiar with selected chronic diseases and conditions.

INTRODUCTION

Disease is an interruption, cessation, or disorder of body functions, systems, or organs.[1] Diseases arise from infectious agents, inherent weaknesses, lifestyle, or environmental stresses. Often a combination of these factors influences the onset of disease. The early development of epidemiology was based on the investigation of infectious disease outbreaks. Today, epidemiology studies also consider diseases that are influenced by noninfectious causes such as genetic susceptibility, lifestyle, and environment.

Identifying the causes of disease and the mechanisms by which disease is spread remains a primary focus of epidemiology. The science and study of the causes of disease and their mode of operation is referred to as **etiology**.[1] Disease processes are complex and require an understanding of several factors, which may include anatomy, physiology, histology, biochemistry, microbiology, and related medical sciences. This book cannot provide a comprehensive foundation of all these fields of study. Thus only the basics of diseases, their classification, and processes will be presented in this chapter.

FUNDAMENTALS OF COMMUNICABLE AND NONCOMMUNICABLE DISEASES AND CONDITIONS

Infectious diseases are caused by invading organisms called pathogens. Infectious diseases may or may not be contagious. When an infectious disease is contagious, or capable of being communicated or transmitted, it is called a **communicable** disease.[1] Examples of infectious communicable diseases are HIV/AIDS, cholera, and influenza. Although all communicable diseases are infectious diseases, not all infectious diseases are communicable diseases. An example of an infectious noncommunicable disease is tetanus, caused by the bacterium *Clostridium tetani*, which is found in the environment. Spores of the bacterium live in the soil, may remain infectious for over 40 years, and are found throughout the world. Similarly, anthrax may be caught by breathing spores that have been in the soil for, in some cases, many years. Another example is Legionnaires' disease, which is caused by inhaling Legionella bacteria from the environment. Noninfectious diseases may be referred to as noncommunicable diseases and conditions, such as heart diseases, most forms of cancer, mental illness, and accidents.

Infectious communicable diseases may be transmitted through vertical or horizontal transmission. **Vertical transmission** refers to transmission from an individual to its offspring through sperm, placenta, milk, or vaginal fluids.[1] **Horizontal transmission** refers to transmission of infectious agents from an infected individual to a susceptible contemporary.[1] Horizontal transmission may involve direct transmission (eg, sexually transmitted diseases), a common vehicle (eg, waterborne, foodborne, or bloodborne diseases), an airborne pathogen (eg, tuberculosis), or a vectorborne pathogen (eg, malaria).

Pathogens are defined as organisms or substances such as bacteria, viruses, or parasites that are capable of producing disease.[1] Infectious diseases are those in which the pathogen is capable of entering, surviving, and multiplying in the host. The ability to get into a susceptible host and cause disease is termed **invasiveness**. The host plays a major part in the ability of a microorganism to cause disease by providing nutrients and a life-sustaining environment. The disease-evoking power of a pathogen is called **virulence**.[1]

Antibiotics work against pathogens because of their toxicity. That is, the antibiotic substance contains elements that are more toxic to bacteria than to the human body. **Tox-**

ins are poisons and consequently kill bacteria or viruses by poisoning them. For example, arsenic is a toxin once used to treat syphilis.[2] The strength of a substance or chemical is measured by how little of it is required for it to work as a poison and how quickly it acts. The shorter the duration and the less of the substance needed to cause the organism to die, the higher the level of toxicity.

Diseases are classified as acute and chronic.

Acute: relatively severe disorder with sudden onset and short duration of symptoms[1]

Chronic: less severe but of continuous duration, lasting over long time periods if not a lifetime[1]

Infectious and noninfectious diseases can be acute or chronic. To help clarify acute and chronic disease classification according to infectivity and communicability, some examples are presented in Table 3.1.

NATURAL HISTORY OF DISEASE

Each disease has a natural history of progression if no medical intervention is taken and the disease is allowed to run its full course. There are 4 common stages relevant to most diseases.

- Stage of susceptibility
- Stage of presymptomatic disease
- Stage of clinical disease
- Stage of recovery, disability, or death

Table 3.1 Examples of diseases and conditions according to selected classifications

	Communicable		***Noncommunicable***	
	Acute	***Chronic***	***Acute***	***Chronic***
Infectious	Influenza/pneumonia	Cancer	Tetanus	
	Lyme disease	Leprosy	Legionnaire's	
	Mumps	Polio	Anthrax	
	Measles	Syphilis		
	Cholera	Tuberculosis		
Noninfectious			Accidents	Alcoholism
			Drug abuse	Cancer
			Homicide	Diabetes mellitus
			Stroke	Heart diseases
			Suicide	Paralysis

The stage of susceptibility precedes the disease and involves the likelihood a host has of developing ill effects from an external agent. The stage of presymptomatic disease begins with exposure and subsequent pathologic changes that occur before the onset of symptoms. This is also typically called the **incubation period**. For noncommunicable chronic diseases, the time from exposure to clinical symptoms is typically called the **latency period**. The stage of clinical disease begins when signs and symptoms manifest. The final stage of recovery, disability, or death is influenced by many factors, including early detection and effective treatment. With regard to prevention, primary prevention may occur during the stage of susceptibility, secondary prevention may occur during the stage of presymptomatic disease or the stage of clinical disease, and tertiary prevention may occur during the stage of clinical disease or in the final stage.

With infectious disease, the natural course of the disease begins with the susceptible person's exposure to a pathogen. The pathogen propagates itself and then spreads within the host. Factors of each disease, each pathogen, and each individual host vary the way a disease responds, spreads, and affects the body. The progress of a disease can be halted at any point, either by the strength of the response of the body's natural immune system or through intervention with antibiotics, therapeutics, or other medical interventions (Figure 3.1). Changes in the body are initially undetected and unfelt. As the pathogen continues to propagate, changes are experienced by the host, marked by the onset of such symptoms as fever, headache, weakness, muscle aches, malaise, and upset stomach. The disease reacts in the body in the manner peculiar to that disease. Possible outcomes are recovery, disability, or death. A generalized presentation of the natural history of disease is shown in Figure 3.2.

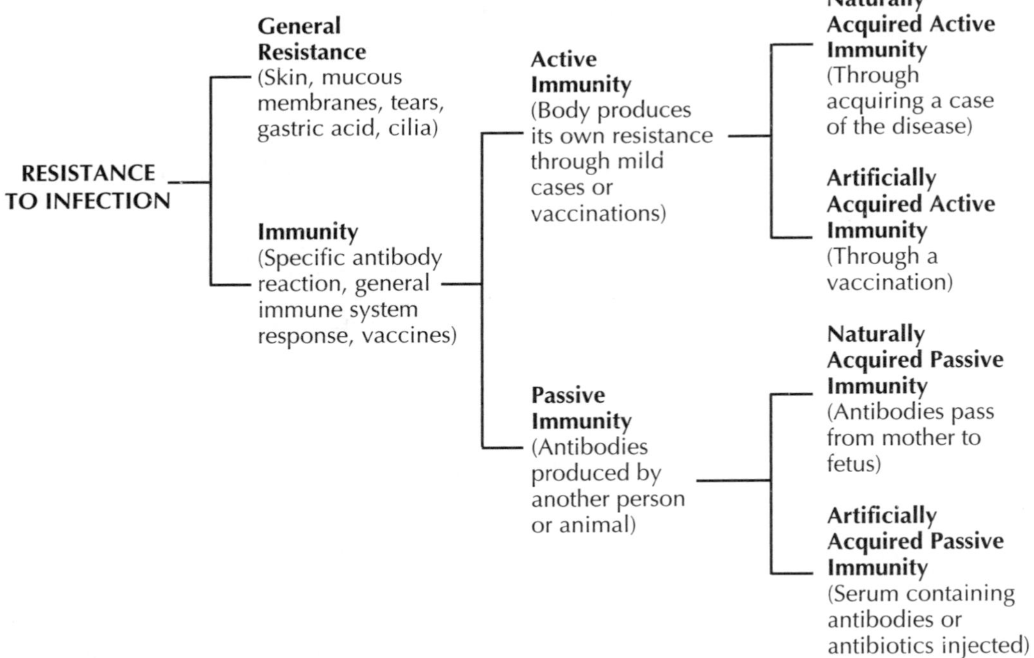

FIGURE 3.1 How the human body resists infections.

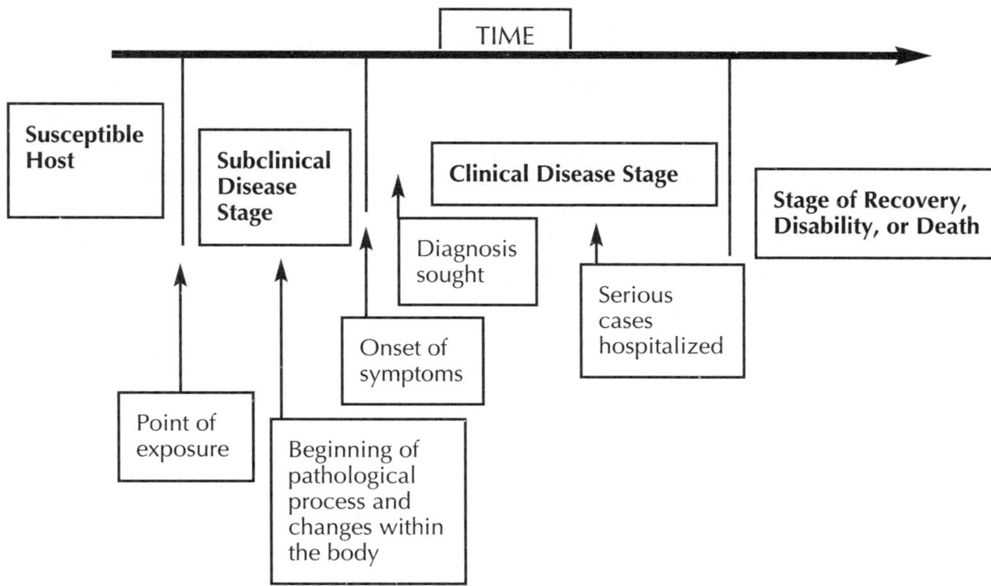

FIGURE 3.2 Natural course of a communicable disease.

CLASSIFYING DISEASES

Diseases can be classified into 5 general categories: congenital and hereditary diseases, allergies and inflammatory diseases, degenerative diseases, metabolic diseases, and cancer. Each of these is defined as follows.

- **Congenital and hereditary diseases** are often caused by genetic and familial tendencies toward certain inborn abnormalities; injury to the embryo or fetus by environmental factors, chemicals, or agents such as drugs, alcohol, or smoking; or innate developmental problems possibly caused by chemicals or agents. They can also be a fluke of nature. Examples are Down syndrome, hemophilia, and heart disease present at birth.[2]
- **Allergies and inflammatory diseases** are caused by the body reacting to an invasion of or injury by a foreign object or substance. Allergies, viruses, bacteria, or other microscopic and microbiological agents can cause an inflammatory reaction in the body. Some inflammatory reactions may result in the body forming antibodies. **Antibodies** are formed as a first line of defense. They are protein substances or globulins derived from B and T lymphocytes that originate in the bone marrow.[2]
- **Degenerative diseases** cause a lower level of mental, physical, or moral state than is normal or acceptable. Degenerative diseases are often associated with the aging process but in some cases may not be age related. Arteriosclerosis, arthritis, and gout are examples of degenerative chronic diseases.[2]
- **Metabolic diseases** cause the dysfunction, poor function, or malfunction of certain organs or physiologic processes in the body, leading to disease states. Glands or organs that fail to secrete certain biochemicals to keep the metabolic process functioning in the body

cause metabolic disorders. For example, adrenal glands may stop functioning properly causing Addison's disease; the cells may no longer use glucose normally, causing diabetes; or the thyroid gland might fail, resulting in a goiter, hyperthyroidism, or cretinism (hypothyroidism).[2]

- **Cancer** is a collective name that refers to a group of many diseases with one common characteristic: uncontrolled cell growth or the loss of the cell's ability to perform apoptosis (cell suicide). The gradual increase in the number of uncontrolled dividing cells creates a mass of tissue called a tumor (neoplasm). When a tumor is malignant, meaning it is capable of spreading to surrounding tissue or remote places in the body, it is called cancer.[3]

Diseases may also be classified according to their source (Table 3.2) or mode of transmission (Table 3.3).

Table 3.2 Classification of sources of disease or illness

Classification	*Examples of Sources*
Allergic	Mold, dust, foods
Chemical	Drugs, acids, alkali, heavy metals (lead, mercury), poisons (arsenic), some enzymes
Congenital	Rubell, cytomegalovirus, syphilis, toxoplasmosis, alcohol abuse
Hereditary	Familial tendency diseases such as alcoholism, genetic or chromosome structure that passes disability, disease, or disorders on to off-spring; syndromes
Infectious	Bacteria, viruses, parasites
Inflammatory	Stings, poison ivy, wounds, slivers or impaled objects, arthritis, serum sickness, allergic reactions
Metabolic	Dysfunctional organs within the body producing hypothyroidism, hyperthyroidism, exophthalmic goiter
Nutritional	Vitamin deficiencies such as scurvy or protein deficiencies such as kwashiorkor
Physical agent	Excessive cold or heat, electrical shock, radiation, injury
Psychological	Biochemical imbalances in the brain as in schizophrenia; loss of or destruction of brain tissue such as in Alzheimer's disease
Traumatic	Wounds, bone fractures, contusions, mechanical injury
Tumors	Environmental or behaviorally stimulated tumors, such as cancer of the lung from smoking
Vascular	Smoking, stress, lack of proper diet, lack of exercise, and other behaviorally related implications that contribute to heart and cardiovascular diseases

Source: Adapted from Green LW, Ottoson JM. *Community Health*. 7th ed. St. Louis, MO: Mosby Publishing Company; 1994.

Table 3.3 Classification of major infectious diseases by mode of transmission

Airborne Respiratory Diseases	***Intestinal Discharge Diseases***	***Open Sores or Lesion Diseases***	***Zoonoses or Vectorborne Diseases***	***Fomiteborne Diseases***
Chickenpox	Amebic dysentery	AIDS	African sleeping sickness	Anthrax
Common colds	Bacterial dysentery (shigellosis) (staphylococcal)	Anthrax	Encephalitis	Chickenpox
Diphtheria	Cholera	Erysipelas	Lyme disease	Common colds
Influenza	Giardiasis	Gonorrhea	Malaria	Diphtheria
Measles	Hookworm	Scarlet fever	Rocky Mountain spotted fever	Influenza
Meningitis	Poliomyelitis	Smallpox	Tularemia	Meningitis
Pneumonia	Salmonellosis	Syphilis	Typhus fever	Poliomyelitis
Poliomyelitis	Typhoid fever	Tuberculosis	Yellow fever	Rubella
Rubella	Hepatitis	Tularemia		Scarlet fever
Scarlet fever				Streptococcal throat infections
Smallpox				Tuberculosis
Throat infections				
Tuberculosis				
Whooping cough				

The ability of a disease to be transmitted from one person to the next or to spread in a population is referred to as the communicability of the disease. The **communicability** of a disease is determined by how likely a pathogen or agent is to be transmitted from a diseased or infected person to another person who is not immune and is susceptible. Five different means of transmission can be used to classify certain infectious diseases. The 5 classifications are airborne or respiratory transmission, transmission through intestinal (alvine) discharge (which includes waterborne and foodborne diseases), transmission through open lesions, zoonotic or vectorborne transmission, and fomiteborne transmission. The 5 classifications and some of the major related diseases and modes of transmission are shown in Table 3.3.[4–8]

Diseases can also be classified by the microbe source from which they come. Table 3.4 presents the different classes of microorganisms along with examples.[2,4,5,6,9–11]

In addition, 3 microscopic animal sources of disease exist. The classifications of the 3 animal sources are presented in Table 3.5. The organism is presented, along with an example of the disease it causes.[2,4,5,6,8–11]

Pathogens are not the only sources of disease, conditions, or death in humans. Many causes of illness, conditions, and injury exist. Some are of man's own doing, some are naturally occurring, and others are environmentally related. Still other conditions are self-inflicted at work, in industry, at home, or in the process of getting to and from work. Table 3.6 presents the different inanimate sources of illness and disability. The source and an example of illness or disability for each are presented, as is the mode of entry into the body.[12,13]

Table 3.4 Classification of microbe sources of disease

Organisms	***Diseases***
Bacteria	
bacilli	Diphtheria (aerobic—*Corynebacterium diphtheriae*)
	Botulism (anaerobic—*Clostridium botulinum*)
	Brucellosis (*Brucella abortus*)
	Legionellosis (*Legionella pneumophila*)
	Salmonellosis (salmonella)
	Shigellosis (*Shigella dysentariae*)
	Cholera (*Vibrio cholerae*)
cocci	Impetigo (*Staphylococcus aureus, streptococci*)
	Toxic shock (*staphylococci*)
	Streptococcal sore throat (*streptococci*)
	Scarlet fever (*streptococci*)
	Erysipelas (*streptococci*)
	Pneumonia (*pneumococci*)
	Gonorrhea (*gonococci*)
	Meningitis (*meningococci*)
spiral organisms	Syphilis (*Treponema pallidum*)
	Rat-bite fever (*Streptobacillusmoniliformis* and *Spirillum minus*)
	Lyme disease (spriochete—*Borrelia burgdorferi*)
acid-fast organisms	Tuberculosis (*Mycobacterium tuberculosis*)
	Leprosy (*Myocobacterium leprae*)
Rickettsia	Rocky Mountain spotted fever (*Rickettsia rickettsii*)
(very small bacteria)	Typhus (*Rickettsia prowazekii*)
Viruses	Chickenpox (herpes virus)
	Influenza
	—Type A: associated with epidemics and pandemics
	—Type B: associated with local epidemics
	—Type C: associated with sporadic minor localized outbreaks
	Measles (*Morbillivirus*)
	Mumps (*Paramyxovirus*)
	Poliomyelitis (Type 1, most paralytogenic; 2, 3, less common)
	Rabies
	Smallpox (*Variola* virus)
Fungi	Mycosis
Molds	Ringworm
Yeast	Biastomycosis
	Dermatophytosis

Table 3.5 Classification of animal sources of disease

Organisms	***Disease***
Protozoa (one celled)	
Amoebae	Dysentery
Plasmodia	Malaria
Worms (metazoa)	
Roundworms	Ascaris (large roundworms)
Pinworms	
Flukes	
Trichinellae	Trichinosis
Arthropods (lice)	Pediculosis
	Scabies (*Sarcoptes scabiei*)

PORTALS OF ENTRY TO THE HUMAN BODY

Different modes of entry into the body have been identified. They are listed here, with the more common sites of entry listed first.

- Respiratory
- Oral
- Reproductive
- Intravenous
- Urinary
- Skin
- Gastrointestinal
- Conjunctival
- Transplacental

INCUBATION PERIODS FOR SELECTED INFECTIOUS DISEASES

To become ill, an individual has to be inoculated with a disease. This brings to mind a picture of an *Anopheles* mosquito biting (inoculation by injection) an unsuspecting susceptible individual on a warm spring evening, infecting the person with a disease such as malaria. The incubation period is the time that elapses between inoculation and the appearance of the first signs or symptoms of the disease. In the case of the victim with the mosquito bite, the incubation for malaria is about 15 days (range 10–35 days) from the time of the bite until the victim starts having shaking chills, fever, sweats, malaise, and a headache. This lasts for about one day and then recurs on and off every 48 hours. Difficulty determining when the exposure occurred (inoculation or exposure to illness)

Table 3.6 Classification of inanimate sources of illness and disability

Source	*Illness/Disability*	*Mode of Entry*
Dusts		
Silica	Silicosis (fibrosis of lung tissue)	Inhalation
Asbestos	Asbestosis (fibrosis of lung tissue)	
	Lung cancer	
Fumes		
Lead	Lead poisoning	Inhalation, Skin
Smoke	Asphyxia from oxygen deficiency	Inhalation
	Smoke poisoning	
	Asphyxia from carbon monoxide	
Gases, mists, aerosols, and vapors	Asphyxia or chemical poisoning (depending on the source)	Inhalation
Electrical energy	Burns, neurologic damage, death	Skin
Noise	Hearing loss, deafness	Nervous system
Ionizing radiation	Cancer, dermatitis	Skin/tissue
Nonionizing radiation	Burns, cancer	Skin/tissue
Thermal energy	Burns, cancer	Skin/tissue
Ergonomic problems	Muscle, skeletal, tissue problems	Skin/tissue
Stress	Mental, emotional physiologic, behavioral problems	Nervous system
Bites	Snakebite poisoning, lacerations, tissue damage	Skin/tissue
Stings	Pain, swelling, redness	Skin/tissue
Chemical ingestion	Cancer, liver damage, respiratory damage	Respiratory, digestive, skin/tissue

makes ascertaining the starting point of the incubation period problematic. Vague prodromal signs of illness make it difficult to determine the end point of the illness, and the signs and symptoms of different diseases are often alike; for example, malaria could initially be mistaken for flu.

Some diseases are transmissible in the last 2 or 3 days of the incubation period, for example, measles and chickenpox. As seen in Table 3.7, incubation periods vary from disease to disease. Incubation periods can also vary with the individual; one who has a more active immune system can retard the pathogen's growth within the body, lengthening the incubation period. It has been observed that diseases with short incubation periods generally produce a more acute and severe illness, while long incubation diseases are less severe, although there are, of course, exceptions.

LATER STAGES OF INFECTION

The **prodromal period** is the second stage of illness and the period in which signs and symptoms of a disease first appear. In most respiratory diseases, this is usually one day. Disease

Table 3.7 Partial list of incubation periods for major communicable diseases

Disease	*Incubation Period*	*Communicability Period*
Botulism	12–36 hours	When exposed
Chickenpox	2–3 weeks	From 5 days before vesicles appear to 6 days after
Common cold	12–72 hours (usually 24)	From 1 day before onset to 5 days after
Conjunctivitis	1–3 days	As long as infection is present and active
Diphtheria	2–5 days	≤2 weeks and not more than 4 weeks
Dysentery (amoebic)	2–4 weeks (wide variation)	During intestinal infection; untreated, for years
Epstein-Barr virus	4–7 weeks	While symptoms are present
Gonorrhea	2–5 days (maybe longer)	Indefinite unless treated
Hepatitis (serum)	45–160 days	Before onset of symptoms
Herpes simplex virus	Up to 2 weeks	As long as 7 weeks after symptoms disappear
Impetigo (contagious)	4–10 days or longer	Until lesions heal
Influenza	1–3 days	Often 3 days from clinical onset
Measles (rubeola)	10 days to onset, rash at 14 days	From prodromal period to 4 days after rash onset
Meningitis	2–10 days	1 day after beginning of medication
Mumps	12–26 days (usually 18 days)	From 6 days before symptoms to 9 days after
Pediculosis	Approximately 2 weeks	As long as lice remain alive
Pneumonia, bacterial	1–3 days	Unknown
Pneumonia, viral	1–3 days	Unknown
Poliomyelitis	3–21 days (usually 7–12 days)	7 to 10 days before and after symptoms
Pinworm (enterobiasis)	2–6 weeks	Up to 2 weeks
Rabies	2–8 weeks or longer	3 to 5 days before symptoms and during the course of the disease
Respiratory viral infection	A few days to a week or more	Duration of the active disease
Ringworm	4–10 days	As long as lesions are present
Rubella (German measles)	8–10 days (usually 14 days)	1 week before and to 4 days after onset of rash
Salmonella food poisoning	6–72 hours (usually 36 hrs)	3 days to 3 weeks (wide variation)
Scarlet fever	1–3 days	24 to 48 hours (treated); 10 to 21 days (untreated)

(continued)

Table 3.7 *(Continued)*

Disease	***Incubation Period***	***Communicability Period***
Staphylococcal food poisoning	2–4 hours	When exposed
Streptococcal sore throat	1–3 days	24 to 48 hours (treated); as long as ill (untreated)
Smallpox	7–17 days (usually 10–12)	Primarily within 7–10 days of onset of rash
Syphilis	10 days–10 weeks (usually 3 weeks)	Variable and indefinite if not treated
Tetanus	4 days–3 weeks	When exposed
Trichinosis	2–128 days (usually 9 days) after ingestion of infected meat	When exposed
Tuberculosis	4–12 weeks (primary phase)	As long as tubercle bacilli are discharged by patient or carriers
Typhoid fever	1–3 weeks (usually 2 weeks)	As long as typhoid bacilli appear in feces
Whooping cough	7–21 days (usually by 10 days)	From 7 days after exposure to 3 weeks after onset of typical paroxysms

transmission is greatest during the prodromal period because of the high communicability of the disease at this stage and because the symptoms are not clearly evident.

The following terms help further characterize disease:

- **Fastigium** is the period when the disease is at its maximum severity or intensity. Diagnosis is easiest at or directly after the differential point. Many respiratory illnesses produce the same symptoms in the prodromal stage, making diagnosis difficult. In the fastigium period, even though the disease is highly communicable, patients do not spread it much. Usually in this phase of the disease, the sick person is home in bed or in the hospital.
- **Defervescence** is the period when the symptoms of the illness are declining. As patients feel they are recovering from a disease in this period, they may not take care of themselves. If the immune system is weakened and cannot effectively fight off the pathogens, a relapse may occur at this stage. This is also a period when the likelihood of transmission of the disease is quite high because patients may be up and about although not yet recovered and still infectious.
- **Convalescence** is the recovery period. Those affected may still be infectious at this point but are feeling much better. They may be out and about, spreading the disease.
- **Defection** is the period during which the pathogen is killed off or brought into remission by the immune system. In some diseases, defection and convalescence may be the same stage. If isolation is required, it is in the defection stage that isolation is lifted.[6]

A factor that affects not only upper respiratory diseases but many others is the strength or virulence of the disease. Recall that virulence is the strength of the disease agent and its ability to produce a severe case of the disease or cause death. Related to the virulence of a pathogen is the viability of the disease-causing agent. **Viability** is the capacity of the pathogen or disease-causing agent to survive outside the host and to exist or thrive in the environment.

When a disease such as a respiratory disease has not yet manifested itself or produces only a mild case of a disease or condition, it is referred to as being **subclinical**. The presence of some diseases can be revealed with clinical tests such as blood analysis. However, clinical symptoms may not be apparent. This state is also referred to as a subclinical infection or subclinical case. In the absence of clinical symptoms, such a condition must be confirmed immunologically.

ZOONOSES

It has long been understood that an animal can be the host, vector, or source of certain infections and diseases (Figure 3.3). Historically, it was recognized that certain diseases can be transmitted from animals to humans. A **zoonosis** is defined as any infection or infectious disease transmissible from animals to humans. The diseases may be endemic or epidemic.

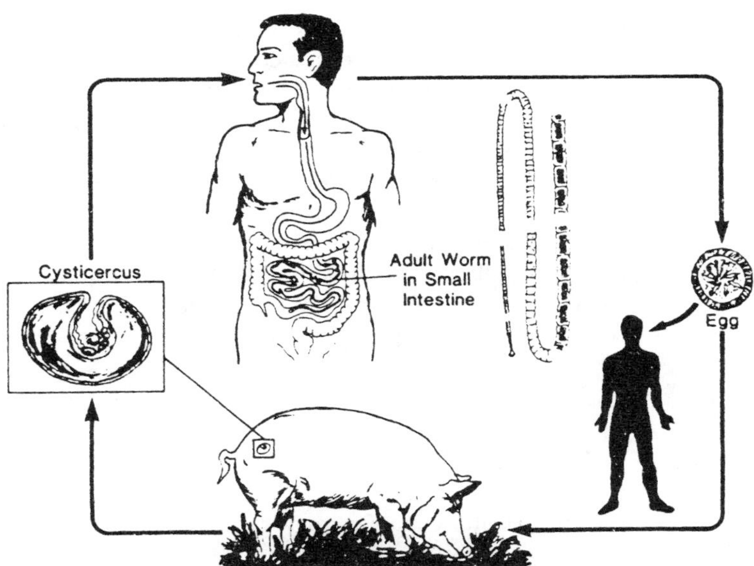

FIGURE 3.3 Example of zoonosis and the disease transmission cycle. The two-host life cycle of *T. solium* involves humans as definitive hosts for the intestinal stage adult tapeworm that is acquired by eating undercooked pork contaminated with cysticerci. Swine, the intermediate host, become infected with the larval stage by ingesting eggs shed in the feces of a human tapeworm carrier. Humans may inadvertently acquire larval-stage infection through the fecal–oral route. (*Source*: Centers for Disease Control and Prevention, "Locally acquired neurocysticercosis—North Carolina, Massachusetts, and South Carolina, 1989–1991." *Morbidity and Mortality Weekly Report*, Public Health Services, U.S. Department of Health and Human Services, Vol. 21, No. 1, Jan. 10, 1992, pp. 1–4)

Thus another way some diseases are classified and studied is based on the ability of the disease to be transmitted to humans from animals. More than 185 diseases have been shown to be transmitted to humans from animals.[11] Common zoonotic diseases include

AIDS
Amebiasis
Anthrax
Bovine papular stomatitis
Brucellosis
California encephalitis
Cat-scratch fever
Colorado tick fever
Cowpox
Dengue fever
Dermatophilosis
Leprosy
Lyme disease
Pasteurellosis
Plague
Q-fever
Rabies
Rat-bite fever
Rickettsial pox
Rocky Mountain spotted fever
Salmonellosis
Shigellosis
Streptococcus infections
Tetanus
Trichinosis
Tularemia
Yellow fever
Zoonotic scabies

Some animals can be carriers of a disease without showing any signs or symptoms. For example, coyotes can carry plague, never becoming sick from the disease, yet spreading it to rodents and humans via a flea vector. Humans may get bitten by a flea while in the woods or at home, get ill a few days later, and not connect their disease to the inoculation by the insect. Historically the animal–flea–human set of events was a connection not easily made. For hundreds of years humans got malaria from mosquito bites and never realized that the disease came from the mosquito. The same was also true for the sequence of events from flea bites to plague.

Humans are most protective of their domestic animals, and any implication that an owner may get a disease from a pet is not well received. Yet the possibility exists and must not be overlooked by the epidemiologist. One of the most common disorders overlooked by pet owners is that of allergies in the family caused by the furry animals in their home. Children or adults may suffer allergies for years and never consider the family pet as the source of the allergic condition until tested by a physician. Tularemia (rabbit fever), cat-scratch fever, worms from dogs, and parrot fever (psittacosis) have long been known to exist and are examples of zoonotic diseases.

INTERNATIONAL CLASSIFICATION OF DISEASES

The World Health Organization (WHO) provides internationally endorsed standard diagnostic classifications for general epidemiologic and health management purposes. These classifications provide a common language of disease for governments, providers of health care, and consumers. In 1990, the 43rd World Health Assembly endorsed International Classification of Diseases 10 (ICD-10). In 1994, it came into use by WHO member states. The first classification of diseases was in the 1850s and was adopted by the International Statistical Institute in 1948. In 1949, the WHO took responsibility for the ICD when the sixth revision was created. For the first time, this revision included causes of morbidity.[14]

The ICD uses death certificates, hospital records, and other sources to classify diseases and health-related problems. The classifications provide a basis for comparing morbidity and mortality statistics among WHO member states. The ICD facilitates the analysis of the general health and well-being of populations. The monitoring of incidence, prevalence, mortality data, and health-related problems is made possible because of standard diagnostic classifications.

NOTIFIABLE DISEASES IN THE UNITED STATES

Beginning in 1961, the Centers for Disease Control and Prevention (CDC) took charge of collecting and publishing data on nationally notifiable diseases. The list of diseases changes from year to year to reflect the emergence of new pathogens or the decline in incidence of certain diseases. Health officials at the state and national levels mutually determine the list of notifiable diseases. Reporting of nationally notifiable diseases to the CDC is no longer required by law but is voluntary. However, reporting of diseases at the state level is required. State regulations specify the diseases that must be reported; who is responsible for reporting; the information required on each case; to whom and how quickly the information is to be reported; and the expected control measures to be taken for specific diseases.[15]

Notifiable diseases are those of considerable public health importance because of their seriousness. As a general rule, a disease is included on a state's list if it (1) causes serious morbidity or death, (2) has the potential to spread, and (3) can be controlled with appropriate intervention. The list of notifiable diseases varies from state to state in order to reflect state-specific public health priorities. Notifiable infectious diseases that are currently reported by most states are presented in Table 3.8. Other reportable diseases may include Alzheimer's disease, animal bites, cancer, disorders characterized by lapses of consciousness, and pesticide exposure.

State health departments also expect reporting of diseases experiencing unusually high incidence and the occurrence of any unusual disease that has public health importance.[15] Reporting of notifiable diseases is required of physicians, dentists, nurses, other health practitioners, and medical examiners. It may also be required or requested of laboratory directors, and administrators of hospitals, clinics, nursing homes, schools, and nurseries.[15]

Individual reports are treated as confidential, and the required timing of reporting the disease may be immediately by telephone, within one day of identification, or within 7 days of identification. For example, anthrax is expected to be reported immediately, whereas AIDS should be reported within a week of identification. Case reports are typically sent to local health departments. The local health department then communicates the information to the state. Where local health departments do not exist or are not in a position to respond to the health problem, or where the state health department has elected to take primary responsibility, case reports are sent directly to the state health department.

The *Morbidity and Mortality Weekly Report* lists on a regular basis a graphic presentation of the trends of occurrence (decrease and increase) of the top notifiable diseases (Figure 3.4).[17]

PROTECTING PUBLIC HEALTH THROUGH IMMUNIZATION

Before the polio vaccine became available in 1955, a peak of 58,000 cases of polio occurred in one year (1952). One of every two cases of symptomatic polio resulted in permanent crippling of the victim. Before the first live virus vaccine for measles was licensed in 1963, the United States had 4 million cases every year. Additionally, there were 4,000 cases of

Table 3.8 Nationally notifiable infectious diseases in the United States[16] in 2005

- Acquired immunodeficiency syndrome (AIDS)
- Anthrax
- Arboviral neuroinvasive and nonneuroinvasive diseases
- Botulism (foodborne infant, wound, and unspecified)
- Brucellosis
- Chancroid
- Chlamydia trachomatis, genital infections
- Cholera
- Coccidioidomycosis
- Cryptosporidiosis
- Cyclosporiasis
- Diphtheria
- Ehrlichiosis
- *Escherichia coli* infections
- Giardiasis
- Gonorrhea
- *Haemophilus influenzae* invasive disease
- Hansen's disease (leprosy)
- Hantavirus pulmonary syndrome
- Hemolytic uremic syndrome, post-diarrheal
- Hepatitis, viral, acute
- Hepatitis, viral, chronic
- HIV infection
- Influenza-associated pediatric mortality
- Legionellosis
- Listeriosis
- Lyme disease
- Malaria
- Measles
- Meningococcal disease
- Mumps
- Pertussis
- Plague
- Poliomyelitis, paralytic
- Psittacosis
- Q Fever
- Rabies
- Rocky Mountain spotted fever
- Rubella
- Rubella, congenital syndrome
- Salmonellosis
- Severe acute respiratory syndrome-associated coronavirus (SARS-CoV) disease
- Shigellosis
- Smallpox
- Streptococcal disease, invasive, Group A
- Streptococcal toxic shock syndrome
- *Streptococcus pneumoniae*, drug resistant, invasive disease
- *S pneumoniae,* invasive in children <5 years
- Syphilis, primary and secondary
- Syphilis, congenital
- Tetanus
- Toxic shock syndrome
- Trichinellosis (trichinosis)
- Tuberculosis
- Tularemia
- Typhoid fever
- Vancomycin-intermediate *S aureus*
- Vancomycin-resistant *S aureus*
- Varicella (morbidity)
- Varicella (deaths only)
- Yellow Fever

encephalitis, which resulted in 400 deaths and 800 cases with irreparable brain damage. The immunization of 60 million children from 1963 to 1972 cost $180 million but saved $1.3 billion by averting 24 million cases of measles. In the end, 2,400 lives were saved, 7,900 cases of retardation were prevented, and 1,352,000 hospital days were saved.[2,4,5,9,18]

The rubella epidemic of 1964–1965 caused 30,000 babies to be born with rubella syndrome, 20,000 of whom lived more than one year. Before the rubella vaccine was licensed in 1969, 58,000 cases per year were reported.[2,4,5,9,18]

Mumps was the leading cause of childhood deafness and juvenile diabetes. Of every 300 cases of mumps, one can result in impaired hearing. For those infected with diphtheria, one of every 10 dies.[2,4,5,9,18]

The immunization process is very important to all individuals in the United States. According to the CDC, if fewer than 80% of the children in a given area have been inoculated

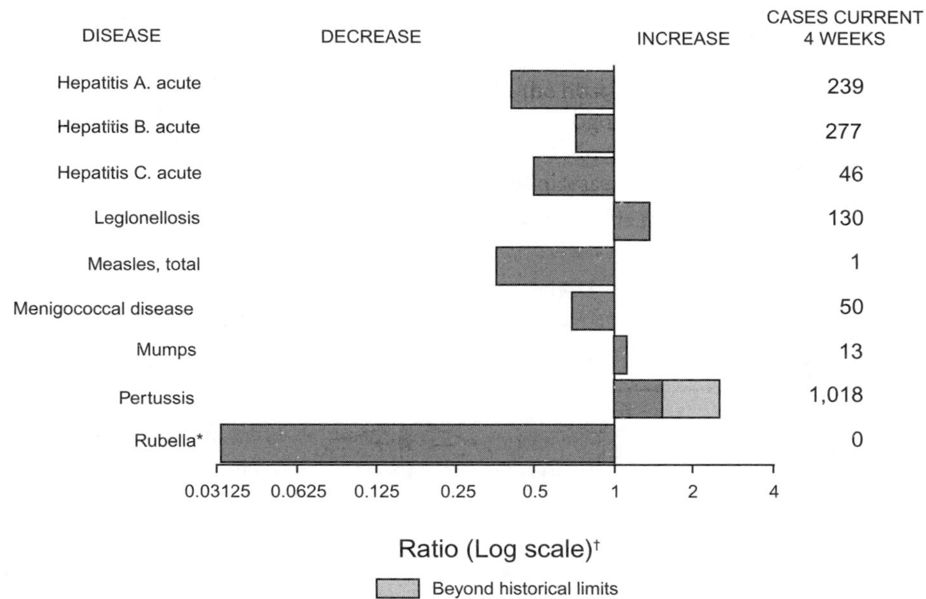

* No rubella cases were reported for the current 4-week period yielding a ratio for 41 of zero (0).
†Ratio of current 4-week total to mean of 15 4-week totals (from previous, comparable, and subsequent 4-week periods for the past 5 years). The point where the hatched area begins is based on the mean and two standard deviations of these 4-week totals.

FIGURE 3.4 Example of selected notifiable disease increase and decrease comparison over a 4-week period ending January 29, 2004, United States. *Source*: Centers for Disease Control and Prevention. Notifiable diseases/deaths in selected cities' weekly information. *MMWR*. 2004;53(41);973–981.

for one of the contagious diseases, the danger of serious outbreaks or localized epidemics remains; every unvaccinated child is at risk.[2,4,5,9,18]

Two classifications of disease immunity are active or passive. With **active immunity** the body produces its own antibodies against a specific invading substance, called an **antigen**, thereby providing very selective protection. This can occur through a vaccine or in response to having a specific disease pathogen invade the body. Active immunity is usually permanent, lasting throughout ones lifetime. **Passive immunity** involves the transfer of antibodies to one person produced by another person. Passive immunity may be acquired through transplacental transfer or breast feeding. Passive immunity can also come from the introduction of already-produced antibodies by another host (eg, immune globulin). Passive immunity is comparatively short lived, usually lasting a few weeks or months.[2,4,5,9,18]

Table 3.9 is a list of the diseases for which vaccines have been developed and that are in current use in the United States. Many well-known diseases still lack vaccines, many are under study, and others are close to completion. One vaccine that is hoped for is an AIDS vaccine, but the possibilities are still limited at this time. Some vaccines are only partially effective and require booster shots, and others, such as the smallpox vaccine, work very well.

Vaccinia is the live virus used in the smallpox vaccine. This vaccine brought about the supposed global eradication of smallpox. The last naturally occurring case of smallpox was

Table 3.9 Diseases for which vaccines are available[19]

Anthrax	Plague
Cholera	Pneumonia
Chicken pox	Polio
Diphtheria	Rabies
German measles (rubella)	Smallpox
Hepatitis A	Rocky Mountain spotted fever
Hepatitis B	Tetanus
Influenza	Tuberculosis
Measles	Typhoid fever
Meningitis	Typhus
Mumps	Whooping cough
Pertussis	Yellow fever

reported in Somalia in 1977. In May of 1980, the World Health Assembly certified that the world was free of naturally occurring smallpox. Even though this report was made worldwide, many public health professionals are skeptical and believe that another epidemic of smallpox is possible. Nonetheless, the vaccine is a good example of the effectiveness of the wide use of immunizations in the eradication of disease.[20]

The introduction of a substance that can cause the immune system to respond and develop antibodies against a disease is what the **immunization** process is all about. Some substances are given orally (polio for example). Most are given by injection or skin pricks. Specific antigens from inactivated bacteria, viruses, or microbe toxins are introduced into the body in the form of a vaccine. The ability of the antigen system to have the strength, activity, and effectiveness to respond to disease is referred to as **antigenicity**. The antigens stimulate the immune system to make the body think it has the disease. The body's immune system responds by developing antibodies and a natural immunity to the disease. If the pathogen later enters the body, the immune system recognizes it, and the body is protected from the disease by the rapid response of the immune system. Some vaccines last a lifetime; others may not. Recent reports indicate that revaccination may be required for some diseases as one gets older. Booster shots keep the immune process active within the body. If antigens and antibodies disappear over time, then a booster shot is needed to strengthen or reactivate the immune response. Booster shots are also given at the outset of an immunization program to help build the body's immune defense systems to the fullest extent possible.[2,4,5,9,18]

When the body cannot respond quickly enough or with enough strength, it is then that help is needed. Antibiotics are used to assist the immune system in its fight against pathogens. Antibiotics are substances such as penicillin, tetracycline, streptomycin, or any other substance that destroys or inhibits the growth of pathogenic microorganisms.[2,5,18]

HERD IMMUNITY

Herd immunity is based on the notion that if the herd (a population or group) is mostly protected from a disease by immunization, then the chance that a major epidemic will occur is limited. Jonas Salk, one of the developers of the polio vaccine, has suggested that if a herd immunity level of 85% is available in a population, a polio epidemic will not occur. Herd immunity is also viewed as the resistance a population has to the invasion and spread of an infectious disease.

Immunizations or past experience with a disease reduces the number of those who are susceptible (susceptibles) in a population. Herd immunity is accomplished when the number of susceptibles is reduced and the number of protected or nonsusceptible persons dominates the herd (population). Herd immunity provides barriers to direct transmission of infections through the population. The lack of susceptible individuals halts the spread of a disease through a group (Figures 3.5 and 3.6).

Figure 3.5 graphically shows how a disease can spread through a population when immunity is low and the number of susceptibilities is high. Figure 3.6 shows how barriers to the spread of a disease are developed when susceptible levels are low and how disease transmission in a population is stopped when an 85% level of immunity exists. Both Figures 3.5 and 3.6 demonstrate the effect that just one diseased person can have on the spread of a disease in a population.

One public health immunization goal would be to have close to 100% immunity in a population so that not even one individual would get the disease. This level of immunity is especially important for life-threatening diseases or those diseases that cause extreme disability, such as polio. The goal of any public health immunization program is to reach 100% of the population, even if herd immunity prevents the occurrence of major epidemics.

COMMUNICABLE DISEASE PREVENTION AND CONTROL

Prevention and control of infectious and contagious diseases are the foundation of all public health measures. Several prevention methods, as well as many control measures, have been developed. There are 3 key factors to the control of communicable diseases.

- Remove, eliminate, or contain the cause or source of infection
- Disrupt and block the chain of disease transmission
- Protect the susceptible population against infection and disease

The methods of prevention and control are used on several fronts. The first front is the environment, the second is the person at risk (host), and the third front is the population or community.[4]

Environmental Control

Environmental control is aimed at providing clean and safe air, water, milk, and food. Also involved in the scope of environmental control is the management of solid waste (trash and garbage), liquid waste (sewage), and control of vectors (insects and rodents) of disease.[4]

Safe air includes the control of infectious pathogens that are airborne. Toxic fumes, ultraviolet light, air pollution, and secondhand smoke are also of concern in air safety control.[4]

Clean and safe water supplies have been key factors in controlling infectious diseases, especially waterborne diseases (enteric or alvine discharge diseases). Maintaining a safe water supply is one of the most basic yet all-important public health activities of the modern age.[4]

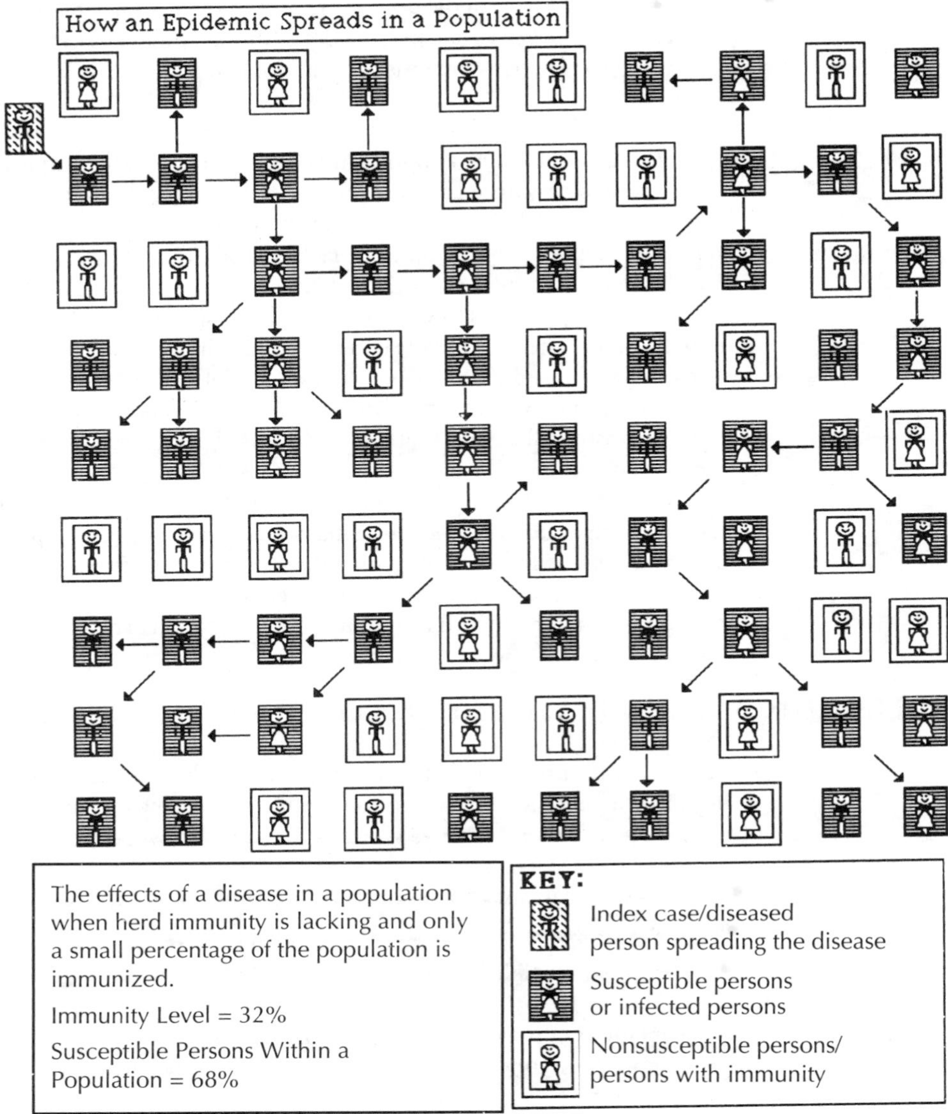

FIGURE 3.5 Diagram of a population, showing a low immunization level which falls short of protecting individuals within the group.

Liquid waste carries pathogens, fecal material, chemical pollutants, industrial waste, and many other pollutants and waste. Sewage and dirty water runoff must be safely conveyed without exposure to the human population; thus, underground sewage systems are of keen importance.[4]

Solid waste management has become one of the greatest public health challenges of modern times. Proper disposal of the massive amounts of garbage and other solid waste,

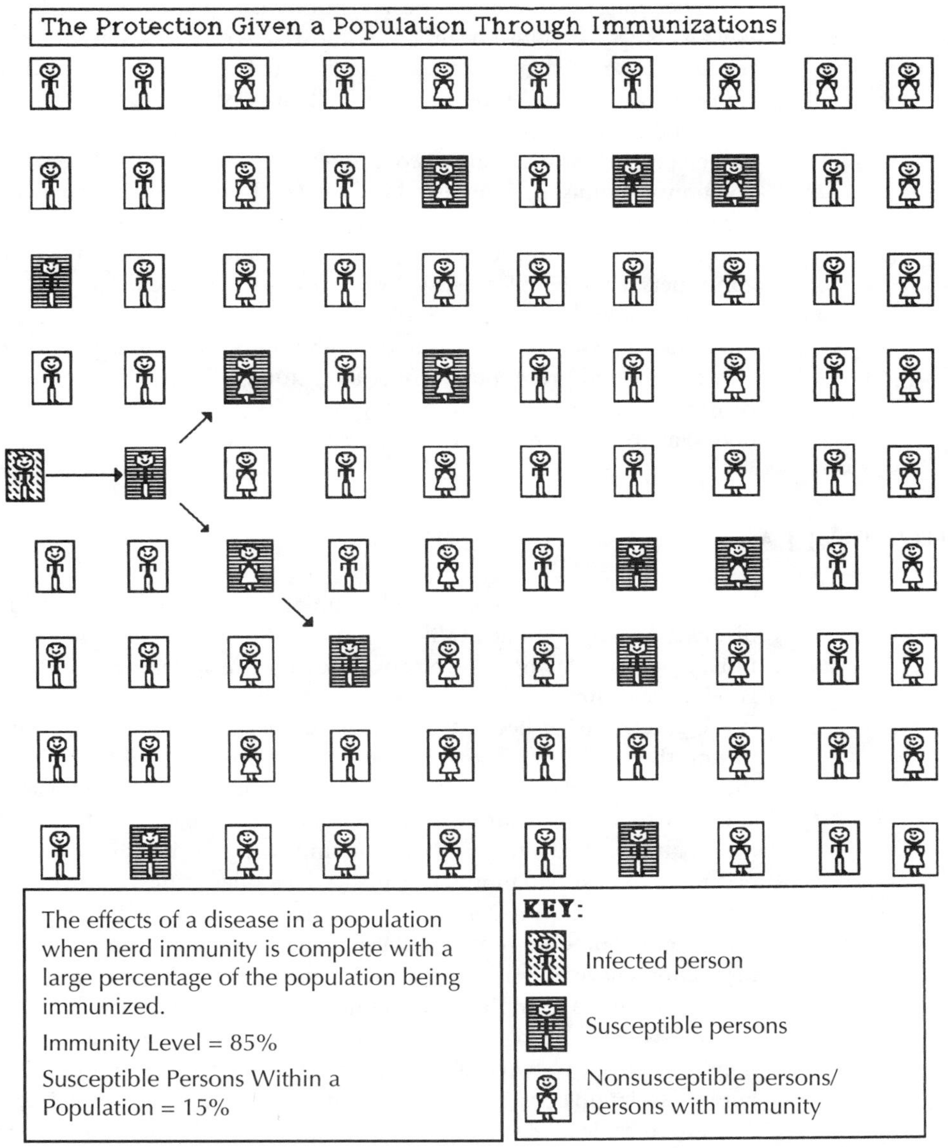

FIGURE 3.6 Diagram of a population showing a high level of immunizations within the group so that it affords a good level of protection to most of the individuals within the group.

such as hazardous and biohazardous materials, continues to be a challenge. Control of garbage odors, flies, and insect problems, from the garbage can at home to the garbage can sitting at the street curb and on to the sanitary landfill, helps prevent the spread of communicable vectorborne disease.[4]

The protection of water, food, and milk is a hallmark of advanced societies. Milk and the cows it comes from must be tested and proved free of infectious diseases. Milk is constantly tested and is treated by heat (pasteurization) to kill pathogens. Proper storage, distribution, transport, and temperature control of milk must be rigorous and continually ensured.[4]

Food must be protected from adulteration, contamination, and spoilage.[4] Food must also be properly stored and served. Proper temperatures for refrigeration, cooking, storage, and transport must be maintained without fail. Proper food handling, including hand washing during preparation, is extremely important to infection control. Many bacteria, especially staphylococci, salmonella, and shigella, can contaminate food and be transmitted to unwary consumers. Food handlers must also be checked and screened to protect the general public.[4]

Animals and insects are sources of disease and infection. The control of animals (both domestic and wild) and insects in the community, both rural and urban, is essential to disease control and prevention. Proper food storage, refrigeration, water protection, garbage control, and sanitation (including lids on garbage cans as well as screening of windows and doors) all help to control insects and related pathogens.[4]

HOST-RELATED CONTROL AND PREVENTION

The host of a disease can be either human or animal, and both are vulnerable to infectious diseases. A goal of public health is to protect the host from contagious diseases and infections by several methods. Protective measures include quarantine, isolation, sanitation, good hygiene, immunizations, and chemoprophylaxis.

Quarantine has been used throughout history to separate ill people from well people to stop the spread of disease. Quarantine was probably the first public health measure to show a marked level of effectiveness in controlling the spread of disease. In the late 1800s and early 1900s, quarantine activities became an organized effort effected by government officials, and this had a major impact on improving the health status of the community, especially with regard to mortality statistics. In modern times quarantine measures are still in use. Currently, the WHO invokes quarantine measures for 3 diseases: cholera, plague, and yellow fever. Some attempts have been made to use quarantine measures against AIDS, but these efforts have been met with much resistance by activist groups.

Isolation is a term that refers to quarantine-type activities but is conducted on an inpatient basis in hospitals or nursing homes. Most state laws as well as accrediting organizations require one or two beds to be kept, designated, and equipped in a hospital or nursing home as isolation beds. The isolation beds are used to segregate and isolate any patient with a communicable disease so that disease will not spread throughout the facility. Isolation is an infection control measure, usually done under the direction and control of the hospital epidemiologist (infection control director) and the infection control committee of a hospital. Isolation measures include:

1. One or two private rooms are used as isolation rooms.
2. Separate infection-control gowns are used.
3. Staff must wear masks.
4. All staff must be gloved when interacting, treating, or working with or on the patient.
5. Hand washing is required on entering and leaving the patient's room.

6. All contaminated articles or possibly contaminated articles, including linen, dressings, syringes, instruments, etc., must be disposed of properly.

Special isolation concerns arise when it comes to dealing with HIV/AIDS patients. The CDC issued procedures for the control of infections including AIDS. Universal blood and body-fluid precautions, or universal precautions, are to be applied to all patients, from the emergency department to outpatient clinics to the dentist's office to the isolation room in the hospital. Barrier techniques are to be implemented, which include gloves, masks, gowns, protective eyewear, and hand washing when in contact with all patients. Gloves are to be used when touching blood or body fluids. Proper disposal of all articles that could be contaminated must be done with care. Care to avoid accidental self-punctures with contaminated needles must be taken. Patients at high risk for AIDS need to be tested. High-risk hospital and clinic personnel also need to be tested for HIV/AIDS on a regular basis.[4]

INFECTION CONTROL AND PREVENTION MEASURES

Personal hygiene is the process of maintaining high standards of personal body maintenance and cleanliness. Cleanliness and health maintenance activities include frequent bathing, regular grooming, teeth cleaning and maintenance, frequent changes of clothes, and hand washing. Family beliefs and practices, food preparation and protection, home environment, and living spaces all contribute to infection control and prevention and are part of hygienic practices (see News File p 68).

Immunizations protect each person from disease and infection. Immunizations are key preventive medicine and public health measures against disease spread in populations or groups.

Chemical and **antibiotic prophylaxis** have shown great success in treating certain infections since 1945 when penicillin was finally mass produced and made available for wide use in the population. In the 1800s, arsenic, a poisonous chemical, was found somewhat effective in treating syphilis, if used in low doses. Sulfa drugs were also found to be effective against many infectious diseases. Use of chemical agents as a means of preventing specific diseases became less common with the development of antibiotic medications.

With the development of both specific antibiotics and broad-spectrum antibiotics, the treatment of individuals and the practice of medicine have greatly changed. The impact of chemical and antibiotic prophylaxis on the health status in the world has been outstanding. Infants and mothers no longer die as a result of the childbirth process in the numbers they formerly did. Wounds heal, surgery is completed without the patient dying later from an infection, streptococcal infections are quickly halted and no longer turn into rheumatic fever, and now it has been shown through research that antibiotics administered within 2 hours of surgery can help prevent surgical wound infections. Many lives have been saved and much suffering has been eliminated because of the development and effective use of chemical and antibiotic prophylaxis.[4]

CHANGING EMPHASIS IN EPIDEMIOLOGIC STUDIES

Although epidemiologic studies originated in the investigation of infectious disease outbreaks, increasing life expectancy in modern times and increasing chronic disease has pro-

NEWS FILE

Disease Transmission and Universal Precautions

Hand Washing Remains Key to Reducing Disease Transmission

Hand washing has long been recognized as one of the most effective ways to reduce the transmission of disease in laypeople and professionals alike. Many serious and life-threatening diseases are transmitted because of inadequate hand washing, especially disease transmitted through the fecal–oral route. Feces remaining on the hands after toilet use may then enter the body when the hands are placed in the mouth or when food becomes contaminated during preparation. *Escherichia coli* 0157:H7, cholera, typhoid fever, salmonella food poisoning, poliomyelitis, and hepatitis A are but some of the diseases transmitted by the fecal–oral route. Dr. Gail Casell, professor and chair of the Department of Microbiology at the University of Alabama, Birmingham, conducted a national survey in Chicago, Atlanta, San Francisco, New Orleans, and New York of 6,333 people, both women and men, directly observed in bathrooms. Although 94% of people asked by telephone say that they always wash their hands after going to the bathroom, direct observation found that only 68% actually did. Generally, women washed their hands more often than men, with women washing 74% of the time and men only 61% of the time (presentation, American Society for Microbiologists, 1996, New Orleans). With the onset of the AIDS/HIV epidemic in the 1980s, universal precautions were developed to protect health care professionals, police, and others who come in direct contact with people who could infect them, especially by blood. Universal precautions are aggressive, standardized approaches to infection control in which all human blood and certain body fluids are treated as if they are known to contain HIV, hepatitis B virus, or other bloodborne pathogens. In universal precautions, hand washing is not enough protection, so personal protective equipment, such as gloves, masks, eye protection, and special equipment for mouth-to-mouth resuscitation and CPR, might be needed for exposure to blood or body fluids.

duced a change in the emphasis of epidemiologic studies. The shift from infectious to chronic disease in the United States is illustrated in Table 1.2 and Figure 3.7.[21,22] In 1998, the WHO estimated that chronic diseases contribute to almost 60% of deaths in the world and 43% of the global burden of disease.[23] On the basis of current trends, by 2020 chronic diseases are expected to be responsible for 73% of deaths and 60% of the burden of disease.[23] Long latency periods between exposure and clinical symptoms are characteristic of chronic diseases. Events related to chronic conditions, including smoking, alcohol drinking, substance abuse, environmental/occupational exposure, diet, physical activity level, and sexual behaviors, have also received considerable attention in epidemiologic studies.

Mental and psychiatric disorders and conditions are noninfectious, noncommunicable, chronic diseases. The understanding of psychiatric disorders and behavioral problems has greatly increased over the last 30–40 years. In 1975, a rough draft of the third edition of the

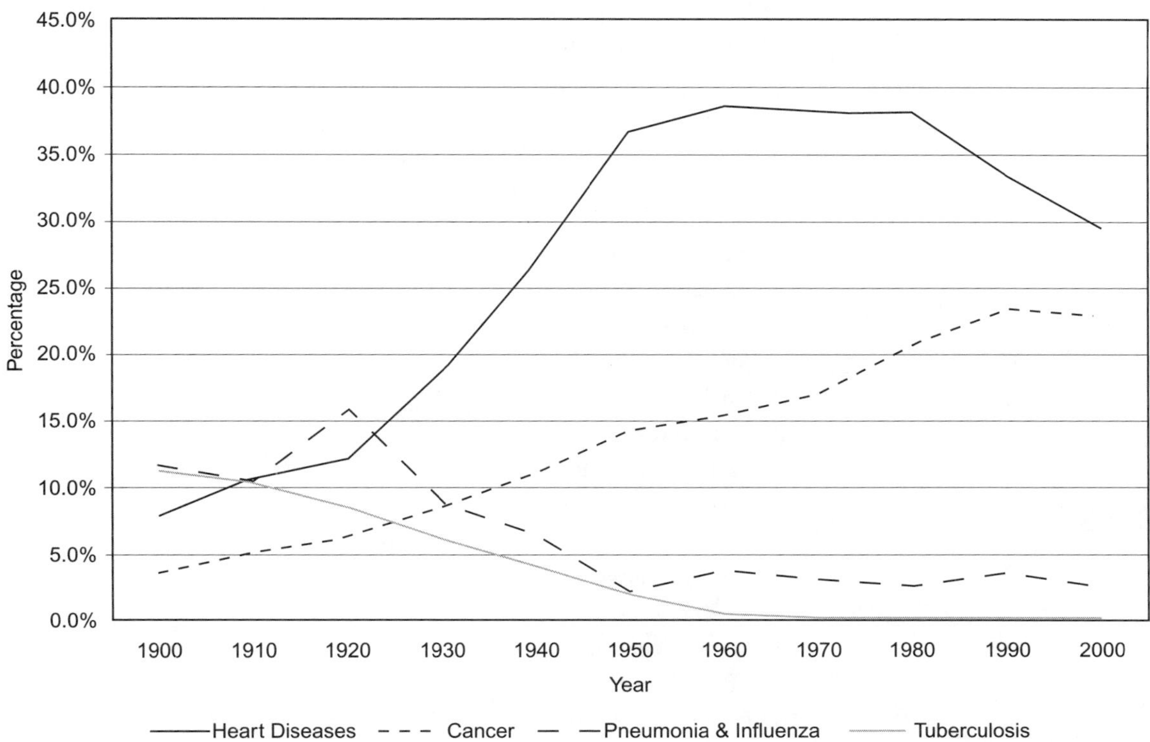

FIGURE 3.7 Percentage of deaths in the United States attributed to selected diseases from 1900 through 2000. *Source:* Centers for Disease Control and Prevention. Leading causes of disease, 1900–1998 (http://www.cdc.gov/nchs/data/statab/lead1900_98.pdf), US Mortality Public Use Data Tape, 2000, National Center for Health Statistics, Centers for Disease Control and Prevention, 2002.

Diagnostic and Statistical Manual of Mental Disorders (DSM) was presented at a special session of the annual American Psychiatric Association conference. Several additional drafts were produced, and meetings were held over the next 5 years. Field trials of the suggested new classifications were made. In 1980 the newly developed classifications of psychiatric disorders were published in the third edition (DSM-III). This revision was a major advancement in the structure and classification of mental conditions. The concept of neurosis was removed from the classification, and stress (posttraumatic)-related issues were included. In 1987 a revised addition of the book, DSM-IIIR, was released.[24] Table 3.10 presents diagnostic categories of mental conditions from DSM-IV (published in 1994), and Table 3.11 presents a "V" code section for behavioral conditions and disorders related to mental illness.[25]

NUTRITIONAL DEFICIENCY DISEASES AND DISORDERS

Nutritional deficiency diseases and disorders can be classified under chronic diseases. The term **malnutrition** literally refers to a condition that arises when the body does not get the

Table 3.10 Diagnostic categories of mental conditions from DSM-IV

1. Disorders usually first evident in infancy, childhood, or adolescence
2. Delirium, dementia, amnestic, and other cognitive disorders
3. Mental disorders due to a general medical condition not elsewhere classified
4. Substance-related disorders
5. Schizophrenia and other psychotic disorders
6. Mood disorders
7. Anxiety disorders
8. Somatoform disorders
9. Factitious disorders
10. Dissociative disorders
11. Sexual and gender identity disorders
12. Eating disorders
13. Sleep disorders
14. Impulse-control disorders not elsewhere classified
15. Adjustment disorders
16. Personality disorders
17. Other conditions that may be a focus of clinical attention
18. Medication-induced movement disorders
19. Relational problems
20. Problems related to abuse and neglect
21. Additional conditions that may be a focus of clinical attention
22. Additional codes for unspecified mental disorders (nonpsychotic)

right amount of vitamins, minerals, and other nutrients to maintain healthy tissues and proper organ function. Malnutrition occurs in people experiencing either undernutrition or overnutrition. **Undernutrition** is a consequence of consuming too little essential vitamins, minerals, and other nutrients or excreting them faster than they can be replenished. Inadequate intake may result from excessive dieting, severe injury, and serious illness. Excessive loss may result from diarrhea, heavy sweating, heavy bleeding, or kidney failure. **Overnutrition** is the consumption of too much food, eating too many of the wrong things, too little physical activity and exercise, or taking too many vitamins or dietary supplements.[1] A list of some malnutrition syndromes with their accompanying causes is shown in Table 3.12.

Primary deficiency diseases can contribute to malnutrition and can result directly from the dietary lack of specific essential nutrients. For example, scurvy results from a dietary deficiency of vitamin C. Secondary deficiency diseases result from the inability of the body to

Table 3.11 V codes for behavioral conditions and related disorders

Malingering
Borderline intellectual functioning
Adult antisocial behavior
Childhood or adolescent antisocial behavior
Academic problem
Noncompliance with medical treatment
Phase of life problem or life circumstance problem
Marital problem
Other specified family circumstance
Other interpersonal problem
Additional codes are for unspecified mental disorders (nonpsychotic) and those in which there is a failure to diagnose a condition by the above classification.

use specific nutrients properly; for example, when food cannot be absorbed into the body while in the alimentary tract or when food is not able to be metabolized.

Obesity is influenced by a number of factors: diet, genetics, development, physical activity, metabolic rate (rate that the body uses food as a source of energy), and psychological problems. Some people choose to overeat (binge) in stressful or depressed states. On the other hand,

Table 3.12 Malnutrition syndromes

Kwashiorkor (protein deficiency)
Marasmus (protein and/or calorie malnutrition, chronic undernutrition)
Iron deficiency anemia
Folic acid deficiency anemia
Vitamin B12 deficiency anemia
Xerophthalmia (vitamin A deficiency)
Endemic goiter (iodine deficiency)
Beriberi (thiamine deficiency)
Ariboflavinosis (riboflavin deficiency)
Pellagra (niacin and amino acid tryptophan deficiency)
Scurvy (vitamin C deficiency)
Rickets (vitamin D deficiency)
Tetany (mineral deficiency)
Osteomalacia and osteoporosis (impaired calcium and phosphorus metabolism affecting bone formation)

anorexia nervosa and bulimia may also result from psychiatric problems. Some of the health problems associated with obesity in epidemiologic research include diabetes, stroke, coronary artery disease, hypertension, high cholesterol, kidney and gallbladder disorders, and some cancers. Obese individuals are also at increased risk of developing osteoarthritis and sleep apnea.

CHRONIC DISEASES AND CONDITIONS

The most prominent chronic diseases are cardiovascular disease, cancer, chronic obstructive pulmonary disease (COPD), diabetes mellitus, and mental health disorders.[23] Chronic diseases are not typically caused by an infectious agent (pathogen) but result from genetic susceptibility, lifestyle, or environmental exposures. Some exceptions are cancers of the cervix, liver, and stomach. Infectious risk factors for cervical cancer, liver cancer, and stomach cancer are human papilloma virus, hepatitis B virus, and the *Helicobacter pylori* bacterium, respectively. Because the human papilloma virus is sexually transmitted and the hepatitis B virus is transmitted via the exchange of body fluids such as blood, semen, breast milk, and in some rare cases saliva, cancers related to these viruses these are classified as chronic infectious communicable diseases.

The latency period for chronic diseases is typically more difficult to identify than is the incubation period for acute infectious diseases. This is explained by the multifactorial etiology that characterizes many chronic diseases. In Chapter 5, "Descriptive Epidemiology According to Person, Place , and Time", per capita cigarette consumption will be compared with lung cancer death rates between 1900 and 2000 (see Figure 5.11). The comparison suggests that the latency period from smoking to lung cancer death is 20–25 years.

Prevention and Control

The development of many chronic diseases is preventable, and some chronic diseases could also be minimized in their severity by changing behavior and moderating exposure to certain risk factors in life. For example, lung cancer and COPD could be greatly reduced if no one smoked. Certain liver diseases could be greatly reduced if alcohol consumption were curtailed. Lifestyle, behavior, and unnecessary exposure to risk factors in life continue to contribute to many chronic diseases in our society. Cardiovascular disease and cancer could be reduced if nutritional and dietary factors were altered. These diseases are also affected by smoking and alcohol.

The main lifestyle and behavior changes needed to prevent and control chronic disease include the reduction, and possibly the elimination, of the use of tobacco and smoking (which includes secondhand smoke); the use of alcohol; and drug abuse. Additional changes include dietary changes (a reduction of fat and empty calories in the diet, lowering cholesterol; maintaining proper calcium levels; limiting certain kinds of protein and red meat), increased fitness and exercise, proper weight maintenance, stress reduction, and increased safety measures.

Prevention measures have made great strides in the area of cancer. Efforts to detect breast cancer at early stages are critical in reducing breast cancer–associated mortality. Early detection programs have been found to be most effective as cancer prevention and control measures. Primary care centers have used early detection programs in order to facilitate cancer screening services. Mammography screening has been done at centers located in shopping centers, and mobile mammography vans have also been used.

Table 3.13 presents the results of a breast cancer screening program in Dade County, Florida, in a Hispanic population. From the screening of the 9,434 patients, 274 biopsies were performed, with 57 of the tests being positive for cancer. Late-stage diagnosis of cancer contributes to the 10% to 15% lower survival rates among women of low socioeconomic status. Early diagnosis and early treatment are the key hallmarks of prevention and control in cancer.[26]

Disability

Disability is the diminished capacity to perform within a prescribed range.[1] The International Classification of Functioning, Disability and Health defines disability as an umbrella term for impairments, activity limitations, and participation restrictions.[27] **Impairment** is any loss or abnormality of psychological, physiologic, or anatomic structure or function.[1] Impairment is often associated with chronic disease because it represents a decrease in or loss of ability to perform various functions, particularly those of the musculoskeletal system and the sense organs. Impairment may also result from a condition, injury, or congenital malformation. **Activity limitations** are difficulties an individual may have in executing activities. **Participation restrictions** are problems an individual may experience in involve-

Table 3.13 Characteristics and results of 9,434 Hispanic patients in the early detection program for breast cancer in Dade County, Florida, 1987–1990

Patient Characteristic	**%**	***Result***	**%**
Race/Ethnicity		Mammography finding (*n* = 11,632)†	
Hispanic	52.8	Not suspicious for cancer	68.0
Non-Hispanic black	40.8	Additional evaluation	27.7
Non-Hispanic white	6.1	Suspicious for cancer	4.3
Unknown	0.3		
		Biopsy result (*n* = 274)	
Age (yrs)		Negative	79.2
<40	15.2	Positive	20.8
40–49	29.0		
50–69	50.1	Histologic result (*n* = 57)	
>70	5.7	In situ	17.5
		Local	36.8
Previous mammogram (*n* = 8,397)*		Regional	35.1
No	74.0	Distant	5.3
Yes	26.0	Unstaged	5.3

*This question was not asked of women at the beginning of the program.
†Includes screening, repeat, and followup mammograms.
Source: CDC. Increasing breast cancer screening among the medically underserved—Dade County, Florida, September 1987–March 1991. *MMWR.* 1991;40:16.

ment in life situations.[27] Some examples of how selected health conditions may be associated with the 3 levels of functioning is shown in Table 3.14.

Many diseases result in disability. For example, polio can cause a whole range of paralysis, from a mild weakness in a leg or arm to a complete loss of function of legs and arms to loss of the ability to breathe. Reye's syndrome can leave a person with neurologic and muscular deficits and disability. Stroke can leave a person paralyzed. Diabetes can lead to amputation of parts of fingers, hands, and limbs, again causing a disability. Each of these diseases is related to impairment, activity limitation, and participation restriction.

Activity limitation data has been collected annually since 1997 in the National Health Interview Survey. Activity limitation in adults (ages 18–64 years) include limitations in handling personal care needs, routine needs, having a job outside the home, walking, remembering, and other activities. From 2000 to 2002, the percentage of activity limitations reported by adults in the United States that were caused by chronic health conditions remained stable.[28] Activity limitation among adults in the United States caused by one or more chronic health conditions is shown for selected variables in Figure 3.8. Activity limitation increases with age, decreases with poverty level, and is lowest for Hispanics, followed by whites only, then blacks only. Activity limitation is slightly higher for females than males. The rate of activity limitation among adults in the United States, arranged by selected chronic health conditions, is shown in Figure 3.9. Rates increased with age for each of the selected chronic health conditions. Arthritis or other musculoskeletal conditions were most frequently identified as causing activity limitation. The next most frequently mentioned causes of activity limitation were mental illness (for ages 18–44 years) and heart/other circulatory problems (for ages 45–54 years and 55–64 years).

Table 3.14 Selected health conditions and disability as related to impairment, activity limitation, and participation restriction[27]

Health Condition	*Impairment*	*Activity Limitation*	*Participation Restriction*
Leprosy	Loss of sensation in extremities	Difficulties in grasping objects	Stigma of leprosy leads to unemployment
Panic Disorder	Anxiety	Not capable of going out alone	Leads to lack of social relationships
Spinal Injury	Paralysis	Incapable of using public transportation	Lack of accommodations in public transportation leads to no participation in social activities
Type I diabetes	Pancreatic dysfunction	None (impairment controlled by medication)	Does not go to school because of stereotypes about disease
Vitiligo	Facial disfigurement	None	No participation in social relations owing to fears of contagion
Person who formally had a mental health problem and was treated for a psychotic disorder	None	None	Denied employment because of employer's prejudice

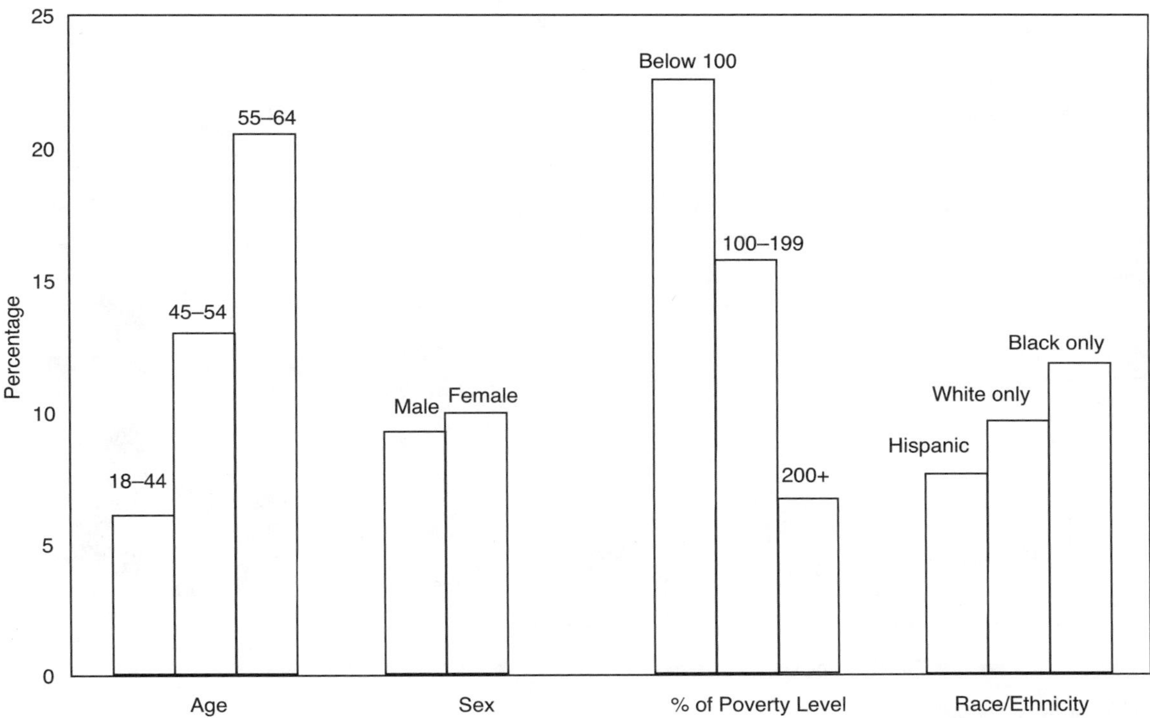

FIGURE 3.8 Activity limitation according to one or more chronic health conditions among adults in the United States, 2000–2002. *Source:* National Center for Health Statistics. *Health, United States, 2004 With Chartbook on Trends in the Health of Americans*. Hyattsville, MD; 2004; 40.

HEALTH GOALS IN THE UNITED STATES FOR THE YEAR 2010

In January 2000, the United States Department of Health and Human Services launched *Healthy People 2010*, a comprehensive, nationwide health-promotion and disease-prevention agenda. *Healthy People 2010* contains 467 objectives designed to serve as a road map for improving the health of all people in the United States during the first decade of the 21st century.[29] *Healthy People 2010* builds on similar initiatives pursued over the past 2 decades. Two overarching goals—to increase quality and years of healthy life and eliminate health disparities—served as a guide for developing objectives that will actually measure progress. The objectives are organized into 28 focus areas (eg, access to quality health services, immunizations and infectious diseases, occupational safety and health, sexually transmitted diseases, and tobacco use), each representing an important public health area. Each objective has a target for improvements to be achieved by the year 2010. The challenge of *Healthy People 2010* is to use scientific knowledge, professional skills, individual commitment, community support, and political influence to enable people to achieve their potential to live full and active lives. Means were set forth for preventing premature death and disability, preserving a physical environment that supports human life, cultivating family and community support, enhancing inherent abilities, and ensuring that all Americans achieve and maintain a maximum level of functioning and overall well-being.

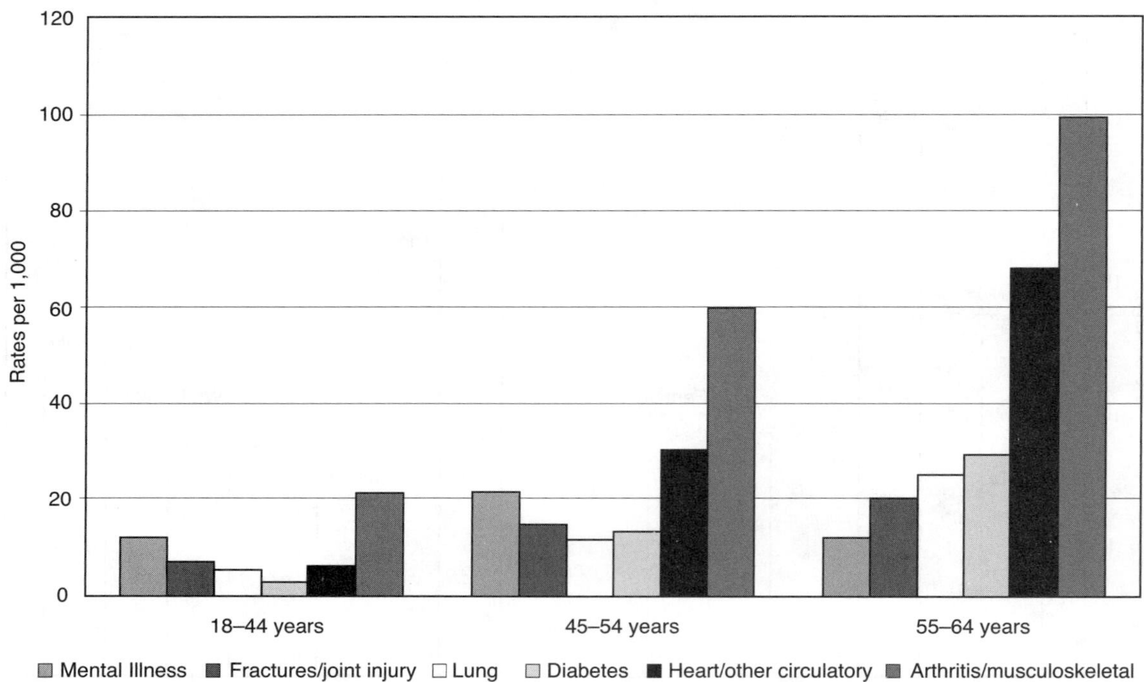

FIGURE 3.9 Activity limitation according to selected chronic health conditions among adults in the United States, 2000–2002. *Source:* National Center for Health Statistics. *Health, United States, 2004 With Chartbook on Trends in the Health of Americans*. Hyattsville, MD; 2004; 41.

EXERCISES

Key Terms

Define the following terms.

Active immunity
Activity limitations
Acute
Antibiotics
Antibodies
Antigen
Antigenicity
Chronic
Communicability
Communicable
Convalescence
Defection
Defervescence
Disability
Disease
Etiology
Fastigium period
Herd immunity
Horizontal transmission
Immunization
Impairment
Incubation period
Invasiveness
Isolation
Latency period
Malnutrition
Overnutrition
Participation restrictions
Passive immunity
Pathogens
Personal hygiene
Prodromal period
Quarantine
Subclinical
Toxins
Undernutrition
Vertical transmission
Viability
Virulence
Zoonosis

Study Questions

3.1 Discuss how infectious and noninfectious diseases relate to communicable and noncommunicable diseases and conditions.

3.2 List and explain the different general classifications of diseases.

3.3 Classifications were given of major infectious diseases. List the 5 modes of transmission and provide examples.

3.4 List the 3 general sources of infectious diseases and provide examples.

3.5 How do incubation periods differ from latency periods?

3.6 Choose 5 infectious diseases and identify the typical incubation periods for these diseases.

3.7 Explain the concept of notifiable diseases.

3.8 Explain and discuss herd immunity.

3.9 What role does increasing life expectancy over the last century have on the types of diseases and conditions affecting mankind?

3.10 Describe how activity limitation is associated with age, sex, poverty level, and race/ethnicity (see Figure 3.8).

3.11 Describe the influence of mental illness and heart disease on activity limitations according to age group (see Figure 3.9).

REFERENCES

1. *Stedman's Medical Dictionary for the Health Professions and Nursing*. 5th ed. New York, NY: Lippincott, Williams & Wilkins; 2005.
2. Crowley LV. *Introduction to Human Disease*. 2nd ed. Boston, MA: Jones and Bartlett; 1988.
3. US National Institutes of Health. National Cancer Institute. Available at: http://www.nci.nih.gov/cancertopics/understandingcancer/cancer. Accessed May 7, 2005.
4. Evans AS, Brachman PS. *Bacterial Infections of Humans: Epidemiology and Control*. 2nd ed. New York, NY: Plenum Medical Book Company; 1991.
5. Bickley HC. *Practical Concepts in Human Disease*. 2nd ed. Baltimore, MD: Williams & Wilkins; 1977.
6. Green LW, Anderson CL. *Community Health*. 4th ed. St. Louis, MO: CV Mosby; 1982.
7. Wigley R, Cook JR. *Community Health*. New York, NY: D Van Nostrand Company; 1975.
8. Grant M. *Handbook of Community Health*. 4th ed. Philadelphia, PA: Lea and Febiger; 1987.
9. Sheldon H. *Boyd's Introduction to the Study of Disease*. Philadelphia, PA: Lea and Febiger; 1984.
10. Berkow R, ed. *The Merck Manual of Diagnosis and Therapy*. 14th ed. Rahway, NJ: Merck and Company; 1982.
11. Acha PN, Szyfres B. *Zoonoses and Communicable Diseases Common to Man and Animals*. 2nd ed. Washington, DC: Pan American Health Organization; 1989.
12. Olishifski JB, McElroy FE. *Fundamentals of Industrial Hygiene*. Chicago, IL: National Safety Council; 1975.
13. Thygerson AL. *Safety*. 2nd ed. Englewood Cliffs, NJ: Prentice Hall; 1986.
14. World Health Organization (WHO). Classifications. Available at: http://www.who.int/classifications/icd/en/. Accessed May 7, 2005.

15. Centers for Disease Control and Prevention (CDC). Epidemiology Program Office. *Principles of Epidemiology: An Introduction to Applied Epidemiology and Biostatistics.* 2nd ed. Atlanda, GA: 1992:353–355.
16. CDC. Epidemiology Program Office. Division of Public Health Surveillance and Informatics. *Nationally Notifiable Infectious Diseases. United States 2005.* Available at: http://www.cdc.gov/epo/dphsi/phs/infdis2005.htm. Accessed May 9, 2005.
17. CDC. Notifiable diseases/deaths in selected cities weekly information. *MMWR.* 2005;54(04): 101–111. Available at: http://www.cdc.gov/mmwr/preview/mmwrhtml/mm5404md.htm#fig1. Accessed May 10, 2005.
18. Shulman S, Phair J, Peterson L, Warren J. *The Biologic and Clinical Basis of Infectious Diseases.* 5th ed. New York, NY: Elsevier; 1997.
19. CDC. Summary of notifiable diseases in the US, 1997. *MMWR.* 1998;46(54):27.
20. CDC. Vaccinia (smallpox) vaccine: Recommendations of the immunizations practices advisory committee (ACIP). *MMWR.* 2001;50(RR10):1–25.
21. CDC. Leading causes of disease, 1900–1998. Available at: http://www.cdc.gov/nchs/data/statab/lead1900_98.pdf. Accessed May 10, 2005.
22. US Mortality Public Use Data Tape, 2000. National Center for Health Statistics, Centers for Disease Control and Prevention, 2002. Available at: http://webapp.cdc.gov/sasweb/ncipc/leadcaus10.html. Accessed September 12, 2005.
23. WHO. Global strategy for the prevention and control of noncommunicable diseases. 1999. Available at: http://ftp.who.int/gb/pdf_files/EB105/ee42.pdf. Accessed May 6, 2005.
24. American Psychiatric Association. *DSM-III: Diagnostic and Statistical Manual of Mental Disorders.* 3rd ed. Washington, DC: American Psychiatric Association; 1987.
25. American Psychiatric Association. *DSM-IV: Diagnostic and Statistical Manual of Mental Disorders.* 4th ed. Washington, DC: American Psychiatric Association; 1994.
26. CDC. Increasing breast cancer screening among the medically underserved—Dade County, Florida, September 1987–March 1991. *MMWR.* 1991;40:16.
27. WHO. *Toward a common language for functioning, disability and health. The International Classification of Functioning, Disability and Health.* Geneva, Switzerland: WHO; 2002:17. Available at: http://www3.who.int/icf/beginners/bg.pdf. Accessed May 8, 2005.
28. National Center for Health Statistics. *Health, United States, 2004 With Chartbook on Trends in the Health of Americans.* Hyattsville, MD; 2004:40–41.
29. US Department of Health and Human Services. *Healthy People 2010: Understanding and Improving Health.* 2nd ed. Washington, DC: US Government Printing Office; 2000.

CHAPTER

4

Design Strategies and Statistical Methods in Descriptive Epidemiology

OBJECTIVES

After completing this chapter you will be able to

- Define descriptive epidemiology.
- Describe uses, strengths, and limitations of descriptive study designs (ecologic study, case report, case series, cross-sectional survey).
- Define the 4 general types of data.
- Define ratio, proportion, and rate.
- Identify ways to describe epidemiologic data according to person, place, and time.
- Distinguish between crude and age-adjusted rates and be able to age-adjust rates using either the direct or the indirect method.
- Define the standardized morbidity (or mortality) ratio.
- Be familiar with the use of tables, graphs, and numerical methods (measures of central tendency and dispersion) for describing epidemiologic data according to person, place, and time.
- Be familiar with selected measures for evaluating the strength of the association between variables.

INTRODUCTION

In Chapter 1, "Foundations of Epidemiology," 2 general areas of epidemiologic study were introduced: descriptive and analytic. **Descriptive epidemiology** involves describing the distribution of health-related states and events by person, place, and time. A descriptive study helps the epidemiologist become familiar with the data, identify the extent of the public health problem, obtain a description of the public health problem that can be easily communicated, identify the population at greatest risk, and provide clues as to the determinants of disease. Analytic epidemiology is appropriate for addressing why and how diseases, conditions, and deaths occur. Analytic epidemiology will be discussed in Chapter 7, "Design Strategies and Statistical Methods Used in Analytic Epidemiology".

Describing data by person allows identification of the frequency of disease and who is at greatest risk. High risk populations can be identified by investigating inherent characteristics of people (age, sex, race, and ethnicity), acquired characteristics (immunity, marital status, education), activities (occupation, leisure, medication use), and conditions (access to health care, environmental state). Identifying the influence of beliefs, traditions, cultures, and societal expectations on acquired characteristics, activities, and conditions is important in providing clues to the causes of disease.

Describing data by place (residence, birthplace, place of employment, country, state, county, census tract, etc.) allows the epidemiologist to understand the geographic extent of disease, where the causal agent of disease resides and multiplies, and how the disease is transmitted and spread.

Finally, describing data by time can reveal the extent of the public health problem according to when and whether the disease is predictable. Assessing whether interactions exist among persons, place, and time may also provide insights into the causes of disease (see Chapter 5, "Descriptive Epidemiology According to Person, Place, and Time").

Descriptive statistics are a means of organizing, summarizing, and describing epidemiologic data by person, place, and time. Descriptive statistics can take on various forms, including tables, graphs, and numerical summary measures. Application of statistical methods makes it possible to effectively describe the public health problem.

DESCRIPTIVE STUDY DESIGNS

There are 4 types of studies commonly used in descriptive epidemiology: ecologic studies, case reports, case series, and cross-sectional surveys. In an ecologic study, the unit of analysis is the population. On the other hand, in a case report, case series, or cross-sectional survey, the unit of analysis is the individual. Descriptive studies are often limited in their ability to test hypotheses. However, they can provide useful information on the extent of the public health problem according to person, place, and time; who is at greatest risk with regard to place and time; possible causal associations; and the need for analytic epidemiologic investigation.

Ecologic Study

An **ecologic study** involves aggregated data on the population level. For example, suppose that the epidemiologist wanted to study whether there is an association between eating 5 or more servings of fruit and vegetables per day and obesity. Figure 4.1 shows the percentage of adults who have a body mass index of at least 30 (are obese) by the percentage of adults who eat 5 or more servings of fruit and vegetables per day. Each dot in the graph represents aggregated data for the state or territory. A linear line fit to the data shows a negative association between obesity and eating 5 or more servings of fruit and vegetables per day. A limitation of ecologic data, however, is that they are often unable to control for potential confounding factors that may explain some or all of the association. For example, it is possible that those who fail to eat 5 or more servings of fruit and vegetables per day are less likely to be physically active and that physical inactivity leads to obesity, not fruit and vegetable intake.

With ecologic data, when interpreting associations between indices, an error may result if the researcher mistakenly assumes that because the majority of a group has a characteristic, the characteristic is definitively associated with those experiencing a health-related state or event in the group. This is called **ecologic fallacy.**[1] It is possible that although higher levels of fruit and vegetable consumption may occur in states and territories with lower levels of obesity, those eating 5 or more servings of fruit and vegetables per day may not be the ones with the lower BMI.

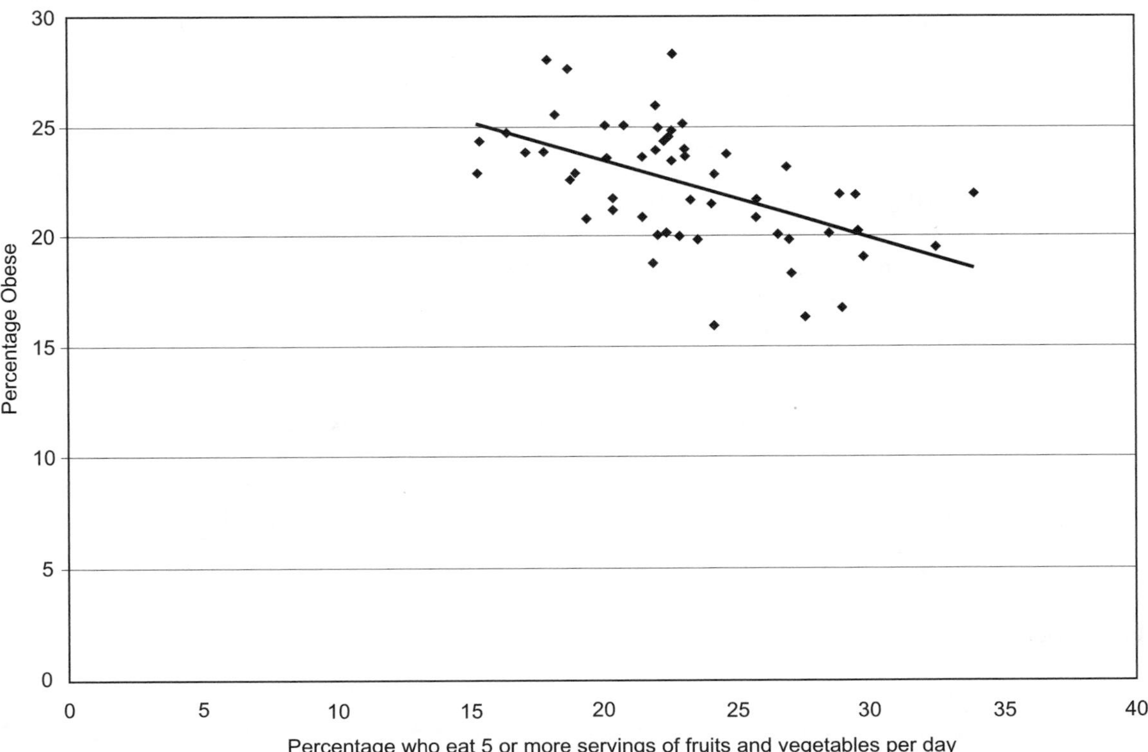

FIGURE 4.1 Correlation between eating 5 or more servings of fruits and vegetables per day and being overweight (in the United States and US territories). *Source:* Centers for Disease Control and Prevention. Prevalence data available at: http://apps.nccd.cdc.gov/brfss/.

Case Reports and Case Series

A **case report** is a profile of a single individual. A recent report described a 74-year-old woman who experienced airway obstruction when a piece of meat became lodged in her trachea.[2] A bystander was unsuccessful at practicing the Heimlich maneuver, and the patient became unconscious. While she was in a supine position, the Heimlich maneuver was again attempted, this time successfully. The woman was then taken to the emergency room where she was complaining of abdominal pain and distention. Further investigation identified a 2-cm rupture of the lesser curvature of her stomach. Contusions were also identified over the fundus and posterior stomach. Surgery corrected the problem, and she was discharged 6 days after surgery without complications. Hence, gastric perforation and other complications resulting from the Heimlich maneuver may exist and patients should be evaluated for such problems.

A **case series** involves a small group of patients with a similar diagnosis. For example, from October 4 to November 2, 2001, the first 10 cases of inhalational anthrax were identified in the United States. These cases were intentionally caused by release of *Bacillus anthracis.* Epidemiologic investigation found that the outbreak consisted of cases in the District of Columbia, Florida, New Jersey, and New York. The *B anthracis* spores were delivered through the mail in letters and packages. The ages of the cases ranged from 43 to 73 years, with 70% being male, and all but one were confirmed to have handled a letter or package containing *B anthracis* spores. The incubation period ranged from 4 to 6 days. Symptoms at the onset included fever or chills, sweat, fatigue or malaise, minimal or nonproductive cough, dyspnea, and nausea or vomiting. Blood tests and chest radiographs were also used to further characterize symptoms.[3] Identifying the symptoms of these patients may lead to earlier diagnosis of future cases.

These 2 examples describe a condition and an infectious disease by person. As a result, information was provided that may be useful for identifying potential complications related to the Heimlich procedure and for early detection of anthrax. Case reports and case series may also suggest the emergence of a new disease or epidemic if the disease exceeds what is expected. For example, on June 4, 1981, the CDC published a report that described 5 young men, all active homosexuals, who were treated for biopsy-confirmed *Pneumocystis carinii* pneumonia at 3 different hospitals in Los Angeles, California, during the period from October 1980 to May 1981. This was the first published report of the disease that would become known as AIDS a year later.[4] By the end of 1982, descriptive epidemiologic study provided strong evidence that the agent causing AIDS was transmitted through homosexual behavior,[5,6] heterosexual behavior,[7,8] blood (needle sharing among drug users) and blood transfusions,[9–11] and from mothers with AIDS to their infants.[12] In 2004, the estimated number of people newly infected with HIV was 4.9 million (4.3 milllion adults and 640,000 children under 15 years).[13]

Cross-Sectional Surveys

Cross-sectional surveys are conducted over a short period of time (usually a few days or weeks), and the unit of analysis is the individual. There is no follow-up period. Cross-sectional surveys are useful for examining associations among health-related states or events and personal characteristics such as age, sex, race and ethnicity, marital status, education, occupation, access to health care, and so on. Hence they reveal who is at greatest risk and provide clues as to the causes of disease. In addition, because cross-sectional surveys are useful for estimating prevalence data, it can also be said that they identify the extent of public health problems.

In 1956 the US Congress passed the National Health Survey Act, which established periodic health surveys to collect information on health-related states or events, use of health care resources, and relevant demographic information. Some such studies conducted in the United States now include the Behavior Risk Factor Surveillance System (BRFSS) Survey, the National Health Interview Survey, the National Hospital Discharge Survey, and the National Health and Nutrition Examination Survey. Another name for cross-sectional surveys such as these, is prevalence surveys. This is because cross-sectional surveys are often effective at obtaining prevalence data. For example, several studies have used cross-sectional surveys to estimate the prevalence of cancer and other chronic diseases.[14–17]

On the basis of a cross-sectional study of 2,531 randomly selected teachers and nonteachers in the public schools from Iowa and Utah, the prevalence of voice disorders (any time when the voice had not worked, performed, or sounded as it normally should) was 57.7% in teachers and 28.8% in nonteachers. The percentage reporting that they currently had a voice disorder was 11.0% of teachers and 6.2% of nonteachers.[18] Survey results also identified that occupation-related voice dysfunction in teachers may have significant adverse results on job performance, attendance, and future career choices.[19] Thus, the magnitude of a public health problem was determined, and teachers were identified as a high risk factor group for voice disorders.

Another example involves a 37-item cross-control sectional survey of 848 non-Hispanic white women in Utah.[20] Utah has relatively low rates of female malignant breast cancer,[21] due in part to the low rates found among women affiliated with the Church of Jesus Christ of Latter-day Saints (LDS or Mormons), who make up a large portion of the female population.[22] Although certain behaviors that protect against breast cancer are already well established, such as parity (number of children born to 1 woman) and breastfeeding,[23,24] the researchers wanted to identify the extent to which religious beliefs and church attendance influenced these and other behaviors. Among their findings parity, prevalence of breastfeeding, and lifetime total duration of breastfeeding were highest among LDS women who attended church weekly.

Some of the strengths of cross-sectional surveys are that they can be used to study several associations at once, they can be conducted over a short period of time, they produce prevalence data, biases resulting from observation and loss to follow-up do not exist, and they can provide evidence of the need for analytic epidemiologic study. They are limited, however, in being able to establish whether an exposure preceded or followed a health outcome. For example, married men may be healthier than nonmarried men. However, it may not be clear whether married men are healthier because of their marriage or because healthier men self-select marriage. Identifying that an association exists between marriage and health in a cross-sectional study says nothing about the causal direction. Other weaknesses include the fact that this method is not feasible for studying rare conditions and has the potential for response bias.

Response bias is a type of selection bias where those who respond to a questionnaire are systematically different from those who do not respond.[25] They may be more likely to be nonsmokers, concerned about health matters, have a higher level of education, be more likely to be employed in professional positions, be more likely to be married and have children, be more active in the community, and so on. Consequently, the results will not be representative of the population of interest.

Serial Surveys

Many of the national health surveys in the United States are conducted annually. Cross-sectional surveys that are routinely conducted are called **serial surveys**. These surveys reveal changing patterns of health-related states or events over time. For example, between 1990 and 2002, the BRFSS survey collected national data on the percentage of adults who are overweight or obese, according to BMI. An increasing trend in both overweight and obese individuals is presented in Figure 4.2.

TYPES OF DATA

Appropriate statistical methods for describing epidemiologic data by person, place, and time depend on the type of data used. **Data** may be thought of as observations or measurements of a phenomenon of interest. Before presenting types of methods for describing data, 4 types of numerical data need defining: nominal, ordinal, discrete, and continuous.

- **Nominal data:** unordered categories or classes (eg, sex, race/ethnicity, marital status, occupation). Nominal data that take on one of 2 distinct values are referred to as **dichotomous**. Nominal data that takes on more than 2 distinct values are called multichotomous.

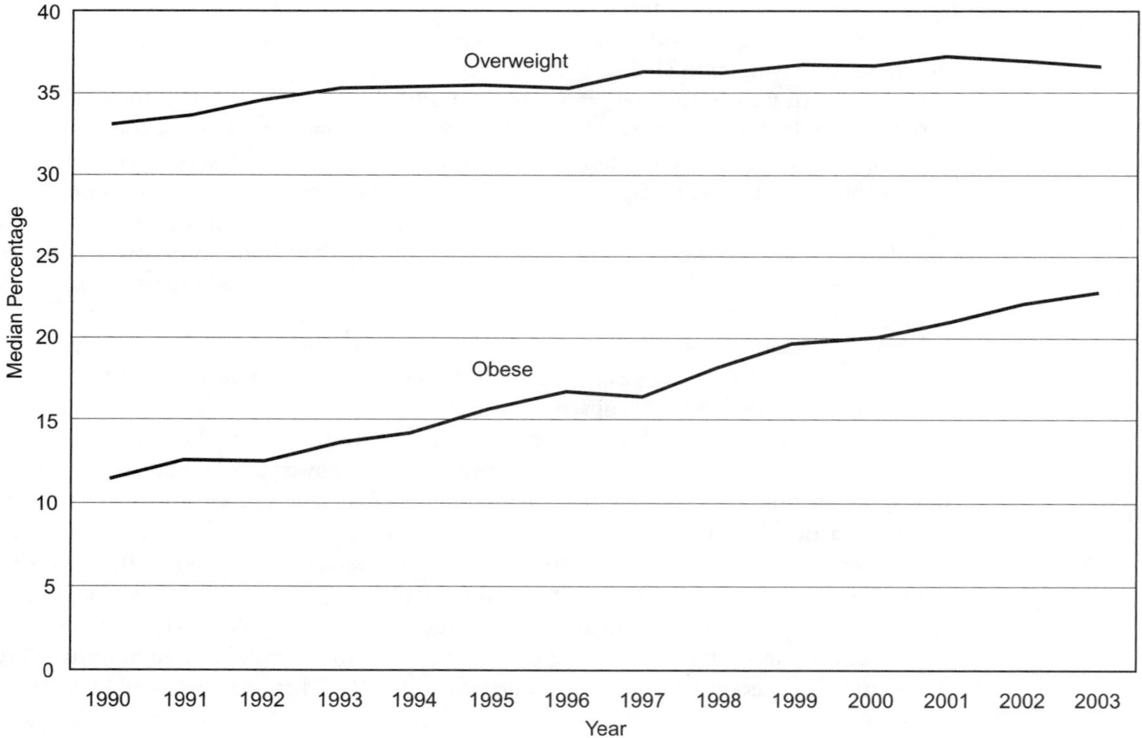

FIGURE 4.2 Percentage of overweight or obese adults in the United States between 1990 and 2003. *Source:* Centers for Disease Control and Prevention. Trends data available at: http://apps.nccd.cdc.gov/brfss/Trends/trendchart.asp?qkey=10010&State=US.

- **Ordinal data:** the order among categories provides additional information (eg, stage or grade of cancer). Ordinal-scale data are commonly used in health behavior research. Suppose health officials want to know if individuals in their area would use an immunization clinic if one was provided in the neighborhood. A cross-sectional survey could be administered with the following 5-point ordinal scale question.

  If an immunization clinic was held in your neighborhood, would you take your children to the clinic for their immunizations? (Check the box that applies most to your intention.)

1 ______	2 ______	3 ______	4 ______	5 ______
Not likely to attend	Will consider attending	May attend	Most likely will attend	Will attend for certain

- **Discrete data:** integers or counts that differ by fixed amounts, with no intermediate values possible (eg, number of new cases of lung cancer reported in the United States in a given year, number of children, and number of sick days taken in a month).
- **Continuous data:** measurable quantities not restricted to taking on integer values (eg, age, weight, temperature).

When data are collected, they are typically entered into a spreadsheet where each row represents a case and each column represents personal characteristics, clinical details, descriptive epidemiologic factors, and so on. A partial **line listing** is shown in Table 4.1. Examples of nominal data are in columns 3, 4, 5, and 8; examples of ordinal data are in column 9; discrete data are in column 6; and continuous data are in columns 2 and 7.

RATIOS, PROPORTIONS, AND RATES

In epidemiology, it is common to deal with data that indicate whether an individual was exposed to an illness, has an illness, experienced an injury, is disabled, or is dead. Ratios, proportions, and rates are commonly used measures for describing dichotomous data. The general formula for a ratio, proportion, or rate is

$$\frac{x}{y} \times 10^n$$

10^n is called the rate base, with typical values of $n = 0, 1, \ldots, 5$.

TABLE 4.1 Partial line listing data[18]

Case	*Age*	*Race*	*Ever Told You Have Breast Cancer*	*One or More Blood Relatives Have Developed Cancer*	*Number of Times Pregnant*	*How Many Years Have You Breastfed*	*What is Your Religious Preference*	*How Often Do You Attend Church*	*Etc.*
(1)	(2)	(3)	(4)	(5)	(6)	(7)	(8)	(9)	
1	59	White	No	Yes	1	0.5	None	Never	
2	39	White	No	No	3	1	Catholic	Weekly	
3	73	White	No	Yes	0	0	LDS	Weekly	

In a **ratio** the values of x and y are independent such that the values of x are not contained in y. The rate base for a ratio is 100 = 1. For example, from the cross-sectional survey exploring breast cancer risk factors in Utah, 704 women indicated that they had one or more children, and 132 said they had never had a child, with 12 not responding to this question. The ratio of parous to nonparous women was 5.3; that is, there were 5.3 times more women who had a child than there were women who never had a child.

In a **proportion**, x is contained in y. A proportion is typically expressed as a percentage, such that the rate base is $10^2 = 100$. For example, 84.2% (704/836 $\times$ 100) of women surveyed in Utah had one or more children.

A **rate** is a type of frequency measure that involves dichotomous data. It may be thought of as a proportion with the added dimension of time:

$$Rate = \frac{Number\ of\ cases\ or\ events\ occuring\ during\ a\ given\ time\ period}{Population\ at\ risk\ during\ the\ same\ time\ period} \times 10^n$$

The selection of the value n in the rate base for a rate is influenced by how common the health-related state or event under consideration is. The size of the rate base influences the clarity of the rate. For example, the female breast cancer incidence rate in 2002 in the United States was 0.000711.21 For the sake of presentation, cancer rates are typically multiplied by a rate base of 105 or 100,000 such that this rate is 71.1 per 100,000.

Historically, the **mortality rate** was commonly used to reflect the risk of disease in the population. Mortality rates usually cover one year and the population denominator is measured at the midyear.

$$Mortality\ Rate = \frac{Deaths\ occuring\ during\ a\ given\ time\ period}{Population\ from\ which\ death\ occurred} \times 10^n$$

As diagnosis and reporting have improved, incidence rates have become increasingly common for describing the occurrence of a health-related state or event.

$$Incidence\ Rate = \frac{New\ cases\ occuring\ during\ a\ given\ time\ period}{Population\ at\ risk\ during\ the\ same\ time\ period} \times 10^n$$

For chronic diseases, incidence rates usually cover one year and the population denominator is measured at the midyear. The rate base for mortality and incidence rates is generally 1,000, 10,000, or 100,000.

When new cases occur rapidly over a short period of time in a well-defined population, the attack rate is used.

$$Attack\ Rate = \frac{New\ cases\ occuring\ during\ a\ short\ period\ of\ time}{Population\ at\ risk\ at\ the\ beginning\ of\ the\ time\ period} \times 100$$

The attack rate is also called the **cumulative incidence rate**. It differs from the conventional incidence rate in that it tends to describe diseases or events that affect a larger proportion of the population of interest. The denominator includes the population at-risk at the beginning of the time period, and because a larger proportion of the population is affected, the rate base is generally $10^2 = 100$.

Sometimes the epidemiologist is interested in the rate of new cases occurring among contacts of known cases. The formula for a **secondary attack rate** is

$$\textit{Secondary Attack Rate} = \frac{\textit{New cases among contacts of primary cases during a short time period}}{(\textit{population at beginning of the time period}) - (\textit{primary cases})} \times 10^n$$

If the denominator of the incidence rate is the sum of the time each person was observed, this is called a **person-time rate**. This measure is also referred to as an **incidence density rate** because the denominator is the time each person is observed instead of the number of people. For example, if 100 people were followed for one year, there are 100 person years in the denominator.

$$\textit{Person-time rate} = \frac{\textit{Number of cases during observation period}}{\textit{Time each person observed totalled for all persons}} \times 10^n$$

Another common measure for describing disease and health-related events is **point prevalence** proportion. The numerator is distinct from the incidence rate in that it contains the number of new and existing cases of a disease or health-related event at a point in time. The denominator is distinct from the incidence rate in that it contains the total study population at a point in time. The rate base is typically $10^2 = 100$.

$$\textit{Point prevalence proportion} = \frac{\textit{New and existing cases of the disease or event at a point in time}}{\textit{Total study population at a point in time}} \times 100$$

This statistic is useful for measuring diseases where it is difficult to know when an individual became a case, such as with arthritis or diabetes. It is also useful for describing the magnitude of a public health problem (burden), whereas the **incidence rate** is more appropriate for describing risk.

It may be informative to think of this statistic as a function of the competing forces of incidence, survival, and cure. High incidence, good survival, and low cure rate reflect high prevalence. Low incidence, poor survival, and high cure reflect low prevalence. Because it is often difficult to say a patient is "cured," most people define prevalence as new and existing cases who are still alive. Only at death are they removed from the prevalent pool. In the context of cancer, breast cancer for women and prostate cancer for men have high incidence and relatively good survival. These are the most prevalent cancers in the United States. On the other hand, pancreatic cancer has low incidence and poor survival; this is among the lowest prevalent cancers in the United States.

Crude and Age-adjusted Incidence and Mortality Rates

The incidence and mortality rates just described produce crude rates. The **crude rate** of an outcome is calculated without any restrictions, such as age or sex or who is counted in the numerator or denominator. However, these rates are limited if the epidemiologist is trying to compare them between subgroups of the population or over time because of potential confounding influences, such as differences in the age distribution between groups. For example, suppose a researcher was interested in knowing whether the death rate for whites differed between Florida and Utah. The National Cancer Institute provides a query system where these rates can be easily generated.[26] In 2002, the crude mortality rate in Florida was 1,096 per 100,000 compared with 579 per 100,000 in Utah. The crude mortality rate ratio is 1.9, meaning the rates in Florida are 1.9 times (or 90%) higher than in Utah. However, the age distribution differs considerably between Florida and Utah. In Florida 6.3% of the population is under 5 years of age, and 16.7% of the population is 65 years and older.[27] Corresponding percentages in Utah are 9.8% and 8.5%.[27] Because death tends to come at a later age, much of the difference in the crude rates could be explained by different age distributions in the 2 populations, not greater risk factors and behaviors resulting in death in Florida. To make a more appropriate comparison of the hazard of death between the 2 populations, it is necessary to adjust for differences in the age distributions. This adjustment allows the researcher to control for the confounding effect of age. Two methods are used in practice for adjusting rates, they are called the direct and indirect methods.

Direct Method for Age-adjusting Rates

The direct method of age adjustment, based on the 2,000 United States standard population, yielded rates of 762 in Florida and 782 in Utah per 100,000. Thus after adjusting for differences in the age distribution, the rate in Florida is 0.97 times that in Utah. In this section, application of the direct method to the age adjustment of rates will be illustrated.

The direct method of adjusting for differences in the age distribution between populations at a point in time or within a population over time involves computing age-specific group rates, such as in 5-year or 10-year age intervals. Rates based on data covering age intervals of 5 or 10 years are generally preferred because they provide more stable rates than those based on single-year age intervals. A standard population is then selected. In the example above, the 2000 US standard population was selected. However, Florida's population, Utah's population, or the sum of both populations could also have been used as the standard. The choice of the standard population is somewhat arbitrary. The key is to select a standard population that is sufficiently large and to apply the standard population consistently between or within groups. The selected standard population is divided into age groups that correspond to the age-specific rates. The age-specific rates are multiplied by the age-specific standard population to give the expected number of cases had the group experienced the same population distribution as the standard population. The expected numbers of cases are summed over each age group. The sum is then divided by the total size of the standard population to give an **age-adjusted rate**.

To illustrate, refer to the data in Table 4.2. Counts were divided by population values to obtain rates. Age-specific rates as well as the overall crude rates were generated for males and females. The crude rate ratio for males to females was 1.09 (376/345). That is, the crude rate was 1.09 times (or 9%) higher for males than females.

Now that the age-specific rates have been calculated, the next step is to select an appropriate standard population for adjustment. If comparing the resulting age-adjusted rates with rates adjusted with a specific standard desired, then that standard should be used. Suppose, however, that knowing the rate for females is desired, assuming they had the same age-distribution as males. To do this, the age-specific female cancer rates are multiplied by the age-specific population values for males to get the expected number of cases for females in each age group, assuming they had the same age distribution as males (Table 4.3). These expected counts are then summed and divided by the total male population. The resulting malignant cancer rate for females age-adjusted to the male population is

TABLE 4.2 Age-specific and overall all-cause malignant cancer incidence rates, 1999–2001, among males and females[28]

	Male			*Female*		
Age	*Counts*	*Population*	*Rate per 100,000*	*Counts*	*Population*	*Rate per 100,000*
<40	8,759	30,560,962	29	9,284	29,211,186	32
40–49	10,628	9,537,477	111	18,455	9,487,526	195
50–59	27,099	7,624,126	355	34,410	7,919,559	434
60–69	49,422	4,535,884	1,090	38,997	4,873,955	800
70–79	64,053	2,984,787	2,146	44,539	3,642,718	1,223
80+	56,609	2,322,377	2,438	57,652	3,861,274	1,493
Total	216,570	57,565,613	376	203,337	58,996,218	345

$$\textit{Age-adjusted rate} = \frac{168{,}930}{57{,}565{,}613} \times 100{,}000 = 294 \textit{ per } 100{,}000$$

The rate ratio for males to females is now 1.28. This means that if females had the same age distribution as males, malignant cancer incidence would be 28% higher for males than females, as opposed to 9% higher found with crude rates.

The magnitude of an adjusted rate does not represent the actual rate of a health-related state or event in the population but is a hypothetical construct useful for comparison. It should be evident that the choice of the standard population is somewhat arbitrary. The key is that once the standard population is selected, it must be consistently applied. For example, if rates are being compared over several years, it is important to age adjust the rates for those years using the same standard population. Researchers generally try to select a standard population that covers the same time period as the data being evaluated as in the next example.

As the life expectancy in the United States continues to increase, comparing the risk of health-related states or events over time without the confounding effect of a changing age

TABLE 4.3 Expected number of all malignant cancer cases in females assuming females have the same age distribution as males

Age	*Male Population*	*Female Rate*	*Expected Counts*
<40	30,560,962	.00032	9,780
40–49	9,537,477	.00195	18,598
50–59	7,624,126	.00434	33,089
60–69	4,535,884	.00800	36,287
70–79	2,984,787	.01,223	36,504
80+	2,322,377	.01,493	34,673
Total	57,565,613		168,930

distribution requires that age-adjusted rates be used. A comparison is made between US crude and age-adjusted rates over time for all-cause mortality and for all malignant cancers shown in Figure 4.3. The crude all-cause mortality rates indicate a decrease in mortality between the years 1969 and 2002. However, when the rates are adjusted for age, the decrease in mortality appears much more pronounced. For all malignant cancers, the crude mortality rate increases more rapidly before the peak in the early 1990s and decreases more slowly after the peak than the age-adjusted all-malignant-cancer mortality rates.

Indirect Method of Age Adjustment

In situations where age-specific rates are unstable because of small numbers or missing numbers, age-adjustment is still possible with the indirect method. As was the case with the direct method, a standard population is selected. This is the larger or more stable and complete of the 2 populations being compared. Age-specific rates are calculated for the standard population. These rates are then multiplied by the age-specific population values in the comparison population to obtain the expected number of health-related states or events in

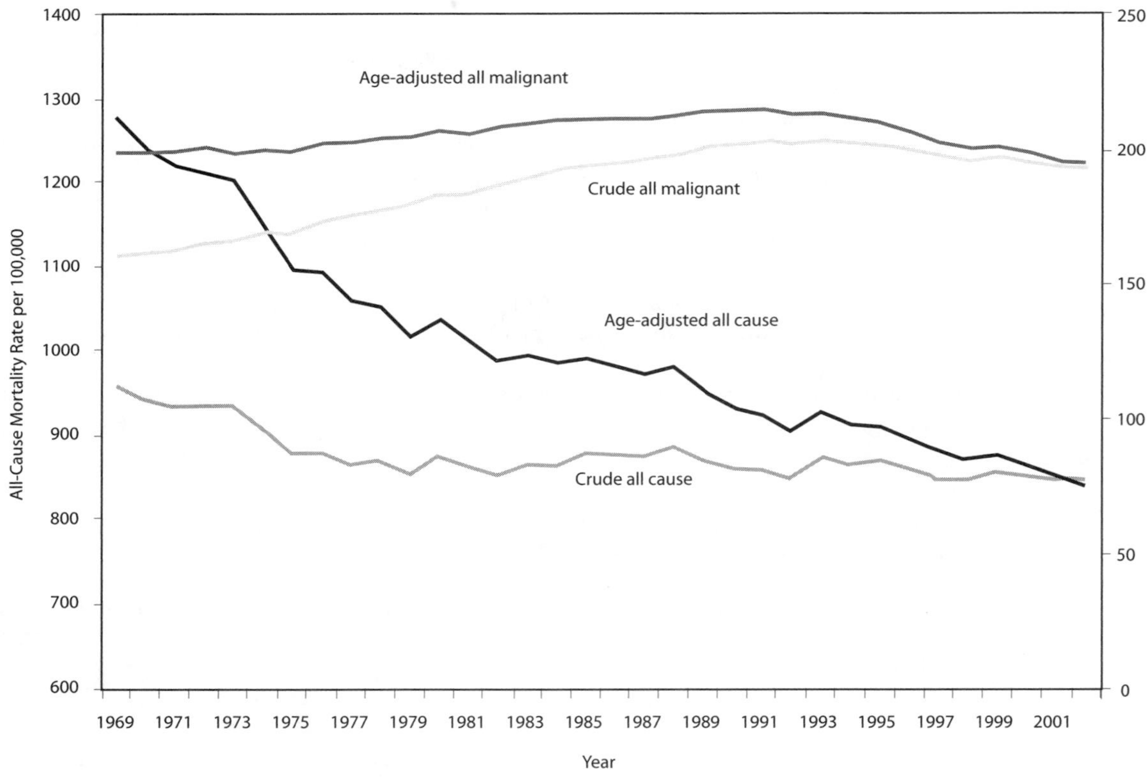

FIGURE 4.3 US crude and age-adjusted (to the 2000 US standard population) rates for all-cause mortality and all malignant cancers according to year. *Source:* National Cancer Institute. SEER. Cancer Query System: US Mortality Statistics available at: http://seer.cancer.gov/canques/mortality.html.

each age group. The total number of health-related states or events observed in the comparison population is then divided by the total number of expected health-related states or events. This ratio is referred to as the standardized morbidity (or mortality when deaths are being considered) ratio (SMR).

$$SMR = \frac{Observed}{Expected}$$

Interpretation:

- SMR = 1 The health-related states or events observed were the same as expected from the age-specific rates in the standard population.
- SMR >1 More health-related states or events were observed than expected from the age-specific rates in the standard population.
- SMR <1 Fewer health-related states or events were observed than expected from the age-specific rates in the standard population.

To illustrate, refer again to the data in Table 4.2. However, suppose that some or all of the female age-specific counts are unavailable but that the total count is available. Further suppose that the age-specific rates for males can be calculated. Now multiply the age-specific rates in the male (standard) population by the age-specific female population values to obtain the expected number of all malignant cancer cases per age-specific group (Table 4.4). Sum the expected counts to obtain the total number of expected malignant cancers in the comparison population

$$SMR = \frac{203{,}337}{272{,}554} = 0.746$$

This ratio indicates that fewer malignant cancer cases (about 25%) were observed in females than expected from the age-specific rates of males.

TABLE 4.4 Data for calculating the age-adjusted malignant cancer rate for females using the indirect method

Age	*Male Rate per 100,000*	*Female Population*	*Expected Counts*
<40	29	29,211,186	8,471
40–49	111	9,487,526	10,531
50–59	355	7,919,559	28,114
60–69	1,090	4,873,955	53,126
70–79	2,146	3,642,718	78,173
80+	2,438	3,861,274	94,138
Total			272,554

Category-Specific Rates

Category-specific rates refer to rates computed for select types of disease (eg, myocardial infarction, stroke, lung cancer) or for select subgroups of the population. Race-specific, age-specific, and gender-specific rates are commonly reported in the literature. Category-specific rates allow researchers to compare the risk and burden of disease occurrence, death, and health-related events among subgroups of the population, such as between blacks and whites, between young and old, and between men and women. Rate ratios are commonly used to compare category-specific rates among subgroups of the population. Geographic-specific rates are also common in epidemiology. Identifying the risk of disease according to characteristics related to place may provide clues to the causes of disease (see Chapter 5).

Confidence Intervals for Rates

When a rate is based on sample data, the sample rate is a point estimate of the population rate. Confidence intervals are used to measure the precision of a sample rate. A confidence interval is the range of values in which the population rate is likely to fall. By convention, 95% confidence intervals are used to indicate a range in which the researchers are 95% confident the true population rate lies. The formula to calculate a 95% confidence interval for an incidence rate or prevalence proportion is

$$Rate \pm 1.96 \sqrt{Rate(1 - Rate)/n}$$

where Rate equals the rate of the cumulative incidence rate or prevalence proportion and where *n* equals the population at risk. For a person-time incidence rate the formula is modified as follows

$$Rate \pm 1.96 \sqrt{Number\ of\ new\ events/(person\text{-}time\ at\ risk)^2}$$

When computing the confidence intervals, the rate or prevalence proportion should be in its decimal form. After the upper and lower limits are derived, multipy these estimates by the appropriate rate base.

TABLES, GRAPHS, AND NUMERICAL MEASURES

Frequency distribution tables, graphs, and numerical measures are common ways to present epidemiologic data.

Tables

A **frequency distribution** is commonly used for presenting the frequency of nominal, ordinal, discrete, or continuous data (grouped into class intervals such that each group covers a range of values). For the level of each of these types of data, the numerical counts associated with the levels of the variable are presented. (Note that a **variable** is any characteristic that can be measured or categorized.) When continuous data are grouped into class intervals, these intervals should not overlap. It is also often useful to present the proportion of counts associated with the level of each variable. The relative frequency is the proportion of counts from the total that appears in each level of the variable.

The numbers of individuals (counts) who have experienced a voice disorder (nominal data) is shown in Table 4.5. The prevalence of individuals who have ever had a voice disorder is 43% [(1088/2531) × 100]. Table 4.6 is more complex because it shows the frequency of individuals in each category of postnasal drip (ordinal data) for those ever having had a voice disorder compared with those who have not. Comparing the 2 distributions shows that ever having had a voice disorder is more likely among individuals with seasonal or chronic postnasal drip. Table 4.7 displays the frequency of individuals across age categories (continuous data) according to status of whether they have ever had a voice disorder. Those reporting ever having had a voice problem were more likely to be aged 40–49 or 50–59 years.

In the study associating breast cancer risk factors with religious preference and church attendance, one variable considered was parity (number of children).[20] Among parous women, parity is associated with LDS status and weekly church attendance in Table 4.8. Parous LDS women who attend church weekly tend to have a greater number of children than all other groups considered. Weekly church attendance has little association with the number of children a women has among parous non-LDS women.

Graphs

Graphs are particularly useful for describing health-related states or events by place and time. Definitions of some common methods for describing data are as follows.

TABLE 4.5 Cases ever having had a voice disorder: nominal data[18]

Ever Had a Voice Disorder	*Number of Individuals*	*Relative Frequency (%)*
Yes	1,088	43.0
No	1,443	57.0

TABLE 4.6 Cases ever having had a voice disorder by classification of postnasal drip: ordinal data[18]

Postnasal Drip	*Number With Voice Disorder*	*Relative Frequency (%)*	*Number Without Voice Disorder*	*Relative Frequency (%)*
Not at all	123	11.3	349	24.2
Occasionally	633	58.2	832	57.7
Seasonally	186	17.1	179	12.4
Chronically	146	13.4	83	5.7
Total	1,088	100.0	1,443	100.0

TABLE 4.7 Cases ever having had a voice disorder by classification of age: grouped continuous data[18]

Age	*Number With Voice Disorder*	*Relative Frequency (%)*	*Number Without Voice Disorder*	*Relative Frequency (%)*
20–29	79	7.3	193	13.4
30–39	227	20.9	330	22.9
40–49	407	37.4	452	31.3
50–59	306	28.1	328	22.7
60+	69	6.3	140	9.7
Total	1,088	100.0	1443	100.0

- **Bar charts** are commonly used for graphically displaying a frequency distribution that involves nominal or ordinal data. The categories in which the observations fall are shown on the horizontal axis, and the vertical bar is drawn above each category, with the height representing the frequency. In some cases, researchers choose to plot the relative frequency such that the height of the bars then represents the percentage in each category. For example, Figure 4.4 is a bar chart that shows the data relating to voice disorders in Table 4.5. Figure 4.5 is a side-by-side bar chart that shows the data from Table 4.6.
- A **histogram** shows a frequency distribution for discrete or continuous data. The horizontal axis displays the true limits of the selected intervals. For example, Figure 4.6 displays the data from Table 4.8.

TABLE 4.8 Number of children among parous women in Utah according to religious preference and church activity in Utah, 2002: discrete data[20]

	LDS				*Non-LDS*				*None*	
	Active		*Less Active*		*Active*		*Less Active*			
Parity	*No.*	*%*	*No.*	*%*	*No.*	*%*	*No.*	*%*	*No.*	*%*
1	41	10.1	11	10.8	8	14.6	16	20.3	17	27.0
2	65	16.0	36	35.3	22	40.0	30	38.0	20	31.8
3	71	17.5	21	20.6	15	27.3	18	22.8	21	33.3
4	91	22.5	18	17.7	3	5.5	9	11.4	3	4.8
5	67	16.5	5	4.9	3	5.5	2	2.5	0	0.0
6+	70	17.3	11	10.8	4	7.3	4	5.1	2	3.2
Total	405	100.0	102	100.0	55	100.0	79	100.0	63	100.0

Active = attends church weekly; Less active = attends church less than weekly.

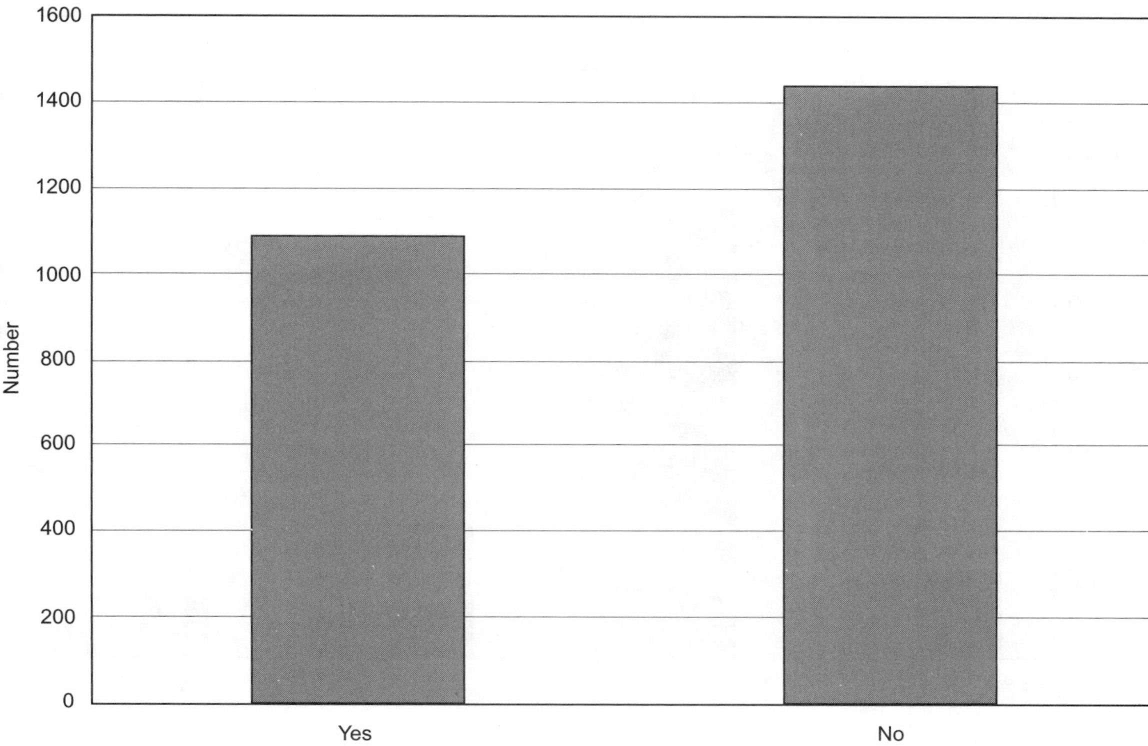

FIGURE 4.4 Frequency of ever having had a previous voice disorder.

- An **epidemic curve** is a histogram that shows the course of an epidemic by plotting the number of cases by time of onset.
- **Box plots** have a single axis and present a summary of the data. Figure 4.7 is a box plot of the percentage of people in each of the 54 states and territories of the United States in 2003 that were obese. The central, vertically depicted box extends from the 25th percentile, 20.2%, to the 75th percentile, 24.4%. The 25th percentile represents the first quartile, and 75th percentile represents the third quartile. The line running between the quartiles is the 50th percentile or median (middle), 22.8%. The asterisk represents the mean (average), 22.4%. The lines projecting out of the box on either side extend to the maximum, 28.4%, and minimum, 16.0%, of the data. Hence, the 54 US states and territories range from 16.0% obese to 28.4% obese. The median state or territory has 22.8% obese. The mean percentage of obesity among the states and territories is 22.4%. The percentage of obesity for the middle half of the states and territories ranges from 20.2% to 24.4%. The lowest percentage of obese adults is in Colorado, and the highest percentage is in Alabama.
- A **two-way (or bivariate) scatter plot** is used to depict the relationship between 2 distinct discrete or continuous variables. Points on the graph represent a pair of values; the value of one variable is listed along the horizontal or *x*-axis, and the value of the other variable is listed along the vertical or *y*-axis. Figure 4.1 is an example of a two-way scatter plot. The point representing the state or territory with the highest percent of its population eating 5 or more servings of fruits and vegetables is the Virgin Islands. The point also represents the 22.0% of their population that are obese.

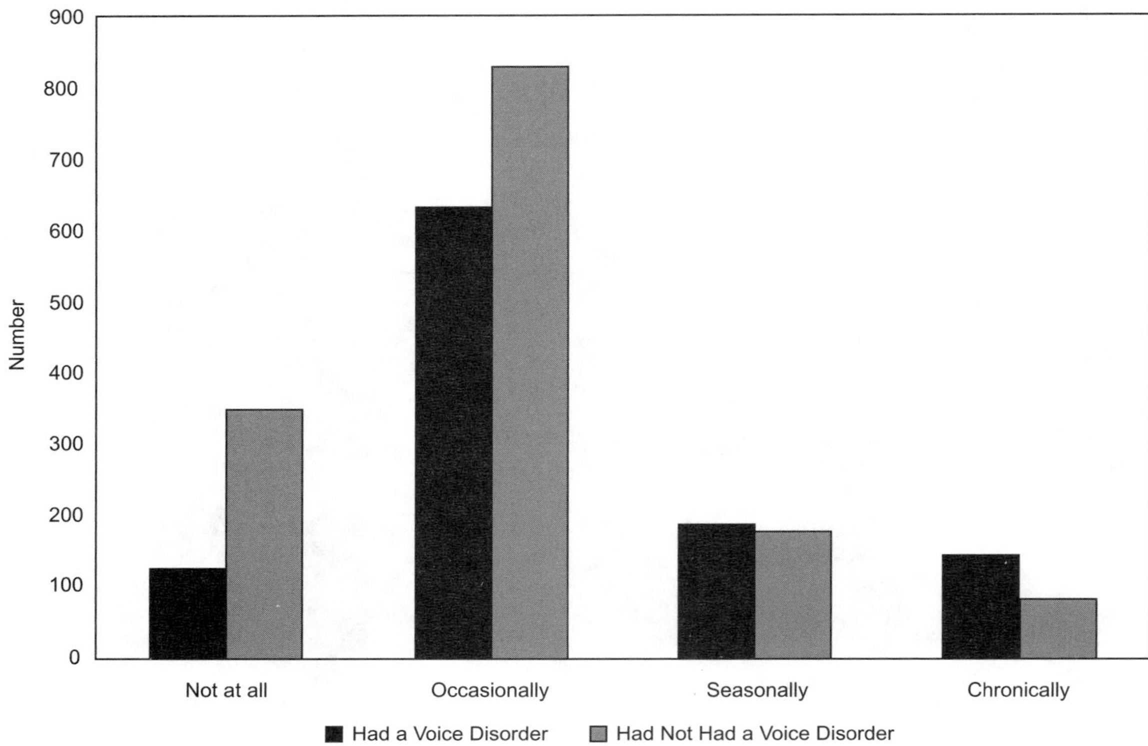

FIGURE 4.5 Frequency of ever having had a disorder or not ever having had a voice disorder, by categories of post-nasal drip.

- A **spot map** is used to display the location of each health-related state or event that occurs in a defined place and time. With rare diseases or outbreaks, each point on the map represents a case. An example of a spot map of Montgomery, Alabama, showing the place of employment of cases in a typhus epidemic in 1922–1925 is shown in Figure 4.8. Some health-related states or events that involve large numbers of cases may be presented on an **area map** with different shadings representing the number or rate of cases in defined geographic areas. For example, Figure 4.9 and Figure 4.10 show maps of the United States with the shading of each state representing fatal occupational injury rates and persons with BMIs over 30, respectively. Figure 4.9 specifically lists fatal occupational injury rates from 1.4 to 14.1 per 100,000 employed workers in 2002.[29] Fatal occupational injury rates exceeded 10 per 100,000 employed workers in Alaska, Wyoming, and Montana. The fatal occupational rate was 4.0 per 100,000 employed workers in the entire country in 2002.
- A **line graph** is similar to a two-way scatter plot in that it depicts the relationship between 2 continuous variables. Each point on the graph represents a pair of values. This graph is distinct from the two-way scatter plot because for each point on the x-axis there is only a single point on the y-axis. Figure 4.2 is an example of a line graph. The graph shows an increasing trend in the percentage of the US adult population who are obese. Line graphs are useful for describing health-related states or events by time. Line graphs will be developed more fully in Chapter 5.

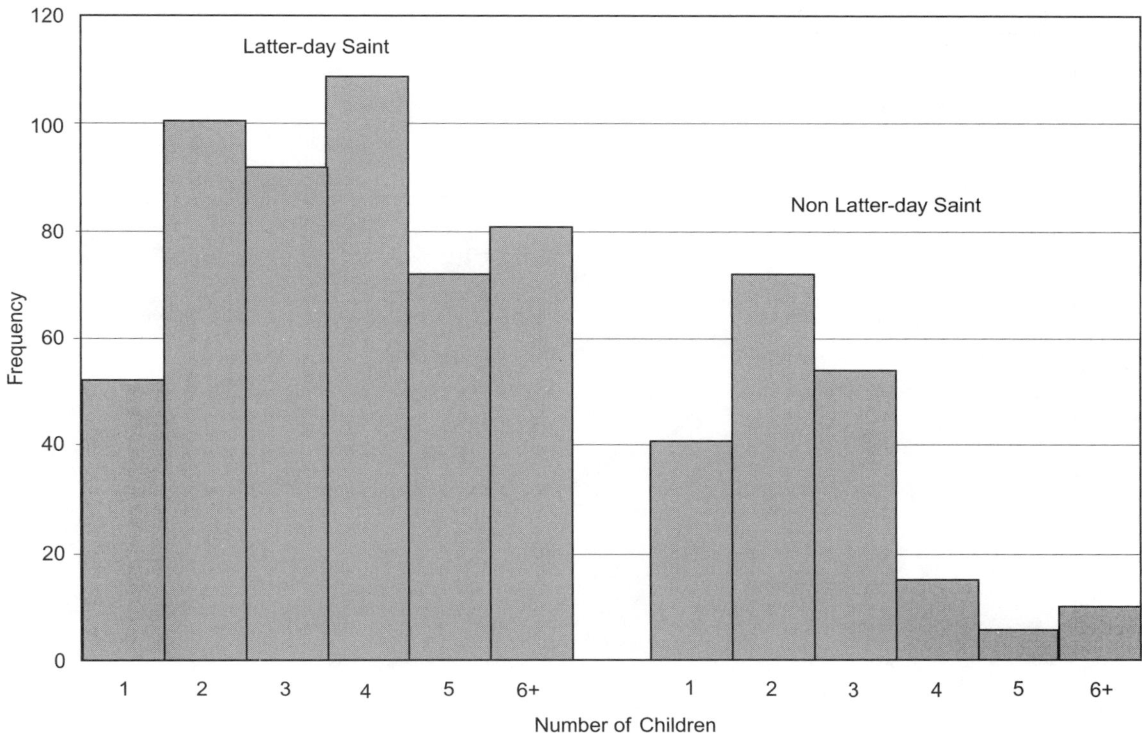

FIGURE 4.6 Frequency of having one-to-six or more children among parous Latter-day Saint (LDS or Mormon) and Non-LDS women in Utah, 2002.

Numerical Methods

It is often informative to summarize and describe discrete and continuous data with measures of central tendency and measures of dispersion. **Measures of central tendency** refer to ways of designating the center of the data. The most common measures are mean, median, and mode.

- **Mean** (arithmetic average) is the sum of all of the values added and then divided by the total number of values. The mean is mathematically responsive to each value in data. The mean is sensitive to extreme values (outliers). Extreme high or low values will cause the mean to not represent the typical values in the frequency distribution because the mean will be pulled in the direction of outliers.
- **Median** is the number or value that divides a list of numbers in half; it is the middle observation in the data set. It is less sensitive to outliers than the mean.
- **Mode** is the number or value that occurs most often; the number with the highest frequency.

Measures of dispersion, also called the spread or referred to as variability, are used to describe how much data values in a frequency distribution vary from each other and from the measures of central tendency. There are several measures of dispersion: range, interquartile range, variance, and standard deviation. These are defined as follows.

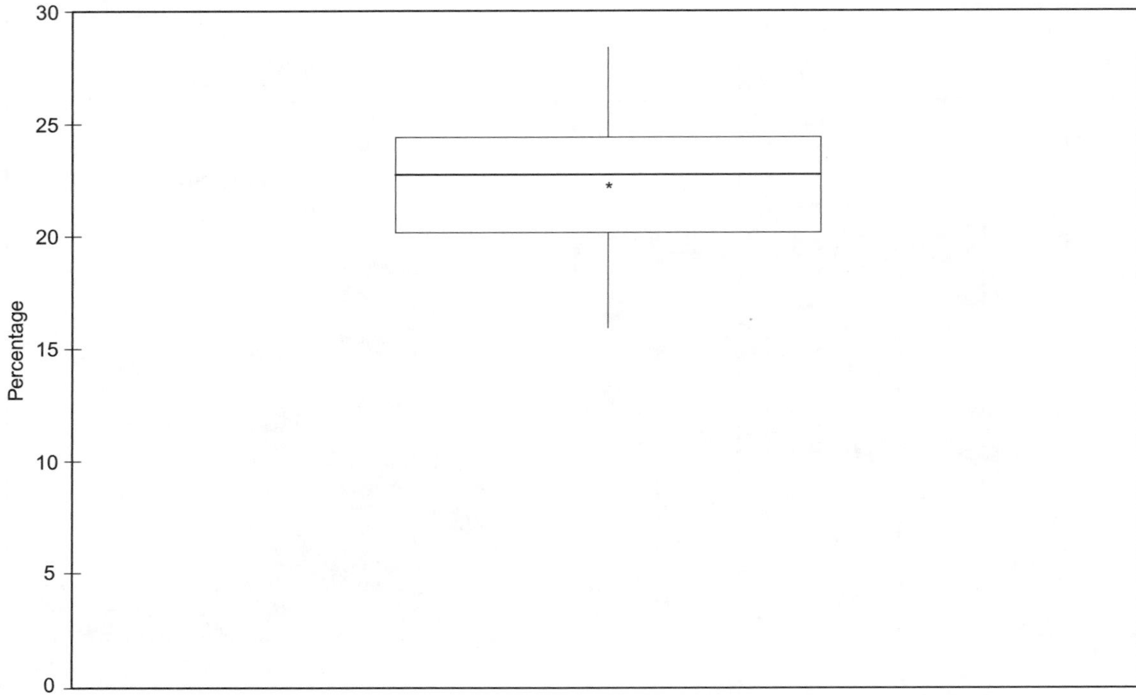

FIGURE 4.7 Box plot displaying the percentage of people obese (BMI 30 or greater) in the United States, 2003.

- **Range** is the difference between the largest (maximum) and smallest (minimum) values of a frequency distribution.
- **Interquartile range** is the difference between the third quartile (75th percentile) and first quartile (25th percentile). Note that the distribution of data consists of 4 quarters. Each quartile represents 25% of the data. Twenty-five percent of the data falls at or below the first quartile, 50% of the data falls below the second quartile (median), 75% of the data fall at or below the third quartile, and 100% of the data fall at or below the fourth quartile.
- **Variance** is the average of the squared differences of the observations from the mean.
- **Standard deviation** is the square root of the variance. The standard deviation has nice mathematical properties that are used in constructing the confidence interval for the mean and in statistical tests for evaluating research hypotheses.

A frequency distribution may be symmetric or skewed. A positive skewed distribution has a tail to the right (also called right skewed). A negative skewed distribution has a tail to the left (also called left skewed). The distribution of parity for women in the breast cancer risk factor study is shown in Figure 4.6. For LDS and non-LDS women in Utah combined, the mean number of children is 3.2; the median number of children is 3; most of the women had 2 children. The distribution is right skewed. The number of children had a range of 13 (0 to 13), with an interquartile range of 2, variance of 3.6, and standard deviation of 1.9.

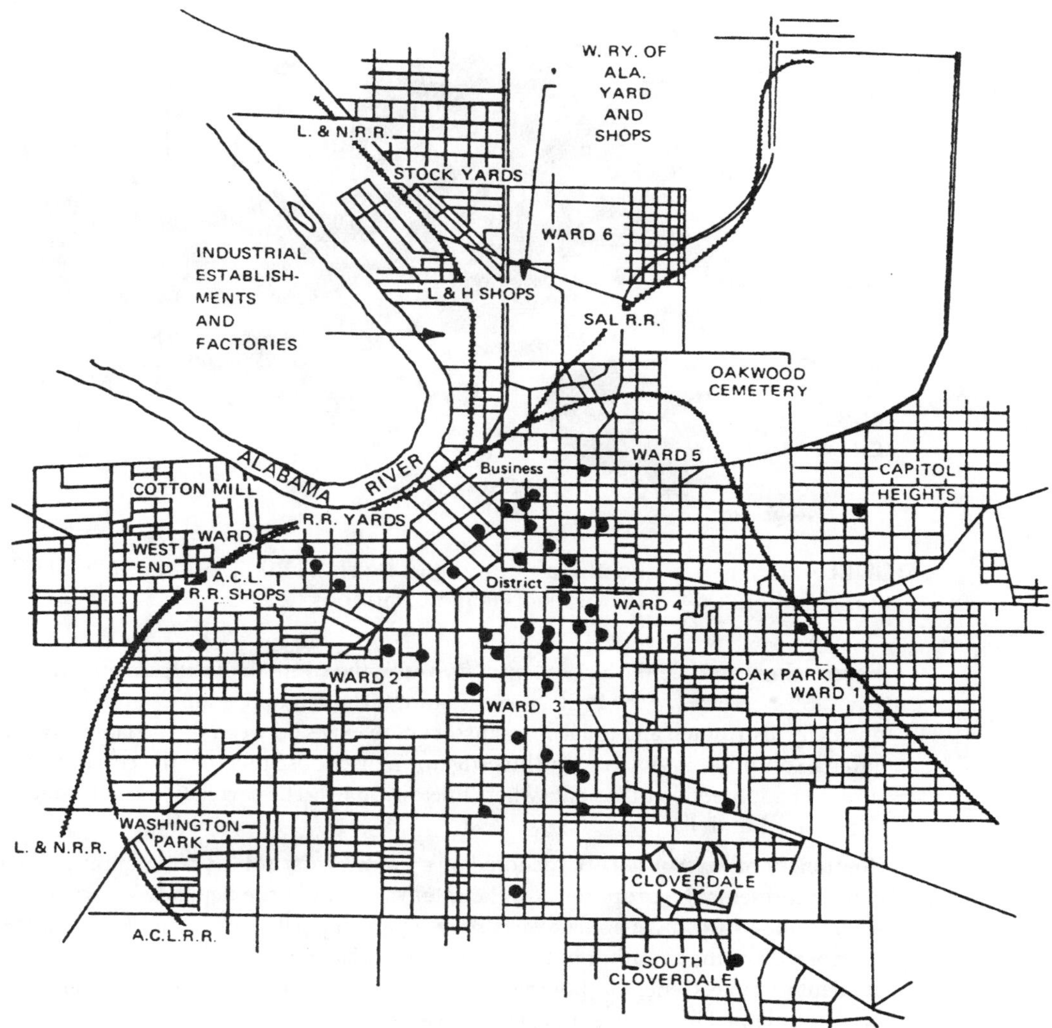

FIGURE 4.8 A spot map showing the place of residence of all cases of typhus in Montgomery, Alabama. *Source*: Adapted from Maxcy, K.F., "An Epidemiological Study of Endemic Typhus (Brill's Disease) in the Southeastern United States," *Public Health Reports,* Vol. 41, pp. 2967–2995, 1926.

MEASURES OF STATISTICAL ASSOCIATION

Epidemiologists are often interested in measuring the strength of association between variables. One approach is to compare the frequency distribution of one variable across the levels of a second variable. The odds ratio or the risk ratio is also commonly used to measure the strength of association between 2 variables (see Chapter 7). For discrete and continuous variables, measuring the association between 2 variables can be achieved by one of the following methods.

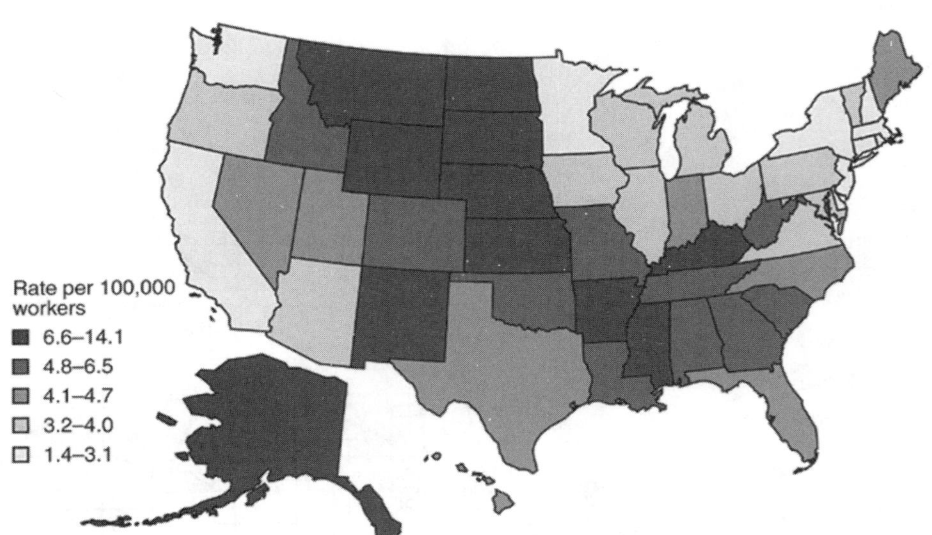

FIGURE 4.9 Fatal occupational injury rates by state, 2002. *Source:* NIOSH Publication Number 2004–146. Worker Health Chartbook, 2004.

- **Correlation coefficient** (denoted by r) measures the strength of the association between 2 variables (also called the Pearson correlation). The method assumes both variables are normally distributed and that a linear association exists between the variables. When the latter assumption is violated, the investigator may choose to apply the correlation measure over a subsection of the data where linearity holds. The correlation coefficient ranges between -1 and $+1$.
- **Coefficient of determination** (denoted by r^2) is the square of the correlation coefficient, and it represents the proportion of the total variation in the dependent variable that is determined by the independent variable. If a perfect positive or negative association exists, then all of the variation in the dependent variable would be explained by the independent variable. Generally, however, only part of the variation in the dependent variable can be explained by a single independent variable.

  Refer again to Figure 4.1 where the scatter plot shows the percentage of adults in each US state and territory who are obese by the percentage of adults who eat 5 or more servings of fruits and vegetables per day. There is a negative association between the variables; that is, as percentage who eat 5 or more servings of fruits and vegetables per day increases, the percentage who are obese decreases. A linear association exists between the data. The correlation coefficient is $r = -0.533$. The coefficient of determination is $r^2 = 0.284$. Thus it can be said that approximately 28% of the variation in obesity is associated with eating 5 or more servings of fruits and vegetables per day. The remaining 72% is associated with other factors, such as exercise, heredity, and age.
- **Spearman's rank correlation coefficient** is an alternative to the Pearson correlation coefficient when outlying data exists such that one or both of the distributions are skewed. This method is robust to outliers.
- **Regression analysis** provides an equation that estimates the change in the dependent variable (y) per unit change in an independent variable (x).This method assumes that for each

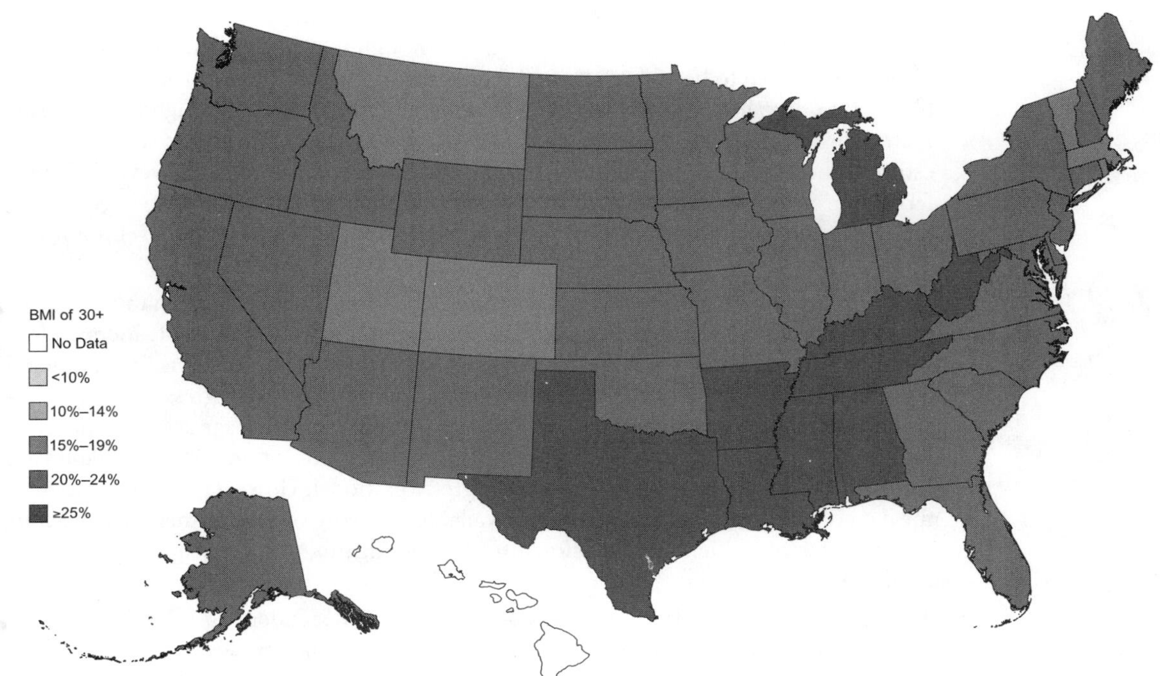

FIGURE 4.10 Obesity (BMI of 30 or above) among United States Adults, 2004. *Source:* Centers for Disease Control. Available at: www.cdc.gov/nccdphp/dnpa/obesity/trend/maps/index.htm.

value of x, y is normally distributed, that the standard deviation of the outcomes y do not change over x, that the outcomes y are independent, and that a linear relationship exists between x and y. Data transformations and other methods are used to respond to violations of these assumptions. In some situations, when outliers exist, the model is estimated after the outliers have been dropped. In situations where a linear relationship between variables does not hold, piecewise linear regression or polynomial regression is employed.

A linear association may be estimated through the use of a procedure called linear regression. This is done by applying the least squares method. This method fits a linear line to the data that minimizes the squared deviations of each point from the straight line. Simple linear regression involves an equation with one independent variable. The equation may be written as

$$y = a + bx$$

The letter a represents the y-intercept of the linear fitted line and the letter b represents the slope. The slope is a measure of association that indicates how y changes when x changes by one unit. For example, using the least squares approach, the estimated linear regression line for the data in Figure 4.1 is

$$Obesity = 30.525 + 0.352 \times Fruit\ Veg$$

For every percent increase in 5 or more servings of fruits and vegetables a day, the percent obese is expected to decrease by 0.352. Although it could be said that the percent obese is estimated to be 30.525 when percent of 5 or more servings of fruits and vegetables is zero, zero lies beyond the range of the data on the *x*-axis. Although *y* can be estimated for any given value of *x*, estimating *y* beyond the range of the *x* values used to estimate the model may result in misleading and nonsensical results. However, it is perfectly appropriate to estimate percent obese for the percent of 5 or more servings of fruits and vegetables per day of 25. This yields an estimated percent of state-level obesity of 21.7%.

- **Multiple regression** is an extension of simple regression analysis in which there are 2 or more independent variables. In multiple regression, the effects of multiple independent variables on the dependent variable can be simultaneously assessed. This type of model is useful for adjusting for potential confounders. For example, in a regression analysis assessing the relationship between heart disease (*y*) and exercise (*x*), age is a potential confounding variable. To control or adjust for this potential confounder, both variables are included as independent variables in the regression model. However, this assumes that the data on the confounding factors are available. In many situations there may be confounding factors which are not known to the investigator, and consequently, data not available for adjustment.
- **Logistic regression** is a type of regression in which the dependent variable is a dichotomous variable. Logistic regression is commonly used in epidemiology because many of the outcome measures considered involve nominal data (eg, ill vs not ill, injured vs not injured, disabled vs not disabled, dead vs alive, and so on).
- **Multiple logistic regression** is an extension of logistic regression in which 2 or more independent variables are included in the model. It allows the researcher to look at the simultaneous effect of multiple independent variables on the dependent variable. As in the case of multiple regression, this method is effective in controlling for confounding factors.

The assumptions for these methods can be evaluated with bivariate scatter plots. It is beyond the scope of this book to explore the methods for evaluating these assumptions with graphical procedures. This is a topic for introductory biostatistics.

The measures of association presented here assume a sufficient sample size. This is because outliers can have large and potentially misleading effects on the statistical measures when the sample size is small. In addition, the measures of association may be used as part of the evidence for establishing a cause-effect association, but they are insufficient in and of themselves. Criteria such as biologic plausibility, consistency among studies, dose-response relationship, and time-sequence of events should also be considered when making judgments about causality.[30]

EXERCISES

Key Terms

Define the following terms.

Age-adjusted rate
Area map
Attack rate
Bar chart
Binary
Bivariate
Box plot
Case report
Case series
Continuous data
Coefficient of determination
Correlation coefficient
Cross-sectional surveys
Crude rate
Cumulative incidence rate
Data
Descriptive epidemiology
Dichotomous
Discrete data
Ecologic fallacy
Ecologic study
Epidemic curve
Frequency distribution
Histogram
Incidence density rate
Incidence rate
Interquartile range
Line graph
Line listing
Logistic regression
Measures of central tendency
Measures of dispersion
Mean
Median
Mode
Mortality rate
Multiple regression
Multiple logistic regression
Nominal data
Ordinal data
Person-time rate
Point prevalence
Proportion
Range
Rate
Ratio
Regression analysis
Secondary attack rateSerial surveys
Spearman's rank correlation coefficient
Spot map
Standard deviation
Two-way scatter plot
Variable
Variance

Study Questions

To answer questions 4.1 to 4.4, refer to the data in Table 4.9.

4.1 The variables in the table represent what type of data?

4.2 Describe the extent of the public health problem of female breast cancer according to place.

4.3 Would age-adjusted rates be more appropriate for comparing the risk of female breast cancer among geographic areas and racial groups? Explain.

For questions 4.4 to 4.6, refer to the data in Table 4.10.

4.4 Describe the extent of the public health problem of female breast cancer according to place.

TABLE 4.9 Female crude malignant breast cancer incidence rates in San Francisco and the metropolitan areas of Detroit and Atlanta according to selected racial groups, 1999–2001[28]

Location	*White Rate*	*Black Rate*	*Asian or Pacific Islander Rate*
San Francisco	171.8	109.8	90.1
Detroit (metropolitan)	160.3	108.7	48.8
Atlanta (metropolitan)	146.9	78.7	43.7
Three areas combined	161.5	96.3	80.7

4.5 The crude rate ratio between whites and Asian or Pacific Islanders is 2.0. The corresponding rate ratio based on the age-adjusted rates is 1.7. What does this tell you about the age distribution between the 2 female populations?

4.6 Does this data provide any clues as to the risk factors for female breast cancer?

4.7 What other descriptive data would be useful for providing clues as to the causes of female breast cancer?

For questions 4.8 to 4.13, refer to the data in Table 4.11.

4.8 Calculate relative frequencies across age-groups for whites, blacks, and Asian or Pacific Islanders. How does the age-specific percentage of breast cancer compare among racial groups?

4.9 Calculate the age-specific rates for each racial group. Graph the age-specific rates for each age group.

TABLE 4.10 Female age-adjusted (to the 2000 US standard population) malignant breast cancer incidence rates in San Francisco and the metropolitan areas of Detroit and Atlanta according to selected racial groups, 1999–2001[28]

Location	*White Rate*	*Black Rate*	*Asian or Pacific Islander Rate*
San-Francisco	155.7	117.7	90.8
Detroit (metropolitan)	140.5	124.4	64.0
Atlanta (metropolitan)	150.0	112.6	58.8
Three areas combined	148.2	119.4	86.3

TABLE 4.11 Female age-specific malignant breast cancer incidence in the combined areas of San Francisco and the metropolitan areas of Detroit and Atlanta according to selected racial groups, 1999–2001

	White		*Black*		*Asian or Pacific Islander*	
	Cases	*Population*	*Cases*	*Population*	*Cases*	*Population*
<50	3,861	7,707,201	1,278	3,204,794	463	1,322,808
50–54 years	2,161	779,208	531	229,532	187	112,795
55–59 years	2,205	577,695	406	153,215	182	74,222
60–64 years	1,858	427,045	396	114,461	168	64,721
65–69 years	1,828	368,091	347	97,741	127	57,622
70+	5,991	1,225,877	936	243,642	291	124,245

4.10 Calculate the 95% confidence interval for the crude female breast cancer rate for each racial group.

4.11 Using the white female population as the standard, use the direct method to calculate age-adjusted rates for blacks and for Asian or Pacific Islanders for age groups 50–54, 55–59, 60–64, and 65–69 years.

4.12 Using the white female population as the standard, use the indirect method to calculate the SMR for blacks and for Asian or Pacific Islanders for the age groups 50–54, 55–59, 60–64, and 65–69 years.

4.13 Describe the age distribution for the 3 racial groups.

4.14 Compare and contrast the incidence rate with the prevalence proportion.

4.15 Compare and contrast the conventional incidence rate with the attack rate.

4.16 If the incidence of disease A is lower than the incidence of disease B, but the prevalence of disease A is higher than the prevalence of disease B, what does that say about the lethality of the 2 diseases? Assume the cure rate is similar between both diseases.

4.17 An accident on the freeway resulted in a chemical leak that exposed several individuals in the nearby community. Many residents complained of respiratory problems. To calculate the probability or risk of illness, describe the statistical measure you would use (including the numerator, denominator, and rate base).

4.18 There were recently 120 people diagnosed in a certain region with disease A. A total of 440 persons lived in the households where these cases resided. If 50 of these diagnosed patients were primary cases, what is the secondary attack rate?

4.19 The mean and median ages for a group participating in a clinical trial are 43 and 51, respectively. What can you say about the distribution of ages?

4.20 Suppose the correlation coefficient measuring the strength of the linear association between exercise (in hours per week) and pulse (per minute) for 1,000 study participants is –0.3. Calculate the coefficient of determination and interpret both these measures.

4.21 Suppose the estimated slope coefficient in a regression model measuring the association between the independent variable exercise (in hours per week) and dependent variable pulse has a slope of –0.05 (per minute). Interpret this result.

4.22 If age was a suspected confounder of the relationship between exercise and pulse, how might you adjust for this factor in your analysis?

4.23 A prospective cohort study showed that 200 new cases of disease X occurred in 2000 person-years. Calculate the person-time incidence rate and 95% confidence interval.

4.24 Refer to Figure 4.10. How might this information be useful in public health planning?

REFERENCES

1. Page RM, Cole GE, Timmreck TC. *Basic Epidemiological Methods and Biostatistics. A Practical Guidebook*. Boston, MA: Jones and Bartlett; 1995.
2. Fearing NM, Harrison PB. Complications of the Heimlich maneuver: Case report and literature review. *J Trauma*. 2002;53:978–979.
3. Jernigan JA, Stephens DS, Ashford DA, et al. Bioterrorism-related inhalational anthrax: the first 10 cases reported in the United States. *Emerg Infect Dis*. 2001;7(6):933–944.
4. Centers for Disease Control (CDC). Pneumocystis pneumonia—Los Angeles. *MMWR*. 1981;30:250.
5. CDC. A cluster of Kaposi's sarcoma and *Pneumocystis carinii* pneumonia among homosexual male residents of Los Angeles and Orange counties, California. *MMWR*. 1982;31:305–307.
6. Jaffe HW, Choi K, Thomas PA, et al. National case-control study of Kaposi's sarcoma and *Pneumocystis carinii* pneumonia in homosexual men: Part 1, epidemiologic results. *Ann Intern Med*. 1983;99:145–151.
7. CDC. Immunodeficiency among female sexual partners of males with acquired immune deficiency syndrome (AIDS)—New York. *MMWR*. 1983;31:697–698.
8. Harris C, Small CB, Klein RS, et al. Immunodeficiency in female sexual partners of men with the acquired immunodeficiency syndrome. *N Engl J Med*. 1983;308:1181–1184.
9. CDC. *Pneumocystis carinii* pneumonia among persons with hemophilia A. *MMWR*. 1982;31:365–367.
10. CDC. Possible transfusion-associated acquired immune deficiency syndrome (AIDS)—California. *MMWR*. 1982;31:652–654.
11. CDC. Acquired immune deficiency syndrome (AIDS): Precautions for clinical and laboratory staffs. *MMWR*. 1982;31:577–580.
12. CDC. Unexplained immunodeficiency and opportunistic infections in infants—New York, New Jersey, and California. *MMWR*. 1982;31:665–667.
13. Joint United Nations Programme on HIV/AIDS and World Health Organization. Global summary of the AIDS epidemic December 2004. Available at: http://www.unaids.org/wad2004/EPI_1204_pdf_en/EpiUpdate04_en.pdf. Accessed May 3, 2005.
14. Byrne J, Kessler LG, Devesa SS. The prevalence of cancer among adults in the United States: 1987. *Cancer*. 1992;68:2154–2159.
15. Hewitt M, Breen N, Devesa S. Cancer prevalence and survivorship issues: Analyses of the 1992 National Health Interview Survey. *J Natl Cancer Inst*. 1999;91(17):1480–1486.
16. Ahluwalia IB, Mack KA, Murphy W, Mokdad AH, Bales VS. State-specific prevalence of selected chronic disease-related characteristics—Behavioral Risk Factor Surveillance System, 2001. *MMWR*. 2003;52(8):1–80.

17. Harris MI, Flegal KM, Cowie CC, et al. Prevalence of diabetes, impaired fasting glucose, and impaired glucose tolerance in US adults. The Third National Health and Nutrition Examination Survey, 1988–1994. *Diabetes Care*. 1998;21(4):518–524.
18. Roy N, Merrill RM, Thibeault S, Parsa RA, Gray SD, Smith EM. Prevalence of voice disorders in teachers and the general population. *J Speech Lang Hear Res*. 2004 Apr;47(2):281–293.
19. Roy N, Merrill RM, Thibeault S, Gray SD, Smith EM. Voice disorders in teachers and the general population: Effects on work performance, attendance, and future career choices. *J Speech Lang Hear Res*. 2004;47(3):542–551.
20. Daniels M, Merrill RM, Lyon JL, Stanford JB, White GL. Associations between breast cancer risk factors and religious practices in Utah. *Prev Med*. 2004;38:28–38.
21. Ries LAG, Eisner MP, Kosary CL, et al. (eds). *SEER Cancer Statistics Review, 1975–2002*. National Cancer Institute. Bethesda, MD. Available at: http://seer.cancer.gov/csr/1975_2002/. Based on November 2004 SEER data submission, posted to the SEER web site 2005.
22. Lyon JL, Gardner K, Gress RE. Cancer incidence among Mormons and non-Mormons in Utah (United States) 1971–1985. *Cancer Causes Control*. 1994;5:149–156.
23. Ewertz M, Duffy SW, Adami HO, et al. Age at first birth, parity and risk of breast cancer: A meta-analysis of 8 studies from the Nordic countries. *Int J Cancer*. 1990;46:597–603.
24. Collaborative Group on Hormonal Factors in Breast Cancer. Breast cancer and breastfeeding: Collaborative reanalysis of individual data from 47 epidemiological studies in 30 countries, including 50,302 women with breast cancer and 96,973 women without the disease. *Lancet*. 2002;360:187–195.
25. Last JM, ed. A dictionary of epidemiology. New York, NY: Oxford University Press; 1995.
26. National Cancer Institute. *Surveillance, epidemiology, and end results. Cancer query system: US mortality statistics*. Available at: http://seer.cancer.gov/canques/mortality.html. Accessed May 21, 2005.
27. US Census Bureau. Fact Sheet. 2003 *American Community Survey Data Profile Highlights*. Available at: http://factfinder.census.gov/servlet/ACSSAFFFacts?_event=&geo_id=04000US49&_geoContext=01000US%7C04000US49&_street=&_county=&_cityTown=&_state=04000US49&_zip=&_lang=en&_sse=on&ActiveGeoDiv=geoSelect&_useEV=&pctxt=fph&pgsl=040. Accessed May 21, 2005.
28. Surveillance Research Program, National Cancer Institute. SEER*Stat software version 6.1.4. Available at: http://www.seer.cancer.gov/seerstat. Accessed May 18, 2005.
29. National Institute for Occupational Safety and Health. *Worker Health Chartbook, 2004*. NIOSH Publication Number 2004-146. Available at: http://www2a.cdc.gov/niosh-Chartbook/imagedetail.asp?imgid=10. Accessed May 17, 2005.
30. Hennekens CH, Buring JE. *Epidemiology in Medicine*. Boston, MA: Little, Brown and Company; 1985.

CHAPTER

5

Descriptive Epidemiology According to Person, Place, and Time

OBJECTIVES

After completing this chapter you will be able to

- Describe the extent of a public health problem according to person, place, and time.
- Easily and effectively communicate a public health problem with the use of tables and graphs.
- Identify who is at greatest risk for selected health-related states or events.
- Use surveillance methods to evaluate the effectiveness of an intervention program.
- Understand how descriptive epidemiology can provide clues as to the causes of disease.

INTRODUCTION

Describing health-related states or events by person, place, and time allows the epidemiologist to identify the extent of the public health problem, describe the public health problem in a way that can be easily communicated, identify who is at greatest risk, evaluate program effectiveness, and provide clues as to the causes of disease. Descriptive data on the **person** characterize who is getting the disease. Descriptors often include age, sex, race/ethnicity, marital and family status, occupation, and education. Descriptive data by **place** address where health-related states or events are occurring most or least frequently. These data often involve comparisons between or among geographic regions, in groups before and after migration, and between twins raised in different settings. Basic to any descriptive epidemiologic study is the analysis and interpretation of the effect of time on the occurrence of health-related states or events. The **time** aspects of epidemiologic investigations range from hours to weeks, years to decades. Short-term disease incubation periods of a few hours can be as important to the epidemiologist as long-term latency periods for chronic diseases that span decades. Another term used occasionally to describe time factors in epidemiology is **temporal**, which means time or refers to time-related elements or issues.

PERSON

Much of the focus of epidemiology is on the "person" aspects of disease, disability, injury, and death. Populations are often characterized according to a number of standard variables and traits, including demographics and the clinical characteristics of disease. From a practical point of view, the traits used to describe the person aspects of epidemiology are limited according to the purpose and resources of concern to a particular study or investigation. Both the information already available from common sources such as public health departments and government agencies, plus the information gathered from investigation, have limitations.

Epidemiologic studies usually concentrate on several major demographic characteristics of the person: age, sex, race/ethnicity, marital status, occupation, education. Comparing health-related states or events over time according to these characteristics, and combinations of these characteristics, can provide clues to the causes of disease. It is also often insightful to compare health-related states or events among and between classifications of these variables.

Age

Because of the strong influence age often has on the outcomes and findings of studies, it has to be considered and, if necessary, controlled for in the study. One approach to control for the potential confounding effect of age over time is to restrict analysis to age-specific categories. For example, female malignant breast cancer rates are presented by 5-year age groups in Figure 5.1. An alternative approach to controlling for age as a potential confounder is to report age-adjusted rates, as described in Chapter 4, "Design Strategies and Statistical Methods in Descriptive Epidemiology." An important assumption for age adjusting rates over time is that the age-specific rates are approximately parallel, as is the case in Figure 5.1.

Scientists have long recognized that the risks of health-related states and events are related to age. For example, the risk of dying from a motor vehicle-related injury is considerably higher for people in the age ranges 15–24 and 75+ years (Figure 5.2).[1] The risk of death

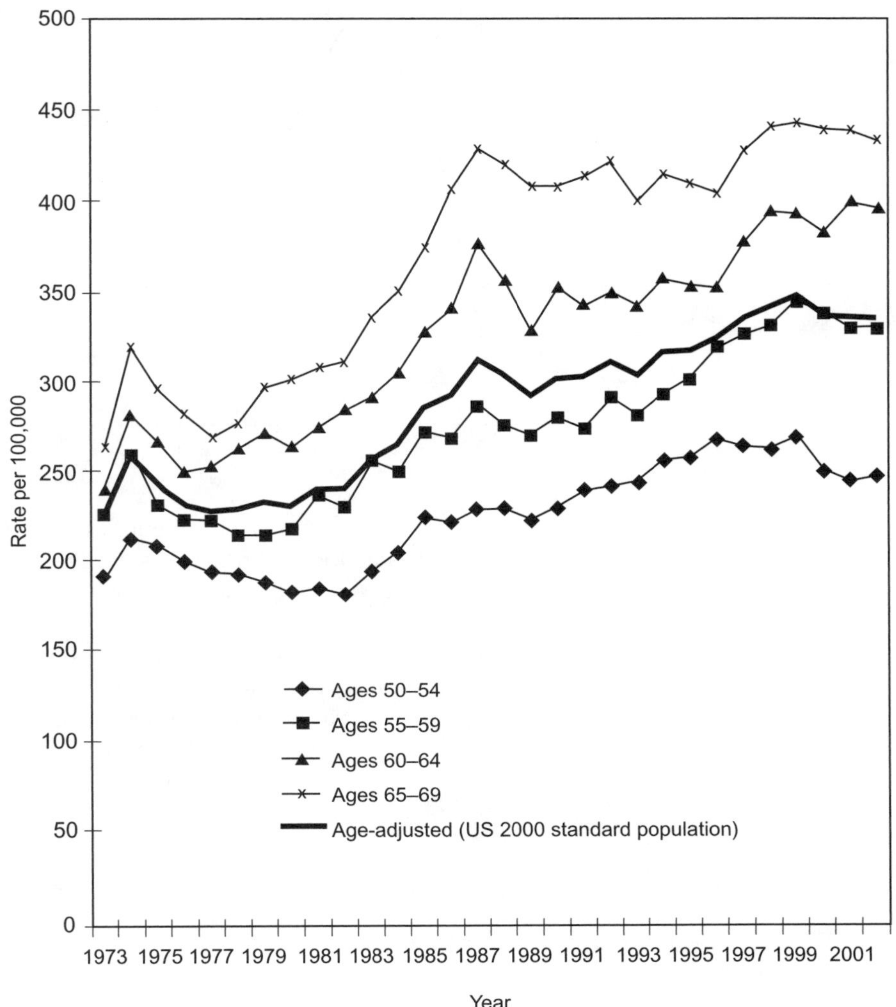

FIGURE 5.1 Female malignant breast cancer incidence rates for ages 50 through 69 in SEER according to calendar year. (Surveillance, Epidemiology, and End Results Program (SEER))

from all causes is higher in the first year of life than any age thereafter until age 55 years, after which the risk sharply increases (Figure 5.3).

Epidemiologists correlate personal characteristics with health-related states or events in order to provide insights into the determinants and causal mechanisms of disease. For example, the incidence of cervical carcinoma in situ increases sharply from about age 15 years, peaks in women aged 25–29, decreases rapidly through ages 50–54, and then gradually decreases thereafter (Figure 5.4).[2] The shape of the age-specific incidence curve suggests that carcinoma in situ of the uterine cervix follows an exposure that affects a substantial number of women close to the same age, and the time from exposure to observable pathologic change is less than 15 years. This pattern is similar to the pattern resulting from an infectious

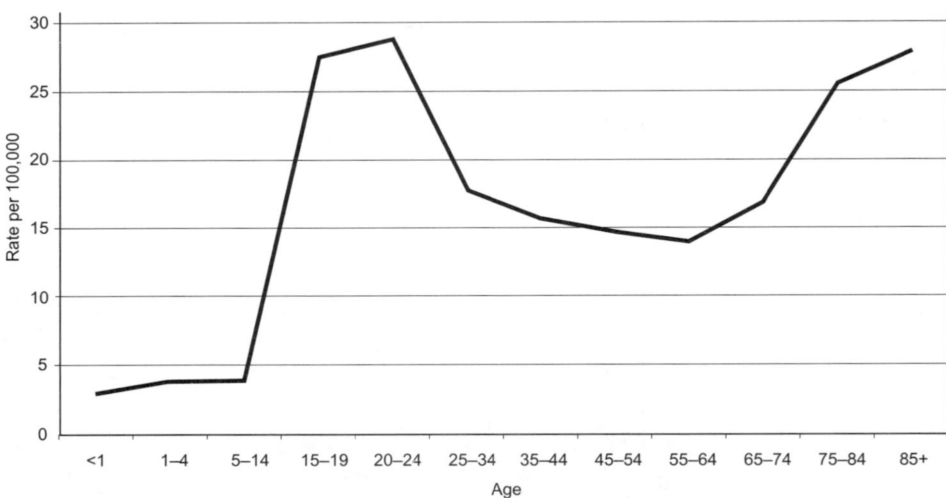

FIGURE 5.2 Death rates for motor vehicle-related injuries in the United States according to age in 2002. (National Center for Health Statistics. *Health, United States, 2004 with Chartbook on Trends in the Health of Americans.* Hyattsville, MD: NCHS; 2004.)

agent. It is now well established that human papillomavirus, transmitted through sexual intercourse, is a primary cause of cancer of the uterine cervix.

Length of life is one of the most basic aspects of the person and one with which epidemiologists are concerned. Longevity or life expectancy continues to be a measure of the

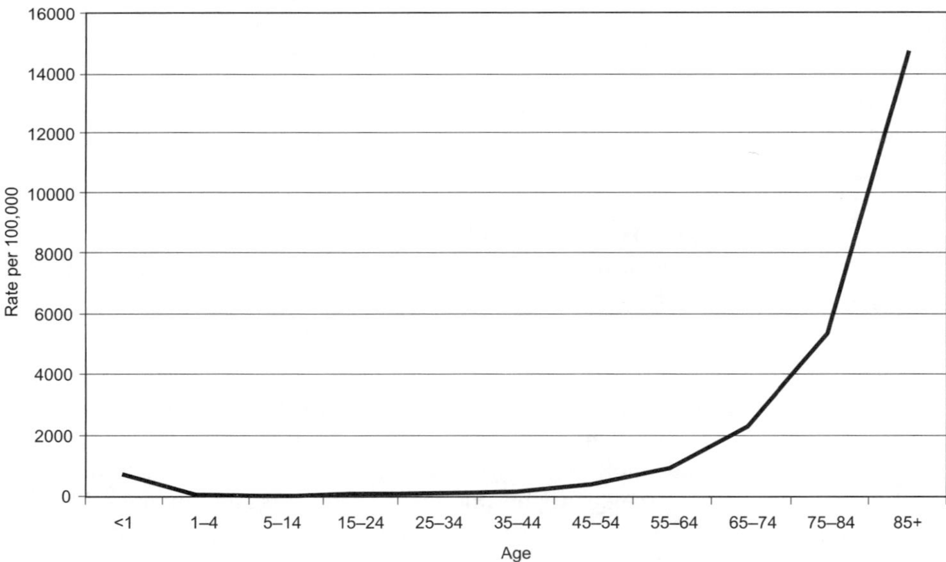

FIGURE 5.3 Death rates for all causes in the United States according to age in 2002. (National Center for Health Statistics. *Health, United States, 2004 with Chartbook on Trends in the Health of Americans.* Hyattsville, MD: NCHS; 2004.)

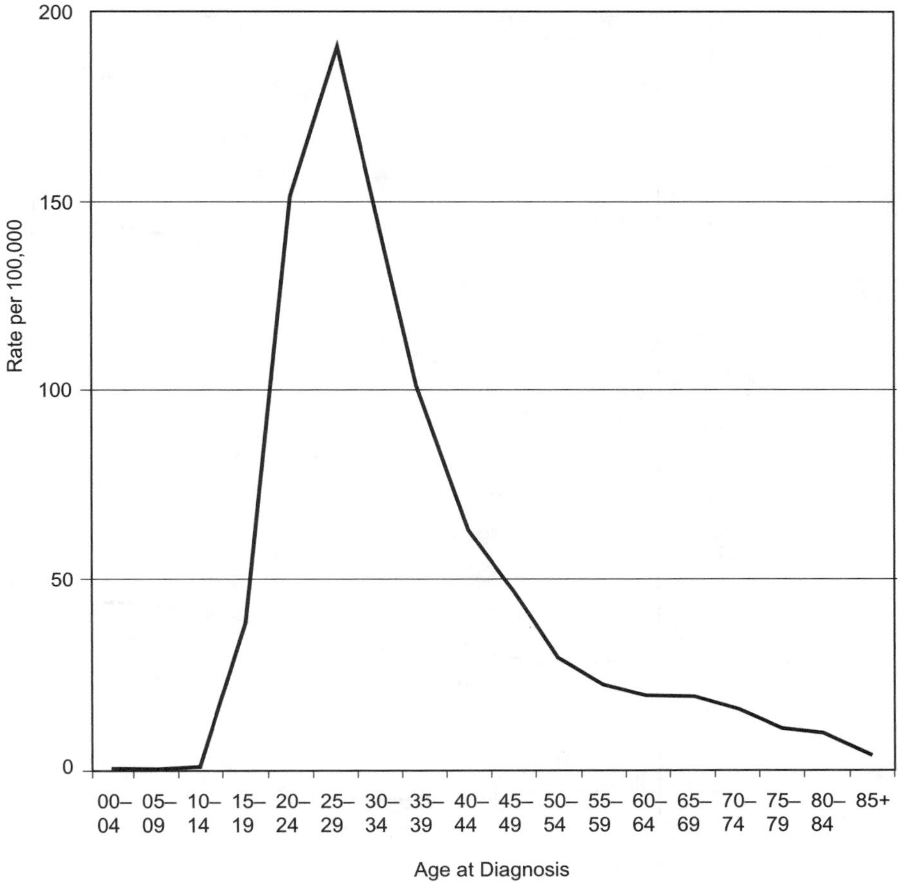

FIGURE 5.4 Age-specific rates of carcinoma in situ of the uterine cervix, 1991–1995. (Surveillance, Epidemiology, and End Results Program (SEER))

health status of specific populations, differing according to demographic and geographic factors. Figure 5.5 shows age-conditional life expectancy in the United States for selected years from 1900 through 2002.[3] In 1900–1902, life expectancy was 49. Life expectancy increased to 77 by 2002. In 2002, years of life remaining, on average, are 58 years for a person alive at age 20, 39 years for a person alive at age 40, 22 years for a person alive at age 60, and 10 years for a person alive at age 90.

Life expectancy is shown across calendar years by sex and race in Figure 5.6. At birth, life expectancy increases over the years for each sex-race combination. The increase is more pronounced for females than males. White females experience the highest life expectancy and black males the lowest life expectancy. In 2002, life expectancy varies considerably by sex and race (75.1 years for white males, 80.1 for white females, 68.8 for black males, and 75.6 for black females). Life expectancy improves across the century for each age-conditional group. Identifying reasons for such differences in life expectancy has been the focus of considerable research in recent years. The causes of death that have contributed most to the

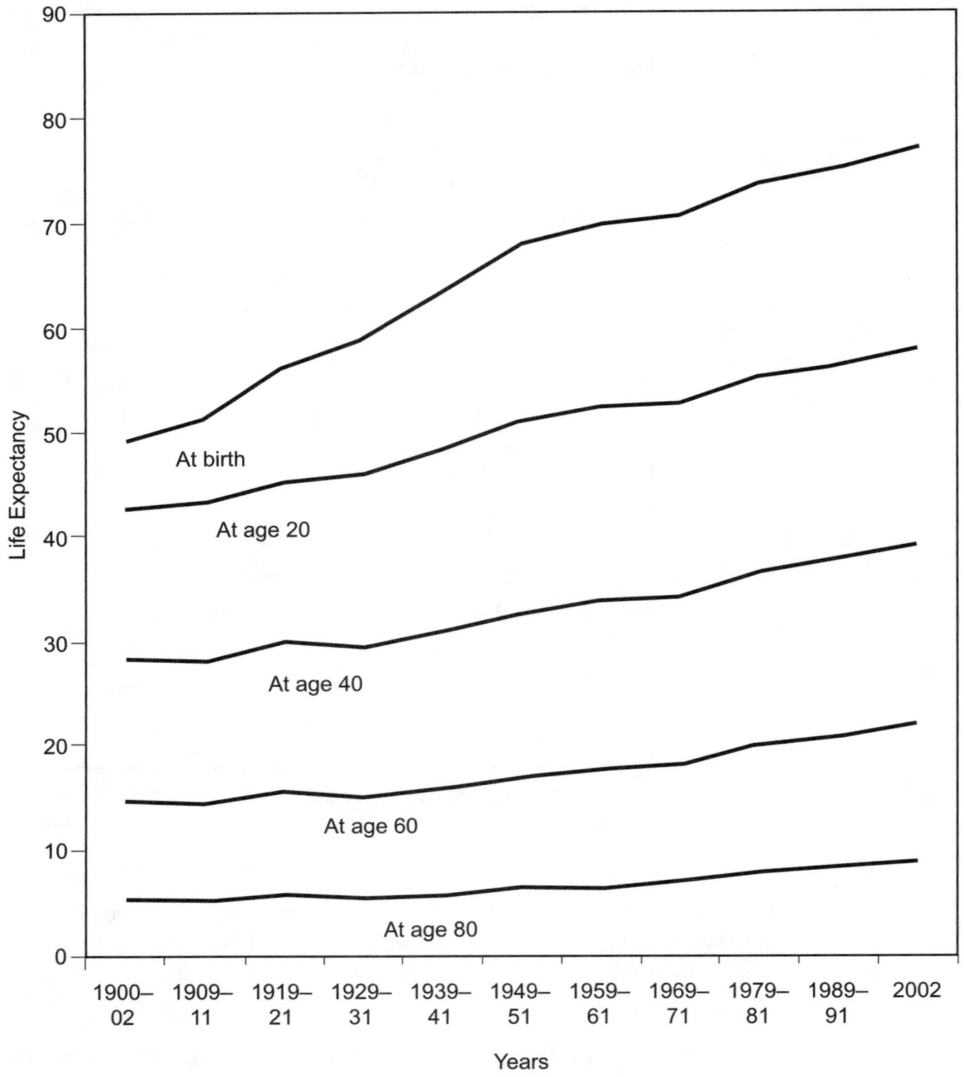

FIGURE 5.5 Life expectancy at birth, age 20, age 40, age 60, and age 80 in the United States from 1900–2002. (Arias E. United States life tables, 2002. *Natl Vital Stat Rep.* 2002;53:6. Available at: http://www.cdc.gov/nchs/fastats/lifexpec.htm. Accessed October 22, 2005.)

disparity in life expectancy between whites and blacks are cardiovascular diseases, homicide, cancer, and infant mortality. These causes of death accounted for about 60% of the differences in life expectancy at birth between blacks and whites, males and females.

Population Pyramids

Population (or **age**) **pyramids** have been used for many years by demographers and epidemiologists to track and compare changes in population age distributions over time. The

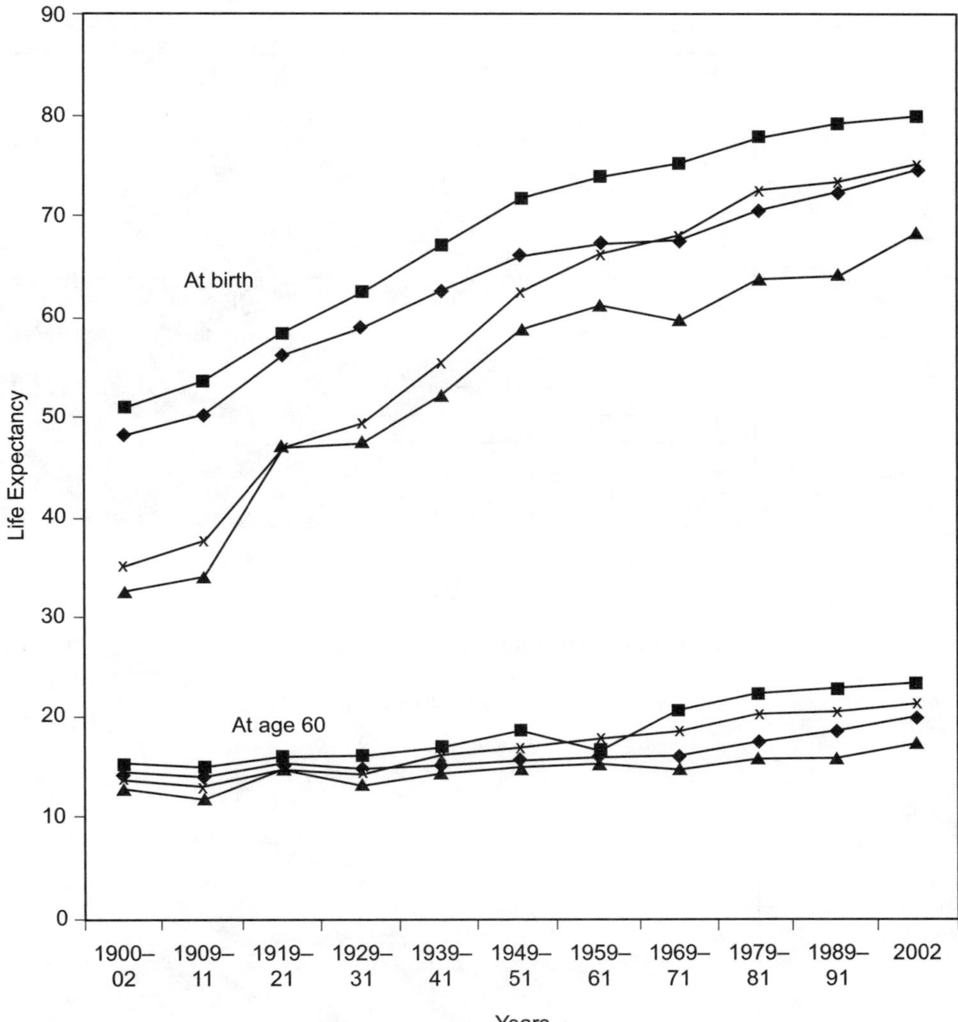

FIGURE 5.6 Life expectancy at birth and age 60 in the United States according to sex and race (white, black) from 1900–2002. (Arias E. United States life tables, 2002. *Natl Vital Stat Rep*. 2002;53:6. Available at: http:// www.cdc.gov/nchs/fastats/lifexpec.htm. Accessed October 22, 2005.)

number of persons in various age groups in a selected population, such as a state or country, is affected by birth rates, fertility levels, wars, death rates, and migration. Thus the population is dynamic and changes over time. Large or small cohorts of people born in the same year can be seen to move up the life span and the population pyramid over time. Percentages of the population in each age group are represented by the height of the bars on the graph, with the sum of the bars equaling 100% (Figure 5.7). The age distribution of males is shown on the left side of the graph, and the age distribution of females is shown on the right side of the graph. A population pyramid uses 2-person characteristics and is an age/sex comparison. The age and sex traits are collected at a specific point in time, usually at the **decennial census**.

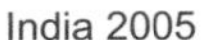

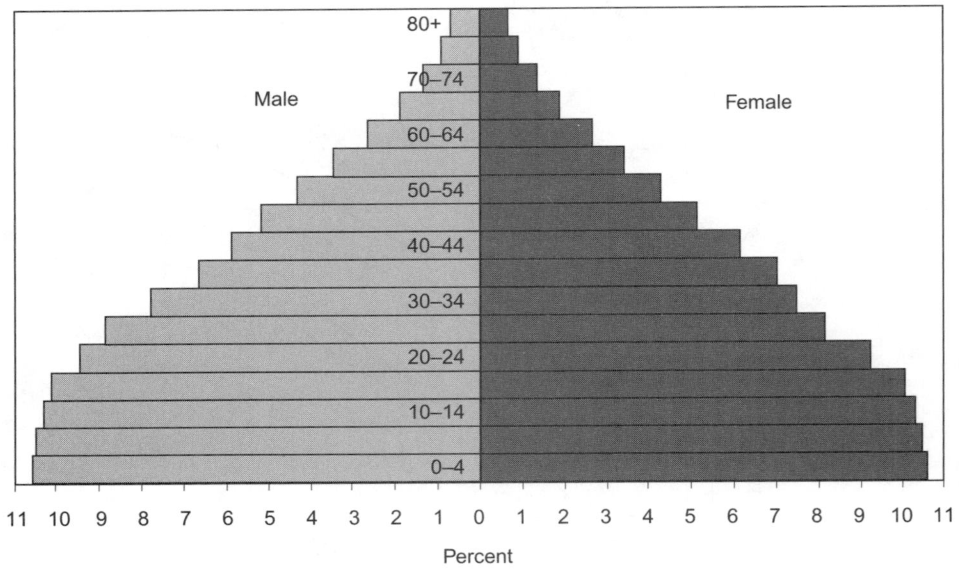

FIGURE 5.7a Population pyramid for the population in India in 2005. (US Census Bureau, Population Division, International Programs Center. Available at: http://www.census.gov/ipc/www/idbsum.html. Accessed October 21, 2005.)

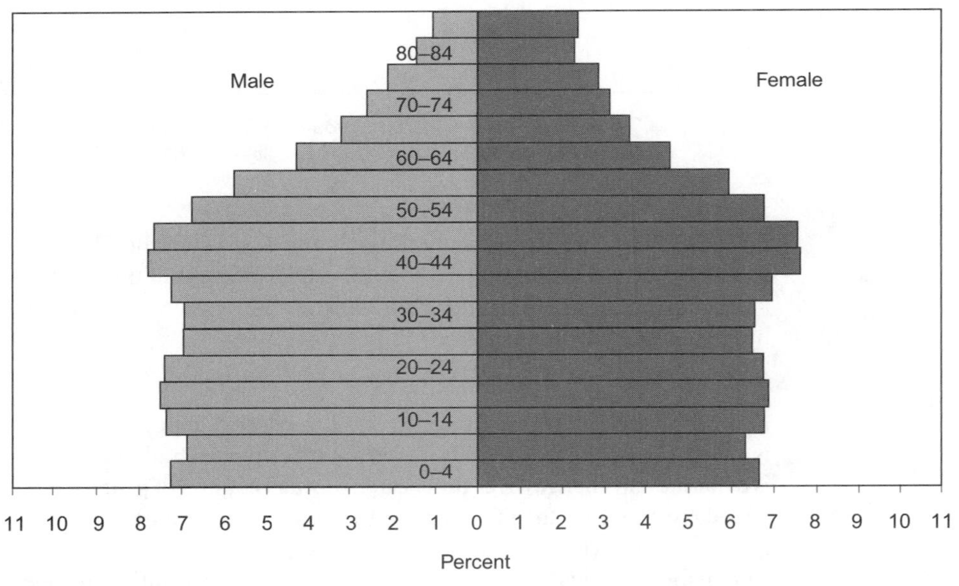

FIGURE 5.7b Population pyramid for the population in the United States in 2005. (US Census Bureau, Population Division, International Programs Center. Available at: http://www.census.gov/ipc/www/idbsum.html. Accessed October 21, 2005.)

Social and health-related changes in populations can be seen in birth cohorts when they are plotted on a population pyramid. Some examples of these changes are the effects of wars, famines, droughts, use of birth control measures, fertility levels (number of females between ages 15 and 45 years available to have children), and the rate of marriage. Poor development of public health systems and little control of infectious disease such as sanitation of water supplies and food, control of sewage and garbage, low levels of immunizations, and poor medical care can lead to increased deaths and fewer people entering older age groups. Not only do all of these factors affect the shape of a population pyramid, but the events of society can also be reflected in the pyramid as time passes. As the events affect a population, the events move up through the different age groups in the pyramid.[4–6]

A tall, pointed pyramid shape represents a population with a high birth rate, a high death rate, and public health, socioeconomic, and medical care conditions that do not allow cohorts to live into old age (Figure 5.7a). This pointed top shape also shows that many persons are dying in each birth cohort each year so that very few persons are in the older age cohorts at the top of the pyramid. The cohorts have rapidly diminished over time, leaving smaller numbers of people in the older age groups. A beehive-shaped pyramid indicates that the population is having low birth rates as well as low death rates. If an hourglass shape is seen, it indicates a much higher proportion of older people. If a large protrusion area is seen, this is a transitional population that has a large birth cohort moving through the population pyramid. If the pyramid is fairly block shaped with only a small point (somewhat close to the beehive shape), this represents a more industrialized society, with effective public health measures in place, good socioeconomic conditions, and good medical care; life expectancy is high with large numbers of age cohorts living into the older age groups. This block-shaped pyramid would be representative of the United States in modern times (Figure 5.7b).[4–6]

The ability of a population to support itself economically is of concern to public health and political officials. How dependent certain segments of a population are on others predicts how well these groups or subgroups can contribute to society. The ability to contribute, or the dependency a group has on others, is measured by a dependency ratio. The dependency ratio reflects the amount of potential dependency in a population and the work life span.[4,5] The **dependency ratio** describes the relationship by age between those who have the potential to be self-supporting and the dependent segments of the population; in other words, those segments of the population not in the workforce. The beginning age of economic self-sufficiency ranges from 15 to 20 years. The upper age for being considered part of the workforce has changed in recent times and will probably be reevaluated because of a continued need for workers as the older cohorts of populations increase in number and the numbers of younger persons entering the workforce decline. Retirement at 65 has already been eliminated in certain work areas of the population. Age 70 is now viewed as the age of retirement by many and will influence the concept of dependency in society in the future.[4,5]

The formula for the dependency ratio is

$$\text{Dependency ratio} = \frac{\begin{array}{c}\text{Population under age 15 and}\\ \text{over retirement age (65+)}\end{array}}{\text{Population ages 15 through 64}} \times 100$$

For example, suppose in a given region 25% of the population are less than 15 years of age and 5% are over 65 years of age. This means that 70% [100 − (25 + 5)] of the people are in the age range of 15 and 64. The dependency ratio equals 43%; that is, there are 43 dependents for every 100 people of working age.

Sex

Sex is biologically founded (ie, a human female has 2 X chromosomes and a human male has one X and one Y chromosome). In contrast, gender is a socially constructed notion of what is feminine and what is masculine (eg, a person is not born a man but, instead, becomes a man). Health-related states or events often differ between males and females. For example, the number of females to males differs across the age span. In the United States in 2000, there were approximately 95 females for every 100 males among those aged 20 years or less (Figure 5.8). In those aged 35–39 years, there were approximately 100 females for every 100 males. At later ages, the ratio of females to males increased such that by ages 100+, there were 400 females for every 100 males.

A few facts point to the differences between males and females. More males are born each year, yet more males than females die within the first year of life (higher infant mor-

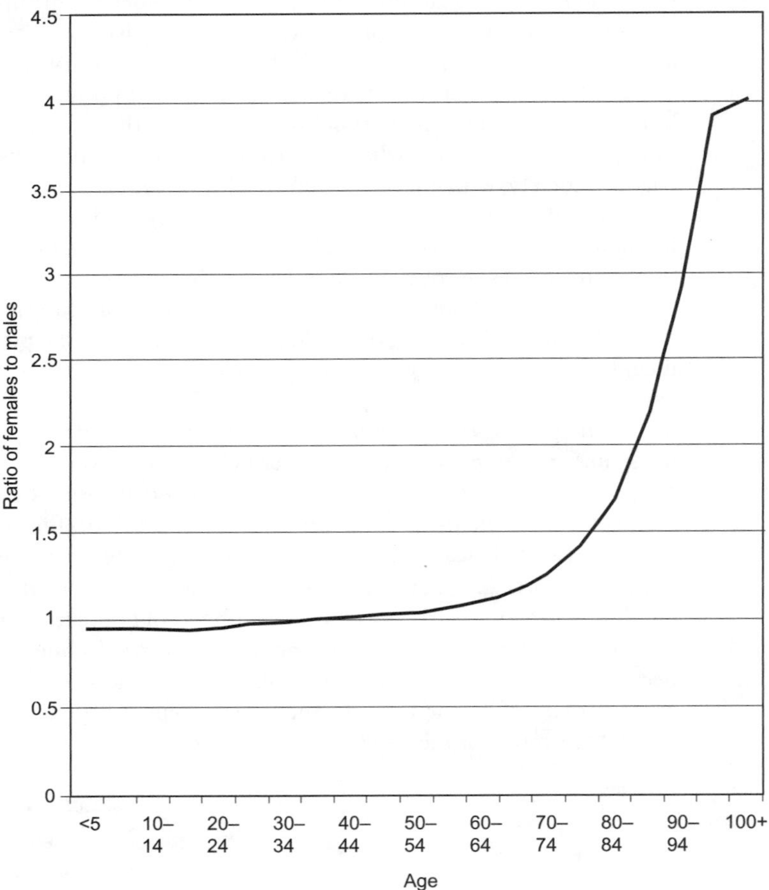

FIGURE 5.8 Ratio of female to male age-specific populations in 2000. (Population Division, US Census Bureau. Available at: www.census.gov/popest/national/asrh/NCEST2003/NC-EST2003-01.pdf. Accessed October 22, 2005.)

tality) and at every stage of life thereafter. Females outlive males by 5 to 7 years. The all-cause death rate is 1.4 times higher for males than females (Table 5.1). This is explained by higher death rates for all of the leading causes of death.

NEWS FILE

The Lifetime Probability of Developing Cancer in the United States

Approximately 1 in 2 Men and 1 in 3 Women will Develop Cancer in Their Lifetime

The lifetime probability of developing invasive cancer is higher in men (45%) than in women (38%). The lifetime probability of developing invasive breast cancer in women is 13%, and the lifetime probability of developing invasive prostate cancer in men is 17%. Other common cancers and their corresponding lifetime probabilities of development are lung and bronchial (8% in men and 6% in women), colon and rectal (6% in men and 5% in women), and bladder (3% in men and 1% in women). The probability of developing invasive cancer is strongly related to age. For example, the probability of developing any invasive cancer from birth to age 39 is 1.4% in men and 1.9% in women, from age 40 to age 59 is 8.0% in men and 9.0% in women, and from age 60 to age 79 is 33.9% in men and 22.6% in women. It should be noted that these estimates are based on the average experience in the population. Hence, for any given individual the risk may be overestimated or underestimated.

(Source: Jemal A, Tiwari RC, Murray T, et al. Cancer Statistics, 2004. CA Cancer J Clin. *2004;54:8–29.)*

TABLE 5.1 Age-Adjusted* Cause-Specific Death Rates per 100,000 for Males and Females in 2002 in the United States[7]

	Males	*Females*	*Ratio*
All causes	1,013.7	715.2	1.4
Diseases of the heart	297.4	197.2	1.5
Cerebrovascular diseases	56.5	55.2	1.0
Malignant neoplasms	238.9	163.1	1.5
Chronic lower respiratory diseases	53.5	37.4	1.4
HIV/AIDS	7.4	2.5	3.0
Motor vehicle-related injuries	22.1	9.6	2.3
Homicide	9.4	2.8	3.4
Suicide	18.4	4.2	4.4
Firearm-related injuries	18.6	2.8	6.6
Occupational injury	6.8	0.7	9.7

*In accordance with the 2000 standard population.

Race/Ethnicity

It is standard practice in epidemiology to describe individuals by race and ethnicity. For example, the decennial census now classifies individuals into 5 racial categories (white, black, American Indian or Alaskan Native, Asian, and Native Hawaiian or Pacific Islander) and 2 ethnic categories (Hispanic origin and not of Hispanic origin). Like sex, these variables may have biological, sociological, and psychological dimensions. Associating risk behaviors and disease outcomes with these variables can provide insights into the causal mechanisms of disease.

Race is a socially constructed variable based on the idea that some human populations are distinct from others according to external physical characteristics or places of origin. Racial or ethnic variations in health-related states or events are explained primarily by "exposure or vulnerability to behavioral, psychosocial, material, and environmental risk factors and resources."[8] Historically, biological explanations have played a limited role in explaining racial disparities.[9,10] Racial prejudice has been proposed as a social stress that can affect health behaviors such as eating, substance abuse, and access to health care services.[11–13] Because of the similarity between race and ethnicity, in that both are determined primarily by their group association and distinction, there is an increasing movement toward use of the term race/ethnicity.[14]

A challenge exists in epidemiologic investigations of racial/ethnic disparities in that broad categories of racial/ethnic groups may be inadequate to capture unique cultural differences. For example, about 52 different tribes of Native Americans are registered in the United States today, representing 52 different cultures, backgrounds, and possible genetic makeups. A similar situation is also true for African-Americans. African-Americans tend to be categorized as blacks. Genetic and genealogic investigations are beginning to show a great deal of diversity among blacks. Like Native Americans, blacks have historically come from different tribes and locations, and all are not the same. Are all whites the same genetically and culturally? Is an Irishman the same as an Italian? Are Swedes the same as Spaniards? Although greater effort to obtain more distinct racial/ethnic groups in research is encouraged, small numbers often limit statistical assessment.

Racial/ethnic population estimates in the United States for 2004 are shown in Table 5.2. Approximately 17.3% of the male population and 15.5% of the female population are Hispanic.

TABLE 5.2 US Population Estimates According to Sex, Race and Hispanic or Latino Ethnicity, July 1, 2004

	Male, Hispanic	*Not Hispanic*	*%Hispanic*	*Female, Hispanic*	*Not Hispanic*	*%Hispanic*
One race	21,057,548	121,294,578	17.4%	19,681,246	127,183,278	15.5%
White	19,793,438	97,039,035	20.4%	18,423,502	100,801,786	18.3%
Black	754,210	17,118,563	4.4%	784,408	18,845,139	4.2%
AIAN	325,732	1,089,209	29.9%	292,271	1,117,539	26.2%
Asian	127,814	5,846,742	2.2%	129,978	6,221,682	2.1%
NHPI	56,354	201,029	28.0%	51,087	197,132	25.9%
Two or more races	289,525	1,895,757	15.3%	293,751	1,959,721	15.0%
Total	21,347,073	123,190,335	17.3%	19,974,997	129,142,999	15.5%

Black, black or African American; AIAN, American Indian and Alaska Native; NHPI, Native Hawaiian and Other Pacific Islander. (Source: US Census Bureau. Available at: http://www.census.gov/popest/national/asrh/NC-EST2004/NC-EST2004-03.xls. Accessed June 10, 2005.)

TABLE 5.3 Age-Adjusted Cause-Specific Death Rates per 100,000 in the United States in 2002 According to Sex and Hispanic Ethnicity*

	Male			***Female***		
	White, not Hispanic or Latino	***Hispanic or Latino***	***Ratio***	***White, not Hispanic or Latino***	***Hispanic or Latino***	***Ratio***
All causes	1,002.2	766.7	1.3	709.9	518.3	1.4
Diseases of the heart	297.7	219.8	1.4	193.7	149.7	1.3
Cerebrovascular diseases	54.4	44.3	1.2	53.9	38.6	1.4
Malignant neoplasms	239.6	161.4	1.5	165.9	106.1	1.6
Chronic lower respiratory diseases	56.5	27.2	2.1	41.2	16.2	2.5
HIV/AIDS						
25–44 years	6.6	11.5	0.6	1.3	3.8	0.3
45–64 years	6.4	20.3	0.3	0.9	5.7	0.2
Motor vehicle-related injuries	22.2	22.2	1.0	10.1	8.1	1.2
Homicide	3.7	11.6	0.3	1.9	2.5	0.8
Suicide	21.4	9.9	2.2	5.1	1.8	2.8
Firearm-related injuries	16.0	13.4	1.2	2.8	1.6	1.8

*In accordance with the 2000 US standard population. (Source: National Center for Health Statistics. *Health, United States, 2004 with Chartbook on Trends in the Health of Americans*. Hyattsville, MD: NCHS; 2004: Table 35–38, 41–42, 44–47.)

The Department of Health and Human Services monitors mortality rates in the United States for several conditions. Death rates for selected causes in the United States in 2002 are presented according to sex and Hispanic ethnicity in Table 5.3. White, not Hispanic or Latino males and females have higher death rates for each of the selected conditions with the exception of HIV/AIDS and homicide. We can now try to discover explanations for these differences in rates by identifying unique behaviors or characteristics in each ethnic group.

Marital and Family Status

Studies have related marital status and health for over a century. Married individuals have been shown to experience lower mortality than do nonmarried individuals, regardless of whether the nonmarried persons were never married, divorced, separated, or widowed.[15,16] Married persons in the United States have also been shown generally to have lower levels of physical, mental, or emotional problems and better health behaviors (more physically active, less smoking, less heavy alcohol drinking).[17] However, married persons, particularly men, were shown to have higher rates of overweight or obesity.

Two theories have been proposed to explain better health among married individuals: marriage protection and marriage selection. Marriage protection refers to married people having more economic resources, social and psychological support, and support for healthy lifestyles. On the other hand, marital selection refers to healthier people being more likely to get married and stay married. It is often difficult, if not impossible, to distinguish the specific influence of these 2 explanations on health.

Family-related factors useful to epidemiologists include family size and placement of members within the family structure. Maternal age is of much concern to the medical and public health community. More Down syndrome babies are born to mothers after age 40. Young teenage births have the highest risk to both the baby and the mother. Considerable health care dollars are spent on premature babies, which are often born to unwed mothers.

The absence of one parent in the family has been a major concern in the last several years. Divorce and cohabitation have risen to the highest levels known in the history of the United States. Disrupted families are common, and children of these families suffer the most in terms of psychological and social problems. More research is needed in the study of the effects of the disrupted family on health status and on ways to prevent the destruction of the family. Table 5.4 presents marital history for people 15 years of age and older in the United States by age and sex in 2001.

Family Structure and Genealogical Research

Studies have shown that family size and marital status can influence physical and mental health. In addition, health behaviors cluster in families. Parental attitudes and behaviors can directly influence their children's health behaviors. Intervention programs aimed at modifying health behaviors and improving health and well-being should focus on the family as the unit of analysis.

TABLE 5.4 Marital History for People 15 Years and Over in the United States by Age and Sex in 2001

	Men			*Women*		
Years	***Ever Married***	***Ever Divorced***	***Ever Widowed***	***Ever Married***	***Ever Divorced***	***Ever Widowed***
15–19	0.9	0.1	—	3.7	0.2	—
20–24	16.1	1.0	—	27.6	2.6	0.3
25–29	49.2	7.5	0.1	62.7	11.9	0.5
30–34	70.5	15.4	0.3	78.3	18.6	0.6
35–39	78.5	22.9	0.5	84.4	28.1	1.1
40–49	85.8	29.5	1.3	89.5	35.4	3.5
50–59	93.7	40.8	2.9	93.6	38.9	9.5
60–69	95.7	30.9	7.6	95.9	28.4	23.3
70+	96.7	18.6	23.1	96.7	17.7	56.3

(Source: Kreider R. Number, timing, and duration of marriages and divorces: 2001. Table 3. Available at: http://www.census.gov/population/www/socdemo/marr-div.html. Accessed June 10, 2005.)

A person inherits many traits, both good and bad, from parents, grandparents, and past family members. Genetically, intelligence levels can be passed down from generation to generation, along with some diseases. For example, some forms of muscular dystrophy are genetically transmitted. Family trees have been used to study the genealogy of both genetically transmitted and communicable diseases. Family trees have been used to confirm hereditary links in many cancers. The Church of Jesus Christ of Latter Day Saints maintains one of the largest genealogy libraries in the world in Salt Lake City, Utah, aiding genealogists and epidemiologists in family history studies.

Occupation

The person characteristic of occupation can be reflective of income, social status, education, socioeconomic status, risk of injury, or health problems within a population group. Selected diseases, conditions, or disorders occur in certain occupations. Brown lung has been associated with workers in the garment industry, black lung with coal miners, and certain accidents and injury to limbs with farm workers.

Occupation is requested on many research questionnaires and is used to measure socioeconomic status. It is also a determinant of risk and is a predictor of the health status of and conditions in which certain populations work. Occupations have been divided into 5 broad classifications. The 5 classifications are

1. Professional
2. Intermediate
3. Skilled
4. Partly skilled
5. Unskilled

Subclassifications of the 5 main classifications have been used in various epidemiologic reports.

Standard mortality ratios (SMRs) for specific occupations have been developed, based on risks that might be associated with the physical and chemical exposures common to certain occupations. For example, coronary artery disease has been found to be less prevalent in several active occupations than it is in sedentary occupations. Persons who work for larger organizations have medical insurance and access to health care providers and medical institutions and thus benefit from better health status.[18,19]

It has also been observed that the health status and mortality of a population can be affected by the levels of employment within the population. The term **healthy worker effect** has been used to describe this observation; that is, employed populations tend to have a lower mortality rate than the general population. Workers tend to be a healthier group to begin with. Persons who are unhealthy or who may have a life-shortening condition are less likely to be employed. As workers go through the life span, the chance of death increases, and the healthy worker effect decreases. Unhealthy workers tend to leave the work environment or retire earlier than healthy employees. Leaving work early in life also reduces exposure to occupational hazards. Instead of exposure to risk factors causing disease, disease causes those at risk to leave work. Absence due to disease produces lower work-related-risk exposure levels than would occur if workers remained at their jobs.[19]

Education

Education, like occupation, can be valuable as a measure of socioeconomic status. Persons with training, skills, and education make substantially more money per year than persons with no training or skills. Persons with higher education levels are more prevention oriented, know more about health matters, and have greater access to health care.

For example, the age-adjusted percentage of current cigarette smoking by those 25 years of age and over in the United States in 2002 was 30.9% for persons with no high school diploma or GED, 28.1% for persons with a high school diploma or GED, 21.6% for persons with some college, and 10.0% for persons with a bachelor's degree or higher.[20] For women aged 40 years and older, the percentage undergoing mammography screening in 2000 was 57.7% for women with no high school diploma or GED, 69.6% for women with a high school diploma or GED, and 76.1% for women with some college or more.[21]

In 2002, the age-adjusted death rate for persons 25–64 years of age with fewer than 12 years of education was 2.9 times higher for males and 2.5 times higher for females than the rate for persons with 13 or more years of education (Table 5.5). Higher death rates for the less educated were observed for chronic and noncommunicable diseases, injuries, and communicable diseases. Education had the largest impact on communicable diseases, followed by injuries, and then chronic and noncommunicable diseases. Infant mortality rates per 1,000 are 7.9 for persons with less than 12 years of education, 7.3 for persons with 12 years of education, and 5.1 for persons with 13 or more years of education.[20]

PLACE

For chronic conditions such as cancer, geographic comparisons of disease frequency among groups, states, and countries can be made to provide insights to the causes of diseases. For example, Utah has the lowest female breast cancer incidence rates in the United States, due in part to low rates among women who are members of the Church of Jesus Christ of Latter-day Saints (LDS or Mormon) who make up a large portion of the female population.[22,23] Researchers compared several reproductive and nonreproductive breast cancer risk factors

TABLE 5.5 Age-Adjusted* Death Rates per 100,000 for Persons 25–64 Years of Age-Selected Causes of Death According to Sex and Educational Attainment in the United States, 2002

	Male				***Female***			
	<12 yrs	***12 yrs***	***13+ yrs***	***Ratio†***	***<12 yrs***	***12 yrs***	***13+ yrs***	***Ratio†***
All causes	726.1	650.2	253.5	2.9	416.6	350.7	168.8	2.5
Chronic and non-communicable diseases	528.9	478.2	193.9	2.7	334.9	288.5	142.6	2.3
Injuries	142.5	129.0	45.4	3.1	49.2	41.0	19.2	2.6
Communicable diseases	53.0	41.6	13.8	3.8	31.8	20.4	6.7	4.7
HIV	23.4	18.6	6.3	3.7	12.6	6.9	1.3	9.7
Other	29.6	23.0	7.5	3.9	19.1	13.5	5.4	3.5

*In accordance with the 2000 US standard population. †The ratio applies to <12 years of education compared with 13+ years of education. (Source: National Center for Health Statistics. *Health, United States, 2004 with Chartbook on Trends in the Health of Americans*. Hyattsville, MD: NCHS; 2004: Table 34.)

between LDS and non-LDS women in the state. LDS women had a comparatively higher number of births, prevalence of breastfeeding, and lifetime total duration of breastfeeding. These results further support the important role parity and breastfeeding play in reducing breast cancer.

Studies of disease among migrants provide insights into the roles of genetics and environment. In one migration study, researchers compared cancer incidence trends among the Japanese in Japan with Japanese and whites in Hawaii between 1960 and 1997.[24] Very strong migrant effects were observed for cancers of the colon and stomach. In general, migration led to lower risks of stomach, esophageal, pancreatic, liver, and cervical cancers and led to higher rates for other cancers. The authors concluded that although environment plays an important role in many of these cancers, the persistent differences in incidence found for some cancers, even several generations after migration, support the presence of a genetic component.

Twin studies also provide a powerful means for assessing the roles of genetics and environment on disease. For example, a recent study assessing the effect of sun exposure on nevus density (a primary risk factor for melanoma) in adolescent twins in the United Kingdom showed that 66% of the total variance of nevus count was associated with genetic effects (eg, eye color, hair color, skin type).[25]

TIME TRENDS

The effect of time is often better understood if presented in graphical form. Chapter 4 defined the line graph. Line graphs are useful for measuring temporal patterns of health-related states or events. There are 4 common temporal trends: secular trends, short-term trends, cyclic trends, and seasonal trends.

Secular trends represent long-term changes in health-related states or events. In the epidemiology literature, another term, *temporal variation* or *trends* (also called *temporal distribution*), has recently emerged and is being used interchangeably with *secular trends.* Changes seen over extended time periods, even several decades in certain diseases, are of concern in epidemiology, especially for prevention and control programs in public health. Secular trends are usually considered to last longer than one year. An example of a major secular trend related to smoking is revealed by the tracking of lung cancer deaths in both males and females over time.

Cancer death rates for most types of cancer in the United States are tracked over time, and secular trends are identified over years and decades. Lung cancer trends provide the most dramatic cancer death rate changes, and they are distinctly visible on line graphs. Figures 5.9 (males) and 5.10 (females) show the secular trends of cancer death rates for 7 different sites in the body. In 1930, the lung was the second-to-least common site of all cancers in males and the least common site of all cancers in females. By 1960 in males and the late 1980s in females, lung cancer death rates had outpaced other cancers. Extensive research has associated cigarette smoking with lung cancer. Increasing, and then decreasing, lung cancer death rates over the century have been associated with cigarette consumption in the United States, allowing for a 20- to 25-year latency period (Figure 5.11). The risk of dying of lung cancer is considerably higher for males than it is for females. Leukemia rates over the years have risen only slightly. Female breast cancer showed little change in incidence through 1990, but a decrease ensued thereafter. The risk of dying from stomach and pancreatic cancers has been consistently higher for males than for females. Also, despite falling mortality rates for colon and rectal cancers in females, the rates remained flat for males between the late 1940s and the 1980s, after which they did start to fall, but not as noticeably as for females.

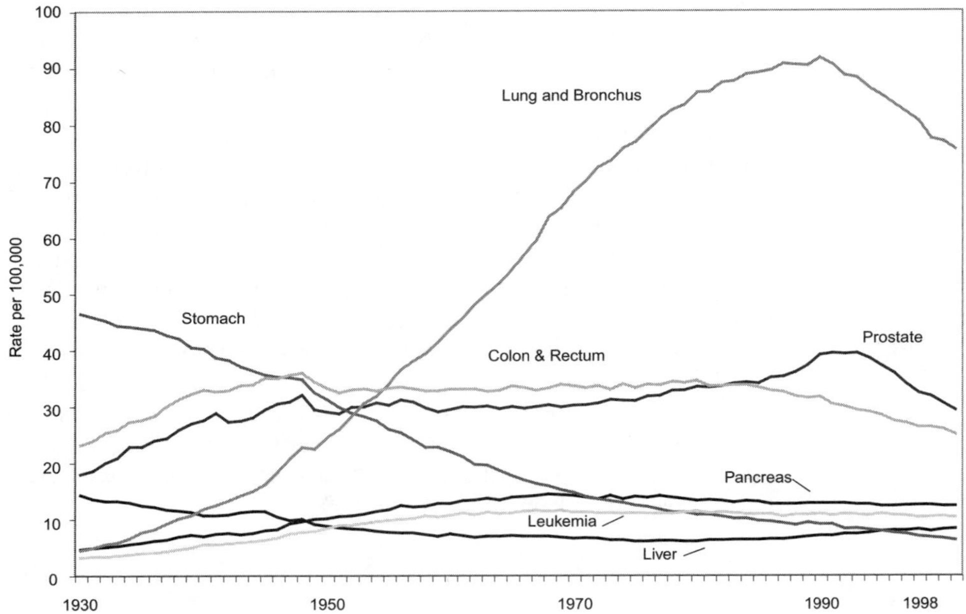

FIGURE 5.9 Site-specific age-adjusted (to the 2000 US standard population) cancer death rates for males, 1930–2001. (US Mortality Public Use Data Tapes 1960–2001, US Mortality Volumes 1930–1959, National Center for Health Statistics, Centers for Disease Control and Prevention; American Cancer Society, *Cancer Facts & Figures 2005*.)

On June 5, 1981, the first cases of acquired immunodeficiency syndrome (AIDS) were reported by health care providers in California and the Centers for Disease Control and Prevention (CDC). Since then AIDS has been a disease of concern not only to medical and public health officials but to almost every member of society. As of May 31, 1991, the CDC had reported 179,136 cases of AIDS in the United States. AIDS has been transmitted mostly by homosexual sex acts, intravenous drug use (contaminated needles), and heterosexual activities in persons with multiple partners. AIDS has also been transmitted from blood transfusions and from mother to child in the process childbirth (perinatally acquired pediatric AIDS cases). Epidemiologists have been concerned about the secular trends of persons infected with AIDS, and public health agencies at local, state, and national levels have been following the trends over the years. Figures 5.12 and 5.13 give 2 examples of the secular trends of AIDS over one decade. Figure 5.12 shows perinatally acquired pediatric AIDS cases, and Figure 5.13 shows AIDS incidence by race.[26]

In the 1990s, researchers identified an unprecedented change in the secular trend in prostate cancer incidence rates in the United States.[27] A gradually increasing secular trend in prostate cancer incidence rates between 1975 and 1989 suddenly increased sharply for both blacks and whites, peaking in 1993 for blacks and 1992 for whites (Figure 5.14).[28] On average, the rates were about 1.5 times higher for whites than blacks. The subsequent fluctuation in prostate cancer incidence rates between 1989 and 1995 has been attributed to rapid and widespread adoption of prostate-specific antigen screening, which began in the

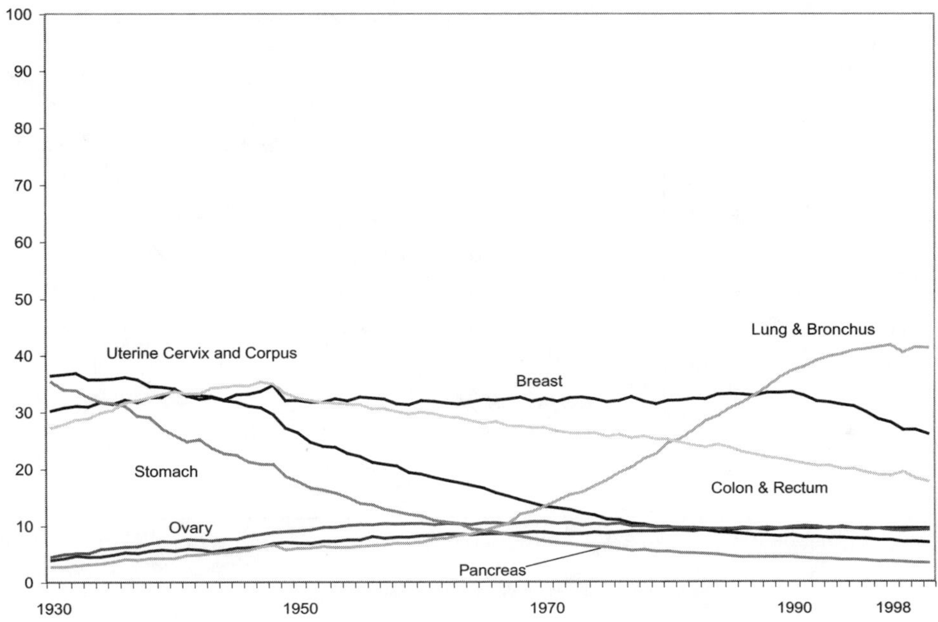

FIGURE 5.10 Site-specific age-adjusted (to the 2000 US standard population) cancer death rates for females, 1930–2001. (US Mortality Public Use Data Tapes 1960–2001, US Mortality Volumes 1930–1959, National Center for Health Statistics, Centers for Disease Control and Prevention; American Cancer Society, *Cancer Facts & Figures 2005*.)

late 1980s.[29] The sharp rise in prostate cancer death rates in the 1990s (see Figure 5.9) has also been shown to be an artifact of prostate-specific antigen screening.[30]

Short-term trends or **fluctuations** are usually brief, unexpected increases in health-related states or events. Short-term trends occur over short time intervals or limited time frames. Even though seasonal and cyclic trends occur within short time frames, because of their unique features they are used as separate categories. Most short-term trends are limited to hours, days, weeks, and months. Thus events of limited duration are included in the short-term trends category. An example of a short-term time frame would be the cholera epidemic studied by John Snow in the early 1800s, presented in Figure 5.15.

A more recent example of an outbreak of gastroenteritis associated with an interactive water fountain occurred in a beachside park in Volusia County, Florida. Since 1989, approximately 170 outbreaks associated with recreational water venues (eg, swimming pools, water parks, fountains, hot tubs and spas, lakes, rivers, and oceans) have been reported, with almost half resulting in gastrointestinal illness. The findings indicate that *Shigella sonnei* and *Cryptosporidium parvum* infections caused illness in persons exposed at an interactive water fountain at a beachside park. The Volusia county health department received reports of 3 children getting a *S sonnei* infection. Of 86 park visitors interviewed, 38 (44%) came down with a gastrointestinal illness. The most common symptoms were diarrhea, abdominal cramps, fever, vomiting, and bloody diarrhea. All ill persons entered the fountain and all but 2 ingested fountain water. The recirculated water passed through a hypochlorite

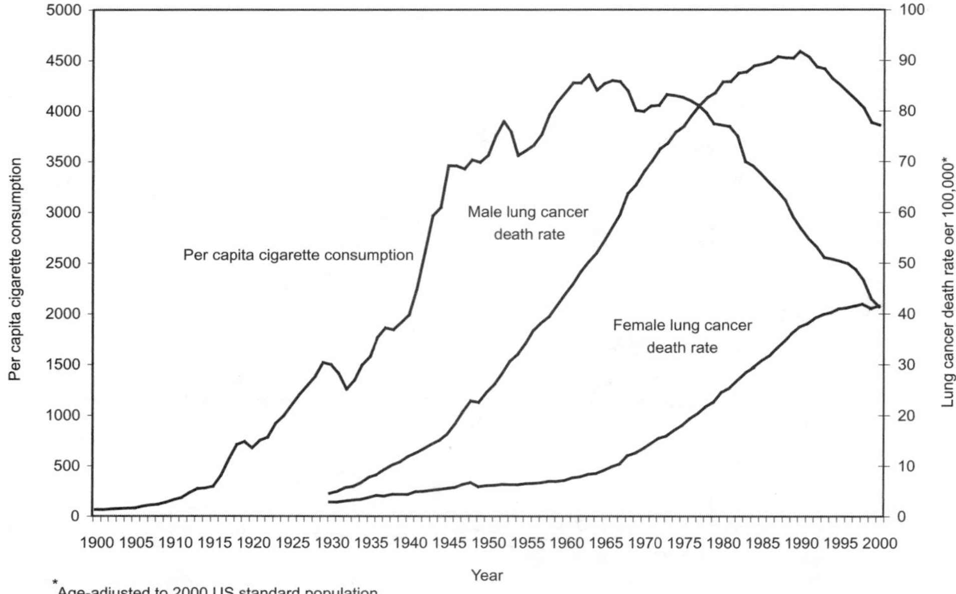

FIGURE 5.11 Lung cancer death rates and per capita cigarette consumption for males and females in the United States during the years 1900 through 2000. (United States Mortality Public Use Data Tapes 1960–2001, US Mortality Volumes 1930–1959, National Center for Health Statistics, Centers for Disease Control and Prevention, 2002 (death rates). US Department of Agriculture, 1900–2000 (cigarette consumption))

tablet chlorination system before being pumped back to the fountain. Several high-pressure fountain nozzles were used throughout the play area. The fountain was popular with children in diapers and toddlers, and they frequently stood directly over the nozzles. Chlorine levels were not monitored, and the tablets that depleted after 7–10 days of use had not been replaced since the park opened August 7. The chart in Figure 5.16 shows that several clinical cases occurred throughout the period.

The health department of Tarrant County reported to the Texas department of health that a group of teenagers attending a cheerleading camp June 9 through 11 became ill with nausea, vomiting, severe abdominal cramps, and diarrhea, some of which was bloody. Two teenagers were hospitalized with hemolytic uremic syndrome (a reduction in red blood cells because of excessive destruction that can lead to jaundice); 2 others underwent appendectomies. Stool cultures were taken and sent to the lab, which showed the teens were infected with *Escherichia coli* 0111:H8. As the shape of the histogram (Figure 5.17) indicates, the outbreak was confined to the camp and lasted only a short while.

Figure 5.18 shows the course of polio, which demonstrates the short-term time factors in this disease. The disease process can cease at any stage, depending on the response of the immune system and the host's ability to resist the disease. Highly infectious, polio has been one of the most devastating and disabling illnesses to beset mankind, and thousands of people have died from it. Polio crippled thousands more until the development and distribution of vaccines in the early 1950s, which finally halted its devastating effects. Polio has a whole range of effects on the human body, from minor muscular involvement to full paral-

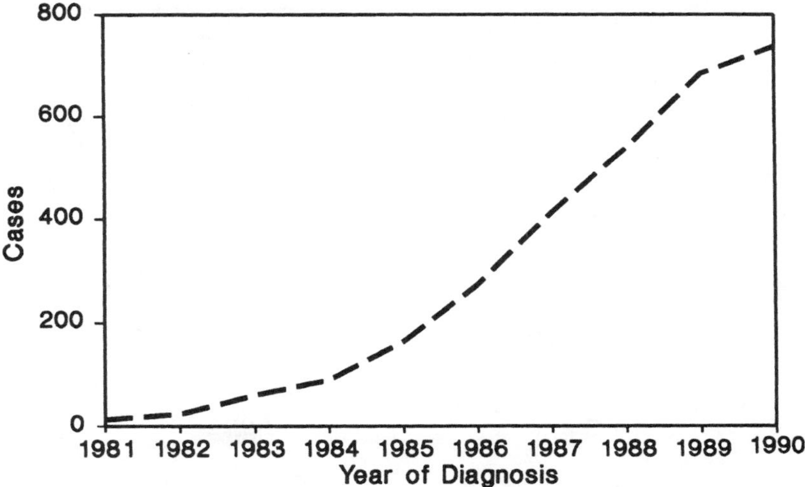

FIGURE 5.12 An example of secular trends in perinatally transmitted AIDS in pediatric cases. [Centers for Disease Control and Prevention, The HIV/AIDS Epidemic: The first 10 years. *MMWR.* 1991;40(22):361.]

ysis of major vital muscle groups. Iron lungs were invented to help those persons who were disabled with paralysis of respiratory muscles. The course of the disease and the time factors of the disease had to be understood in order to intervene through control and prevention measures.

Cyclic patterns represent periodic increases and decreases in the occurrence of health-related states or events. These patterns are often predictable. Some disease cycles are

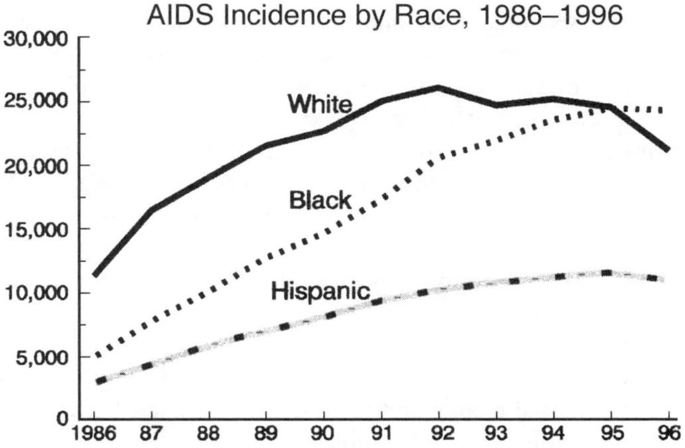

FIGURE 5.13 An example of secular trends which shows AIDS incidence by race, 1986–1996. (Centers for Disease Control and Prevention. Trends in the HIV and AIDS epidemic, 1998. Available at: http://www.cdc.gov/nchstp/od/Trends.htm. Accessed October 22, 2005.)

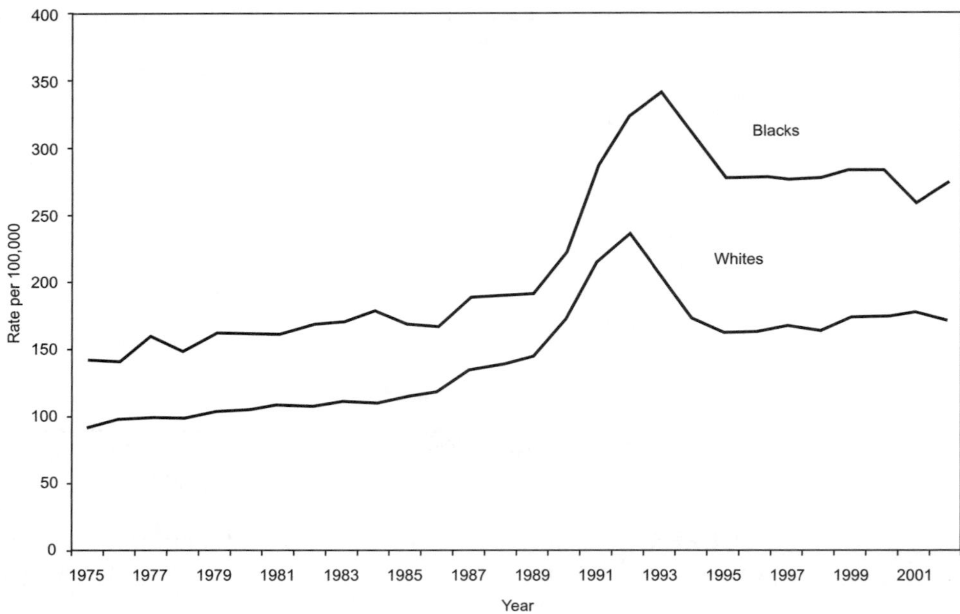

FIGURE 5.14 Age-adjusted (to the 2000 US standard population) prostate cancer incidence rates for white and black men by year of diagnosis. (Surveillance, Epidemiology, and End Results (SEER))

seasonal, while cycles of other diseases may be controlled by other cyclic factors such as the school calendar, immigration patterns, migration patterns, duration and course of diseases, placement of military troops, and wars. Other phrases used to describe trends of disease cycles are *secular* and *seasonal* cyclical patterns. Cyclic changes refer to recurrent alterations in the occurrence, interval, or frequency of diseases. Seasonal trends are presented in the paragraphs that follow. Some disease outbreaks occur only at certain times but in predictable time frames or intervals over long terms; thus epidemiologists track cyclic changes over time. The study approach is quite straightforward. Cases of the disease under study are followed and tabulated by time of onset according to a diagnosis or proof of occurrence. Short-term fluctuations should use shorter time elements.

One disease that is very cyclic on a short-term basis is chicken pox (varicella). When outbreaks of chicken pox are viewed over time, major cyclic variations are seen throughout the year. Chicken pox is one of the notifiable diseases and is more easily and accurately tracked than some others. Figure 5.19 presents the cyclic nature of chicken pox.[31] A similarly and dramatically portrayed annual cycle is seen in outbreaks of salmonella food poisoning.

Seasonal trends and variations are interesting to study and provide dramatic visual presentations when epidemiologic activities are plotted on a chart or graph. Extremes in difference are readily seen. For example, influenza peaks in January and February and occurs least frequently in the middle of the summer. In contrast, aseptic meningitis peaks in the summer, which may be related more to behaviors of the populations than to the weather. More people go swimming in the summer, exposing themselves to contaminated water in

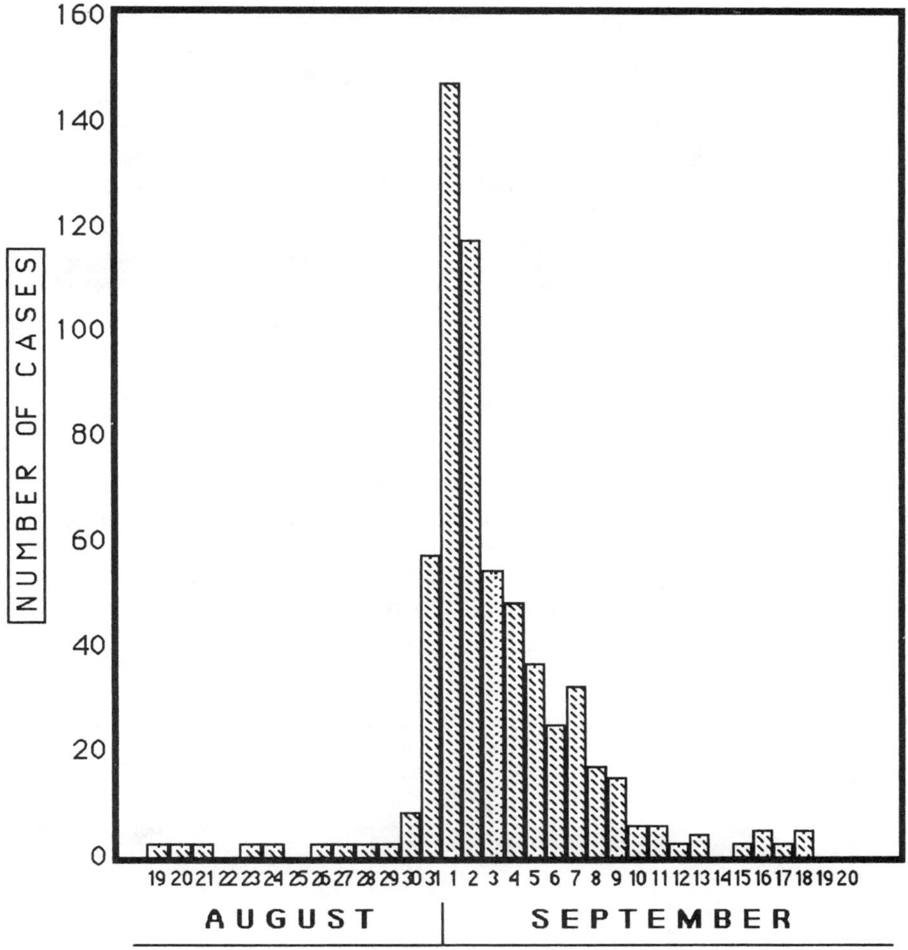

FIGURE 5.15 Example of the time factor in the cholera epidemic in the Broad Street–Golden Square area of London in the 1800s, showing the epidemic curve of the outbreak. (Snow, J. *Snow on Cholera.* New York, NY: The Commonwealth Fund; 1936.)

swimming pools, ponds, and lakes, all of which may have high bacteria levels or other abundant pathogens such as amoebas.

Seasons show many factors of health interest, such as the fact that children born in the summer achieve higher mean scores on IQ tests than winter-born children. High cholesterol readings in accountants are related to the tax calendar. Suicide rates are tied to seasonal variation and times of year. Mental retardation varies some with season. Births of children with mental retardation peak in February, with the lowest rates seen in the summer. Admission rates to hospitals are cyclic and seasonal. Figure 5.20 is a chart comparing seasonal fluctuations of 2 different communicable diseases, meningococcal infections and encephalitis. Figure 5.20 is an example of the observed dramatic seasonal fluctuations of diseases (as is Figure 5.19).[18]

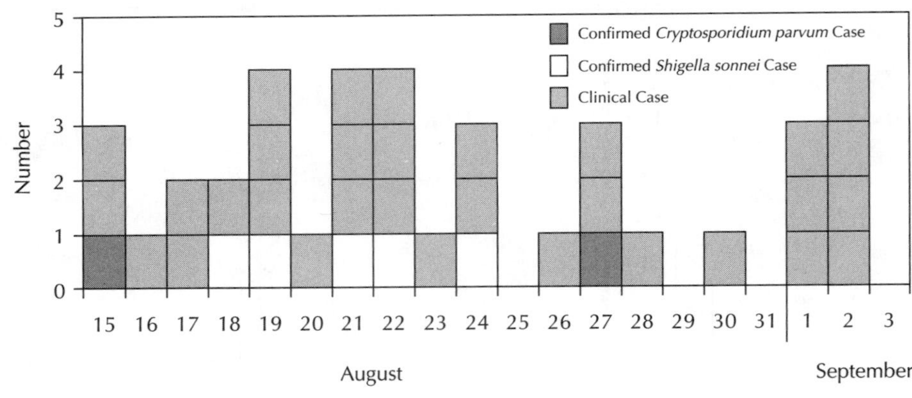

FIGURE 5.16 An example of short-term trends, this chart shows the number of gastroenteritis cases associated with an interactive fountain by date of illness onset—Volusia County, Florida, 1999. [Centers for Disease Control and Prevention. Outbreak of gastroenteritis associated with an interactive water fountain at a beachside park—Florida, 1999. *MMWR*. 2000;49(25):565–568.]

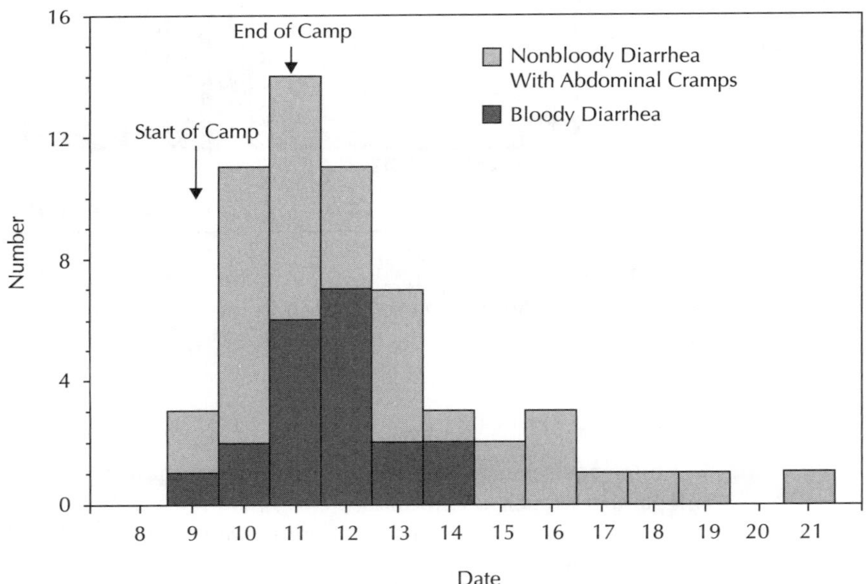

FIGURE 5.17 An example of short-term trends, this chart shows the number of *Escherichia coli* 0111:H8 cases associated with a foodborne illness at a cheerleading camp, by date of onset in Tarrant County, Texas. [Centers for Disease Control and Prevention. *Escherichia coli* 0111:H8 outbreak among teenage campers—Texas, 1999. *MMWR*. 2000;49(15):321–324.]

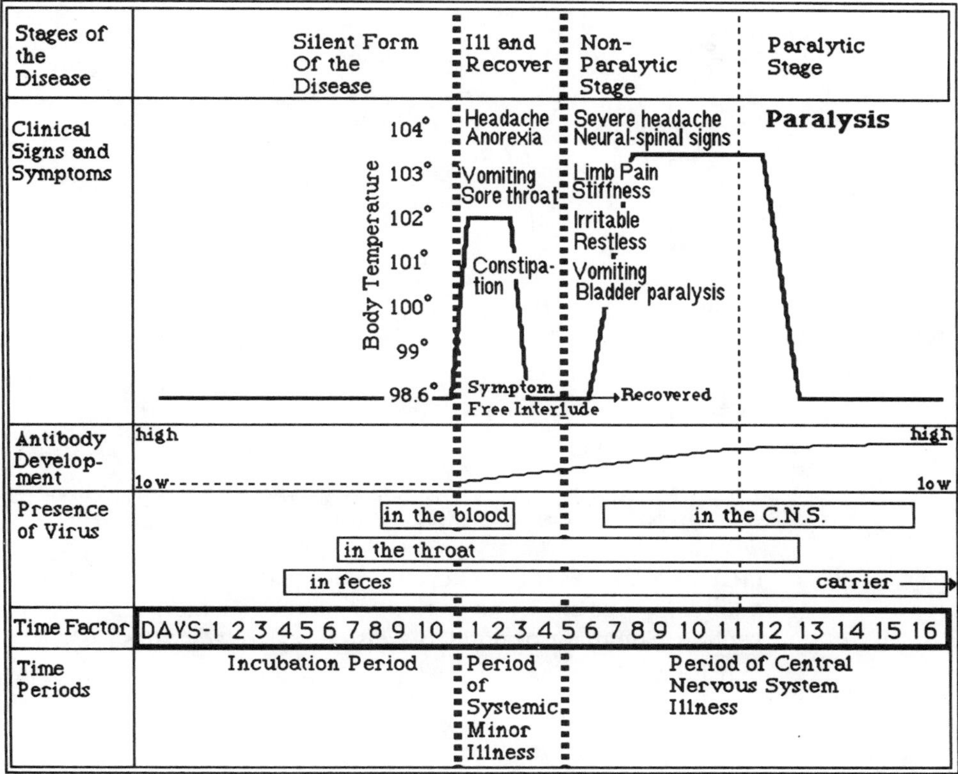

FIGURE 5.18 Graphic representation of time factors in the course of the disease poliomyelitis. (Adapted from: Reagan H. *Schematic Representation of Major Findings in the Typical Course of Clinically Biphasic Poliomyelitis.* Unpublished handout.)

Birth Cohort Plots

William Farr (1807–1883) first described the birth cohort analysis of mortality data in 1870. A **birth cohort analysis** plots the distribution of age at incidence or death for a selected disease or event by year of birth rather than year of death. To illustrate, suppose death rates of white males from diseases of the heart in the United States interests the researcher. Analysis shows increasing risk of death over the age span for each birth cohort, only at higher levels for older birth cohorts (Figure 5.21). In the age group 55–64 years, the death rate for those in the 1910 cohort is 34% higher than for those in the 1920 cohort, 90% higher than for those in the 1930 cohort, and 152% higher than for those in the 1940 cohort. Higher smoking prevalence likely explains, at least in part, the higher burden of diseases of the heart in successively older cohorts.

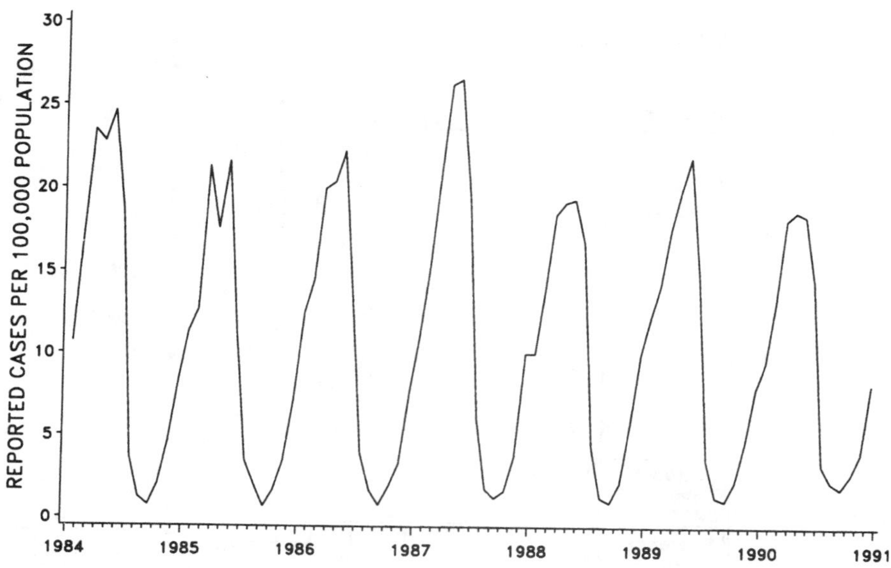

FIGURE 5.19 Example of cyclic trends of disease—cycles of chickenpox (varicella) outbreaks over an 8-year period by month. [Centers for Disease Control and Prevention. Summary of notifiable diseases, United States—1990. *MMWR.* 1991;39 (53):1–61.]

EVALUATION

When a program is initiated to change health behaviors and, ultimately, the risk of developing and dying from disease, the monitoring of behaviors, disease risk, and death rates between groups and over time is important in order to determine the effectiveness of the program. Health programs can be aimed at improving prevention behaviors (eg, increasing vaccination levels, reducing smoking, increasing fruit and vegetable consumption, increasing physical activity, decreasing obesity, increasing screening) and subsequent disease risk. On the national level, the CDC provides an extensive monitoring system and statistical databases for evaluating the nation's health in terms of prevention and health outcomes.[32] Monitoring efforts have identified considerable progress in reducing smoking prevalence in the United States (Figure 5.11). Consequently, declining rates of heart disease and smoking-related cancers have been observed (Figures 6.4 and 5.11). Figures 5.9 and 5.10 also show considerable progress in the war against cancer.

State public health officials monitor vaccine-preventable disease rates in order to assess whether vaccination programs are effectively reaching the appropriate people. If a vaccine-preventable disease rate begins to rise, this may signal that the vaccination program is not reaching specific at-risk populations. Monitoring these disease rates by racial/ethnic groups, for example, may show that the increasing rate only exists among a given minority group. The public health official should then investigate whether barriers related to culture, language, and access to care are present. The vaccination program should then be altered to address and overcome these barriers.

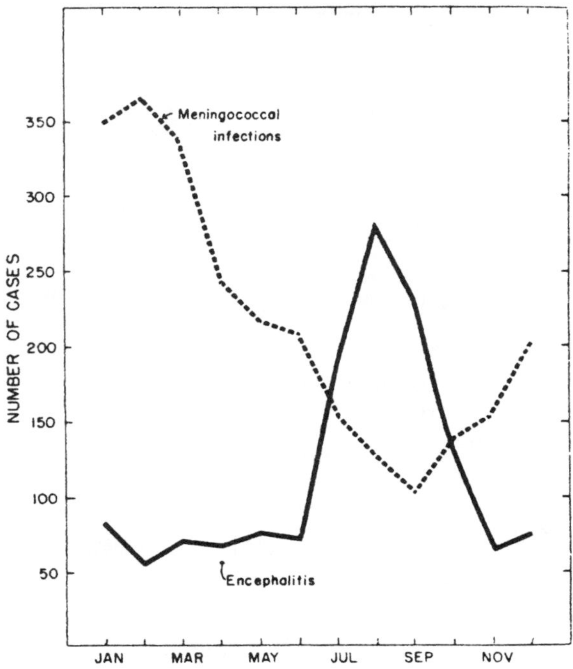

FIGURE 5.20 Example of seasonal variation of different diseases. Meningococcal disease occurs most in the winter months and encephalitis, transmitted by the mosquito, is highest in summer months. (Centers for Disease Control and Prevention. Reported cases of meningococcal infections and of primary encephalitis by month: United States—1968. *MMWR.* 1971;17(32).

CAUSAL INSIGHTS

Plotting health-related states or events over time can give the epidemiologist insights into the probable determinants of disease. If a disease occurs only in the summer, then that is when the epidemiologist searches for causal factors. Some of the questions an epidemiologist might ask are

- Is the increase a result of exposure to new water sources, for example, drinking from a stream in the mountains?
- Is it from summertime swimming in a contaminated public swimming pool or a lake?
- What vectors are available for disease transmission in the given time period and are missing at other times of the year (or in other seasons)?
- Are vehicles of transmission present during some but not other time periods?
- Are the cases exposed to certain environmental elements, situations, places, or circumstances during this time period that are not available at other times of the year or in other seasons?

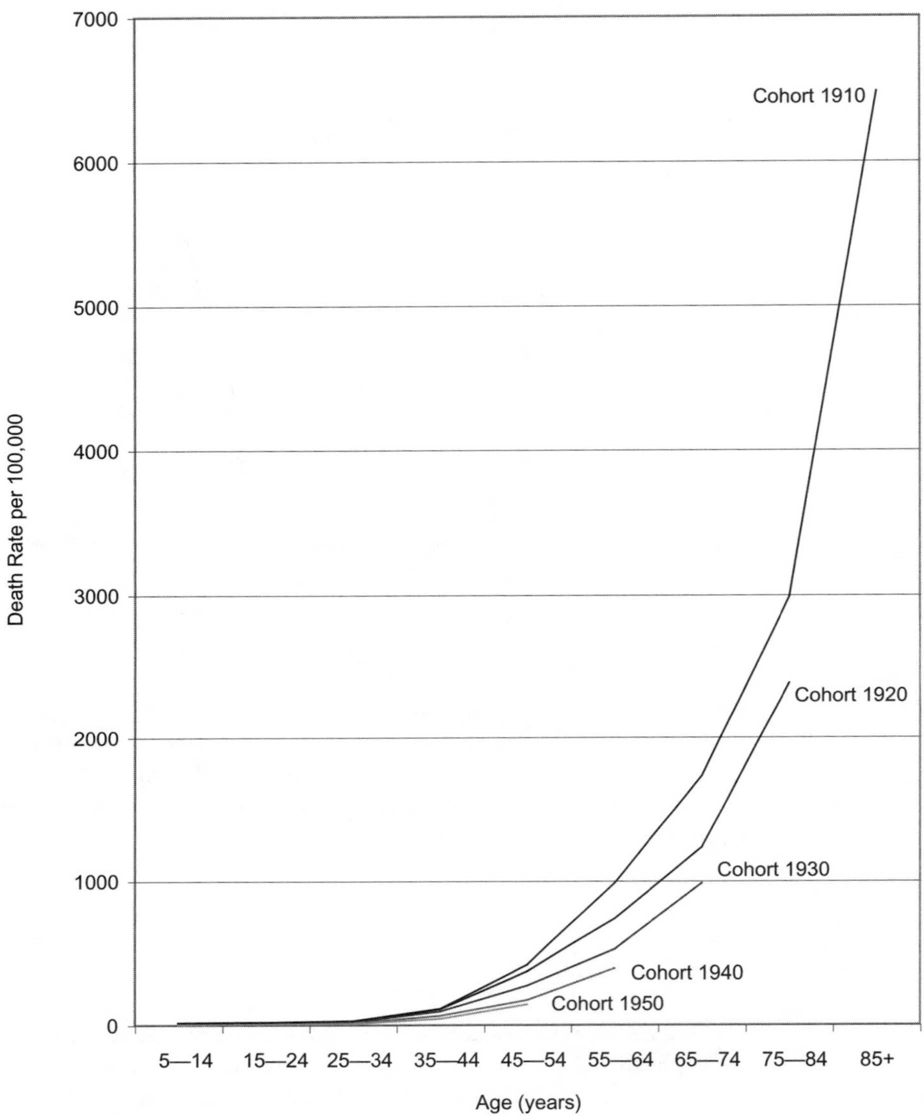

FIGURE 5.21 Death rates from diseases of the heart for white males in the US according to birth year. (National Center for Health Statistics. *Health, United States, 2004 with Chartbook on Trends in the Health of Americans*. Hyattsville, MD: NCHS; 2004.)

- Are those affected hiking or camping in the woods in the summer when insects are present that have been implicated in vectorborne diseases?
- Have foodborne diseases from summertime camping, hiking, fishing, hunting trips or picnics been considered?
- Are certain fomites used during certain time periods that might not be used during other seasons, such as shared drinking glasses or containers?

Studies involving geographic comparisons of disease frequency between groups, states, and countries, along with migration studies and twin studies have further yielded important insights into the respective roles genetic and environmental forces have on disease. Some of the questions an epidemiologist might ask include

- What are the geographic areas of highest and lowest disease incidence/mortality?
- What is the relative risk of disease incidence/mortality among selected migrant groups compared with a reference population?
- What are the unique environmental and behavioral characteristics of these areas?
- How does time among migrant groups influence change in risk of disease incidence/mortality?
- What is the time of separation and unique environmental and behavior characteristics among twins?

Confounding factors are always a threat in descriptive studies, thereby limiting the ability to establish cause-effect relationships. Although analytic epidemiologic studies are better for establishing cause-effect relationships, descriptive studies are a good first step in the search for causes of health-related states or events.

SURVEILLANCE IN EPIDEMIOLOGY

Surveillance was defined in Chapter 1 as the ongoing, systematic collection, analysis, interpretation, and dissemination of health data. Much of the information presented in the current chapter involves surveillance data. In epidemiology, persistent monitoring and assessment of changes in populations related to disease, conditions, injuries, disabilities, or death is done mostly to initiate investigations and to develop and evaluate public health prevention and control programs. The most common approach to surveillance is the survey. The federal government recognized early the importance of using surveys to monitor health; thus, the US approved the National Health Survey Act in 1956. Many national health surveys are now routinely administered, including the Behavior Risk Factor Surveillance System Survey, the National Hospital Discharge Survey, the National Health Interview Survey, and the National Health and Nutrition Examination Survey.

EXERCISES

Key Terms

Define the following terms.

Birth cohort analysis
Cyclic patterns
Decennial census
Dependency ratio
Person
Place
Healthy worker effect
Population (age) pyramid
Seasonal trends
Secular trends
Short-term trends or fluctuations
Surveillance
Temporal
Time

Study Questions

5.1 Refer to the cause-specific death rates in Table 5.1 and discuss possible reasons for the differences between males and females.

5.2 Refer to Table 5.3 and discuss possible reasons for the observed differences in death rates between those of Hispanic origin and those not of Hispanic origin.

5.3 Go to the US Census Bureau's site on international demographic data, http://www.census.gov/ipc/www/idbsum.html. Calculate the dependency ratio for Afghanistan and for the United States using 2005 data. Discuss potential reasons for differences in the results.

5.4 Refer to US data for 2005 and 2025 available at the Web site listed under question 5.3. Use a computer spreadsheet to construct population pyramid plots for the 2 time periods. Describe the 2 plots and discuss possible reasons for the observed differences.

5.5 Refer to the mortality trends shown in Figure 5.10. What role might screening have had on the observed rates for cancers of the (a) uterine cervix and corpus and (b) breast?

5.6 What does the data in Figure 5.11 tell you about the latency period between smoking and lung cancer for males?

5.7 Refer to Table 5.5 and discuss why higher education is associated with lower risk from the selected causes of death shown in the table.

5.8 Discuss how descriptive epidemiology by person, place, and time can contribute to each of the following: (a) identifying the extent of the public health problem, (b) describing the public health problem in a way that can be easily communicated, (c) identifying who is at greatest risk, (d) evaluating program effectiveness, and (e) providing clues as to the causes of disease.

REFERENCES

1. National Center for Health Statistics. *Health, United States, 2004 with Chartbook on Trends in the Health of Americans*. Hyattsville, MD: NCHS; 2004: Table 44.
2. Ries LAG, Kosary CI, Hankey BF, Miller BA, Edwards BK, eds. *SEER cancer statistics review, 1973–1996*. Bethesda, MD: National Cancer Institute; 1999.
3. Arias E. United States life tables, 2002. Table 11. *Natl Vital Stat Rep*. 2002;53:6. Available at: http://www.cdc.gov/nchs/fastats/lifexpec.htm. Accessed June 7, 2005.
4. Mausner JS, Kramer S. *Epidemiology: An Introductory Text*. Philadelphia, PA: Saunders; 1985.
5. Weeks JR. *Population*. 2nd ed. Belmont, CA: Wadsworth; 1981.
6. Hartley SF. *Community Populations*. Belmont, CA: Wadsworth; 1982.
7. National Center for Health Statistics. *Health, United States, 2004 with Chartbook on Trends in the Health of Americans*. Hyattsville, MD: NCHS; 2004: Tables 35–38, 41–42, 44–47, 49.
8. Williams DR, Lavizzo-Mourey R, Warren RC. The concept of race and health status in America. *Public Health Rep*. 1994;109:26–41.
9. Senior PA, Bhopal R. Ethnicity as a variable in epidemiologic research. *BMJ*. 1994;309:327–330.
10. Lewontin RC, Rose S, Kamin LJ. *Not in Our Genes: Biology, Ideology, and Human Nature*. New York, NY: Pantheon Books; 1984.
11. Krieger N. The making of public health data: Paradigms, politics and policy. *J Public Health Policy*. 1992;13:412–427.

12. LaVeist TA. Beyond dummy variables and sample selection: What health services researchers ought to know about race as a variable. *Health Serv Res.* 1994;29:1–16.
13. Schulman K, Berlin J, Harless W. The effect of race and sex on physicians' recommendations for cardiac catheterization. *N Engl J Med.* 1999;340:619–626.
14. Committee on Pediatric Research. Race/ethnicity, gender, socioeconomic status—research exploring their effects on child health: A subject review. *Pediatrics.* 2000;105(6):1349–1351.
15. Berkman J. Mortality and marital status. Reflections on the derivations of etiology from statistics. *Am J Public Health.* 1962;52(8):1318–1329.
16. Verbrugge LM. Marital status and health. *J Marriage and Fam.* 1979;41(2):267–285.
17. Schoenborn CA. Marital status and health: United States, 1999–2002. Advanced Data From Vital and Health Statistics. 2004;351:1–36. Available at: http://www.cdc.gov/search.do?action=search&queryText=health+marital+status. Accessed June 11, 2005.
18. MacMahon B, Pugh TF. *Epidemiology: Principles and Methods.* Boston: Little, Brown and Company; 1970.
19. Monson RR. *Occupational Epidemiology.* 2nd ed. Boca Raton, FL: CRC Press; 1990.
20. National Center for Health Statistics. *Health, United States, 2004 with Chartbook on Trends in the Health of Americans.* Hyattsville, Maryland: NCHS; 2004: Table 20.
21. National Center for Health Statistics. *Health, United States, 2004 with Chartbook on Trends in the Health of Americans.* Hyattsville, MD: NCHS; 2004: Table 81.
22. Daniels M, Merrill RM, Lyon JL, Standford JB, White GL Jr. Associations between breast cancer risk factors and religious practices in Utah. *Prev Med.* 2004;38:28–38.
23. Merrill RM, Folsom JA. Female breast cancer incidence and survival in Utah according to religious preference, 1985–1999. *BMC Cancer.* 2005;5:49.
24. Maskarinec G, Noh JJ. The effect of migration on cancer incidence among Japanese in Hawaii. *Ethn Dis.* 2004;14(3):431–439.
25. Wachsmuth RC, Turner F, Barrett JH, Gaut R, Randerson-Moor JA, Bishop DT, et al. The effect of sun exposure in determining nevus density in UK adolescent twins. *J Invest Dermatol.* 2005;124(1):56–62.
26. Centers for Disease Control and Prevention. The HIV/AIDS Epidemic: The first 10 years. *MMWR.* 1991;40(22):361.
27. Merrill RM, Potosky AL, Feuer EJ. Changing trends in US prostate cancer incidence rates. *J Natl Cancer Inst.* 1996;88(22):1683–1685.
28. Surveillance Research Program, National Cancer Institute SEER*Stat software (www.seer.cancer.gov/seerstat) version 6.1.4. Also available at: http://seer.cancer.gov/csr/1975_2002/results_merged/sect_23_prostate.pdf. Accessed May 23, 2005.
29. Merrill RM, Feuer EJ, Warren JL, Schussler N, Stephenson RA. Role of transurethral resection of the prostate in population-based prostate cancer incidence rates. *Am J Epidemiol.* 1999;150(8):848–860.
30. Feuer EJ, Merrill RM, Hankey BF. Cancer surveillance series: Interpreting trends in prostate cancer—Part II: Cause of death misclassification and the recent rise and fall in prostate cancer mortality. *J Natl Cancer Inst.* 1999;91(12):1025–1032.
31. Centers for Disease Control and Prevention. Summary of notifiable diseases, United States—1990. *MMWR.* 1990;39:53.
32. Centers for Disease Control and Prevention. Data and Statistics. Available at: http://www.cdc.gov/scientific.htm. Accessed June 10, 2005.

CHAPTER

6

General Health and Population Indicators

OBJECTIVES

After completing this chapter you will be able to

- Identify common indices used in identifying the health status of populations.
- Calculate, interpret, and apply selected health status measures.
- Understand the vital statistics registration system in the United States.

INTRODUCTION

On July 1, 2005, the estimated world population was 6,451,058,790.[1] This number represented a net increase of 74,195,672 over the previous year, with an average increase in the world population of 6,182,973 per month, 203,276 per day, 8,470 per hour, and 141 per minute. The estimated population of the United States on the same date was 296,346,455. In the United States there is currently one birth every 8 seconds, one death every 13 seconds, one international migration (net) every 26 seconds, and a net gain of one person every 12 seconds. Various indicators or indices of population dynamics, such as crude birth and mortality rates influence population growth.

Descriptive epidemiology makes use of several indices to identify the health status of populations. These indices are typically related to births and deaths because such data have been more readily available than have morbidity data. The indices are also often expressed as rates. A rate is the frequency of an event, disease, or condition, in relation to a unit of population, with a time specification (see Chapter 4, "Design Strategies and Statistical Methods in Descriptive Epidemiology"). This chapter will present many of the common indices used in epidemiology for measuring health status.

BIRTH

Birth rate represents the number of live births per 1,000 population. It is calculated as follows.

$$\text{Birth Rate} = \frac{\text{Number of live births in a population during a specified time period}}{\text{Population from which births occurred}} \times 1{,}000$$

The denominator is measured at the midpoint of the specified time period. For years in which there is no census (eg, 1991–1999), rates are based on national estimates of the population on July 1. In census years (eg, 2000), the population on April 1 is used. Birth rates are expressed as the number of live births per 1,000 population. The birth rate may be expressed according to factors such as the mother's age, race/ethnicity, or marital status (specific rate), or it may represent the entire population (crude rate).

A related measure is the fertility rate, which represents the number of live births per 1,000 females of childbearing age (15–44 years). It is calculated as follows.

$$\text{Fertility Rate} = \frac{\text{Number of live births in a population during a specified time period}}{\text{Population of women ages 15–44 years}} \times 1{,}000$$

The denominator is the midpoint of the specified time period. Monitoring trends in birth and fertility rates is important for effective planning because changes in the population composition can then be accommodated. For example, high birth and fertility rates result in a large population of dependent children who will require schools and affordable child care. On the other hand, low birth and fertility rates may result in an inadequate number of younger workers supporting a dependent elderly population.

MORTALITY

As discussed in Chapter 2, "Historic Developments in Epidemiology," John Graunt (1620–1674) developed a system of tracking and understanding causes of death that was called the Bills of Mortality. William Farr (1807–1883) was appointed registrar general in England and built on the ideas of Graunt. Farr's registration system for vital statistics laid the foundation for data collection and for the use of vital statistics in epidemiology. The foundations of the work of both Graunt and Farr were death-related statistics.

Mortality is the epidemiologic and vital statistics term for death. In our society there are generally three things that cause death: (1) degeneration of vital organs and related conditions; (2) disease states; and (3) society or the environment (homicide, accidents, disasters, etc.).[2]

In many countries, laws require the registration of vital events: births, deaths, marriages, divorces, and fetal deaths. All deaths have to be certified by a physician or a coroner. If any foul play is involved in a death, most states require an autopsy, and the results of the autopsy are recorded. An autopsy provides objective data that accurately certify the cause of death. Some physician diagnoses of cause of death are not completely correct because of the difficulty of making such a diagnosis without an autopsy. The physician signing the death certificate may not be the attending physician. Thus he or she might not have complete information on the cause of death and may record only what he or she knows about the death. All deaths are recorded and reported to local health departments and to the state office of vital statistics. Reports of vital event statistics, including deaths, are reported to the National Center for Health Statistics at the Centers for Disease Control and Prevention (CDC).[2–5]

In the United States, legal authority for the registration of births, deaths, marriages, divorces, and fetal deaths resides individually with the 50 states, Washington, DC, and the 5 territories (Puerto Rico, the Virgin Islands, Guam, American Samoa, and the Commonwealth of the Northern Mariana Islands). Each of these jurisdictions is responsible for maintaining registries of vital events and for issuing copies of birth, death, marriage, and divorce certificates. The laws of each state provide for a continuous and permanent vital registration system. Each system depends on the conscientious efforts of physicians, hospital personnel, funeral directors, coroners, and medical examiners in preparing or certifying information needed to complete the original death records (Figure 6.1).

Causes of Death

The National Center for Health Statistics developed and recommends the use of a standard certificate of death. Each state is expected to include the minimum information required as set forth on the US standard certificate of death. Some states include additional information that they deem important. Death statistics are of great importance to epidemiologic activities. **Death certificates** not only provide information on the total numbers of deaths, but they also provide demographic information and other important facts about each person who dies, such as date of birth (for cohort studies) and of death (for accurate age), stated age, place of death, place of residence, occupation, sex, cause of death, and marital status. Other information may include type of injury, place and time of injury, etc. See the sample certificate of death for the state of California (Figure 6.2). A separate certificate is used for fetal deaths (Figure 6.3).

<table>
<tr><th>Responsible Person or Agency</th><th>Birth Certificate</th><th>Death Certificate</th><th>Fetal Death Report (Stillbirth)</th></tr>
<tr><td>Hospital authority</td><td>1. Completes entire certificate in consultation with parent(s).
2. Files certificate with local office or State office per State law.</td><td>When death occurs in hospital, may initiate preparation of certificate: Completes information on name, date, and place of death; obtains certification of cause of death from physician; and gives certificate to funeral director.
NOTE: If the attending physician is unavailable to certify to the cause of death, some States allow a hospital physician to certify to only the fact and time of death. With legal pronouncement of the death and permission of the attending physician, the body can then be released to the funeral director. The attending physician still must complete the cause-of-death section prior to final disposition of the body.</td><td>1. Completes entire report in consultation with parent(s).
2. Obtains cause of fetal death and other medical and health information from physician.
3. Obtains authorization for final disposition of fetus.
4. Files report with local office or State office per State law.</td></tr>
<tr><td>Funeral director</td><td></td><td>1. Obtains personal facts about decedent and completes certificate.
2. Obtains certification of cause of death from attending physician or medical examiner or coroner.
3. Obtains authorization for final disposition per State law.
4. Files certificate with local office or State office per State law.</td><td>If fetus is to be buried, the funeral director is responsible for obtaining authorization for final disposition.
NOTE: In some States the funeral director, or person acting as such, is responsible for all duties shown above under hospital authority.</td></tr>
<tr><td>Physician or other professional attendant</td><td>For in-hospital birth, verifies accuracy of medical information and signs certificate. For out-of-hospital birth, duties are the same as those for hospital authority, shown above.</td><td>Completes certification of cause of death and signs certificate.</td><td>Provides cause of fetal death and other medical and health information.</td></tr>
<tr><td>Local office* (may be local registrar or city or county health department)</td><td>1. Verifies completeness and accuracy of certificate and queries incomplete or inconsistent certificates.
2. If authorized by State law, makes copy or index for local use.
3. Sends certificates to State registrar.</td><td>1. Verifies completeness and accuracy of certificate and queries incomplete or inconsistent certificates.
2. If authorized by State law, makes copy or index for local use.
3. If authorized by State law, issues authorization for final disposition on receipt of completed certificate.
4. Sends certificates to State registrar.</td><td>If State law requires routing of fetal death reports through local office, the local office performs the same functions as shown for the death certificate.</td></tr>
<tr><td colspan="4">City and county health departments use data derived from these records in allocating medical and nursing services, following up on infectious diseases, planning programs, measuring effectiveness of services, and conducting research studies.</td></tr>
<tr><td>State registrar, office of vital statistics</td><td colspan="3">1. Queries incomplete or inconsistent information.
2. Maintains files for permanent reference and is the source of certified copies.
3. Develops vital statistics for use in planning, evaluating, and administering State and local health activities and for research studies.
4. Compiles health-related statistics for State and civil divisions of State for use of the health department and other agencies and groups interested in the fields of medical science, public health, demography, and social welfare.
5. Sends data derived from records or copies of records to the National Center for Health Statistics.</td></tr>
<tr><td>Public Health Service, National Center for Health Statistics</td><td colspan="3">1. Prepares and publishes national statistics of births, deaths, and fetal deaths; constructs the official US life tables and related actuarial tables.
2. Conducts health and social-research studies based on vital records and on sampling surveys linked to records.
3. Conducts research and methodological studies in vital statistics methods, including the technical, administrative, and legal aspects of vital records registration and administration.
4. Maintains a continuing technical assistance program to improve the quality and usefulness of vital statistics.</td></tr>
</table>

* Some States do not have local vital registration offices. In these States, the certificates or reports are transmitted directly to the State office of vital statistics.

FIGURE 6.1 Vital Statistics Registration System in the United States. [US Department of Health and Human Services. *Medical Examiners' and Coroners' Handbook on Death Registration and Fetal Death Reportings.* Hyattsville, MD: US Department of Health and Human Services, Public Health Service, National Center for Health Statistics; October 1987. DHHS Publication No. (PHS) 87-1110.]

CERTIFICATE OF DEATH
STATE OF CALIFORNIA
USE BLACK INK ONLY/NO ERASURES, WHITEOUTS OR ALTERATIONS
VS-11 (REV. 1/00)

STATE FILE NUMBER — LOCAL REGISTRATION NUMBER

DECEDENT PERSONAL DATA
1. NAME OF DECEDENT—FIRST (GIVEN) | 2. MIDDLE | 3. LAST (FAMILY)
4. DATE OF BIRTH MM/DD/CCYY | 5. AGE YRS. | IF UNDER 1 YEAR: MONTHS, DAYS | IF UNDER 24 HOURS: HOURS, MINUTES | 6. SEX | 7. DATE OF DEATH MM/DD/CCYY | 8. HOUR
9. STATE OF BIRTH | 10. SOCIAL SECURITY NO. | 11. MILITARY SERVICE: YES / NO / UNK | 12. MARITAL STATUS | 13. EDUCATION—YEARS COMPLETED
14. RACE | 15. HISPANIC—SPECIFY: YES / NO | 16. USUAL EMPLOYER
17. OCCUPATION | 18. KIND OF BUSINESS | 19. YEARS IN OCCUPATION

USUAL RESIDENCE
20. RESIDENCE—(STREET AND NUMBER OR LOCATION)
21. CITY | 22. COUNTY | 23. ZIP CODE | 24. YRS IN COUNTY | 25. STATE OR FOREIGN COUNTRY

INFORMANT
26. NAME, RELATIONSHIP | 27. MAILING ADDRESS (STREET AND NUMBER OR RURAL ROUTE NUMBER, CITY OR TOWN, STATE, ZIP)

SPOUSE AND PARENT INFORMATION
28. NAME OF SURVIVING SPOUSE—FIRST | 29. MIDDLE | 30. LAST (MAIDEN NAME)
31. NAME OF FATHER—FIRST | 32. MIDDLE | 33. LAST | 34. BIRTH STATE
35. NAME OF MOTHER—FIRST | 36. MIDDLE | 37. LAST (MAIDEN) | 38. BIRTH STATE

SAMPLE

DISPOSITION(S)
39. DATE MM/DD/CCYY | 40. PLACE OF FINAL DISPOSITION

FUNERAL DIRECTOR AND LOCAL REGISTRAR
41. TYPE OF DISPOSITION(S) | 42. SIGNATURE OF EMBALMER | 43. LICENSE NO.
44. NAME OF FUNERAL DIRECTOR | 45. LICENSE NO. | 46. SIGNATURE OF LOCAL REGISTRAR | 47. DATE MM/DD/CCYY

PLACE OF DEATH
101. PLACE OF DEATH | 102. IF HOSPITAL, SPECIFY ONE: IP / ER/OP / DOA | 103. FACILITY OTHER THAN HOSPITAL: CONV. HOSP. / RES. CARE / OTHER | 104. COUNTY
105. STREET ADDRESS—(STREET AND NUMBER OR LOCATION) | 106. CITY

CAUSE OF DEATH
107. DEATH WAS CAUSED BY: (ENTER ONLY ONE CAUSE PER LINE FOR A, B, C, AND D) | TIME INTERVAL BETWEEN ONSET AND DEATH | 108. DEATH REPORTED TO CORONER: YES / NO; REFERRAL NUMBER
IMMEDIATE CAUSE (A)
DUE TO (B) | 109. BIOPSY PERFORMED: YES / NO
DUE TO (C) | 110. AUTOPSY PERFORMED: YES / NO
DUE TO (D) | 111. USED IN DETERMINING CAUSE: YES / NO
112. OTHER SIGNIFICANT CONDITIONS CONTRIBUTING TO DEATH BUT NOT RELATED TO CAUSE GIVEN IN 107
113. WAS OPERATION PERFORMED FOR ANY CONDITION IN ITEM 107 OR 112? IF YES, LIST TYPE OF OPERATION AND DATE.

SAMPLE

PHYSICIAN'S CERTIFICATION
114. I CERTIFY THAT TO THE BEST OF MY KNOWLEDGE DEATH OCCURRED AT THE HOUR, DATE AND PLACE STATED FROM THE CAUSES STATED. DECEDENT ATTENDED SINCE MM/DD/CCYY | DECEDENT LAST SEEN ALIVE MM/DD/CCYY | 115. SIGNATURE AND TITLE OF CERTIFIER | 116. LICENSE NO. | 117. DATE MM/DD/CCYY
118. TYPE ATTENDING PHYSICIAN'S NAME, MAILING ADDRESS, ZIP

CORONER'S USE ONLY
I CERTIFY THAT IN MY OPINION DEATH OCCURRED AT THE HOUR, DATE AND PLACE STATED FROM THE CAUSES STATED. | 120. INJURY AT WORK: YES / NO | 121. INJURY DATE MM/DD/CCYY | 122. HOUR | 123. PLACE OF INJURY
119. MANNER OF DEATH: NATURAL / SUICIDE / HOMICIDE / ACCIDENT / PENDING INVESTIGATION / COULD NOT BE DETERMINED | 124. DESCRIBE HOW INJURY OCCURRED (EVENTS WHICH RESULTED IN INJURY)
125. LOCATION (STREET AND NUMBER OR LOCATION AND CITY, ZIP)
126. SIGNATURE OF CORONER OR DEPUTY CORONER | 127. DATE MM/DD/CCYY | 128. TYPED NAME, TITLE OF CORONER OR DEPUTY CORONER

STATE REGISTRAR
A | B | C | D | E | F | G | H | FAX AUTH. # | CENSUS TRACT

FIGURE 6.2 Example of a Standard Certificate of Death for the State of California. (Revision January 2000)

Cause of Death on the Death Certificates

The International Classification of Diseases (ICD) is the standard diagnostic classification for mortality statistics. ICD-10 is the latest classification in a series that dates back to the 1850s. It was endorsed by the Forty-third World Health Assembly in May 1990. ICD is designed to promote consistency among countries in the way they collect, process, classify, and present mortality statistics, including a format for reporting causes of death on the death certificate.

CERTIFICATE OF FETAL DEATH
STATE OF CALIFORNIA
STATE FILE NUMBER — USE BLACK INK ONLY MAKE NO ERASURES, WHITEOUTS, OR OTHER ALTERATIONS — LOCAL REGISTRATION DISTRICT AND CERTIFICATE NUMBER

THIS FETUS: 1A. NAME—FIRST (GIVEN) | 1B. MIDDLE | 1C. LAST (FAMILY)
2. SEX | 3A. THIS FETUS, SINGLE, TWIN, ETC. | 3B. IF MULTIPLE THIS FETUS 1ST, 2ND, ETC. | 4A. DATE OF EVENT—MONTH, DAY, YEAR | 4B. HOUR—24 HOUR CLOCK TIME

PLACE OF DELIVERY: 5A. PLACE OF EVENT—NAME OF HOSPITAL OR FACILITY | 5B. STREET ADDRESS—STREET, NUMBER, OR LOCATION
5C. CITY | 5D. COUNTY | 5E. PLANNED PLACE OF DELIVERY

SAMPLE

FATHER: 6A. NAME OF FATHER—FIRST (GIVEN) | 6B. MIDDLE | 6C. LAST (FAMILY) | 7. STATE OF BIRTH | 8. DATE OF BIRTH—MONTH, DAY, YEAR

MOTHER: 9A. NAME OF MOTHER—FIRST (GIVEN) | 9B. MIDDLE | 9C. LAST (MAIDEN) | 10. STATE OF BIRTH | 11. DATE OF BIRTH—MONTH, DAY, YEAR

CERTIFICATION: I CERTIFY THAT THIS FETUS WAS BORN DEAD AT THE HOUR, DATE AND PLACE STATED FROM THE CAUSES STATED. | 12A. SIGNATURE OF PHYSICIAN, CORONER, OR DEPUTY CORONER | 12B. DEGREE OR TITLE AND TYPED NAME | 12C. DATE SIGNED | 12D. LICENSE NUMBER

FUNERAL DIRECTOR AND LOCAL REGISTRAR: 13A. DISPOSITION(S) | 13B. PLACE OF DISPOSITION—NAME AND ADDRESS | 13C. DATE MO, DAY, YEAR | 14A. SIGNATURE OF EMBALMER | 14B. LICENSE NUMBER
15A. NAME OF FUNERAL DIRECTOR (OR PERSON ACTING AS SUCH) | 15B. LICENSE NUMBER | 16. SIGNATURE OF LOCAL REGISTRAR | 17. REGISTRATION DATE

CONFIDENTIAL HEALTH AND MEDICAL INFORMATION

CAUSE OF DEATH: 18. FETAL DEATH WAS CAUSED BY: IMMEDIATE CAUSE (A) | DUE TO (B) | DUE TO (C)
19. WAS DEATH REPORTED TO CORONER? REFERRAL NUMBER — YES / NO
20A. WAS AUTOPSY PERFORMED? YES / NO
20B. WAS IT USED IN DETERMINING CAUSE OF DEATH? YES / NO
21. OTHER SIGNIFICANT CONDITIONS OF FETUS OR MOTHER—CONTRIBUTING TO FETAL DEATH BUT NOT RELATED TO CAUSE GIVEN IN 18.

FATHER: 22. RACE | 23. HISPANIC SPECIFY — YES / NO | 24A. USUAL OCCUPATION | 24B. USUAL KIND OF BUSINESS OR INDUSTRY | 24C. EDUCATION—YRS. COMPLETED

MOTHER: 25. RACE | 26. HISPANIC SPECIFY — YES / NO | 27A. USUAL OCCUPATION | 27B. USUAL KIND OF BUSINESS OR INDUSTRY | 27C. EDUCATION—YRS. COMPLETED
28A. RESIDENCE—STREET, NUMBER, OR LOCATION | 28B. CITY | 28C. STATE | 28D. ZIP | 28E. COUNTY

MEDICAL DATA (ENTER THE APPROPRIATE CODE(S) FOR ITEMS 29D AND 32A-35 FROM THE VS 12A SUPPLEMENTAL WORKSHEET.):
29A. DATE LAST NORMAL MENSES BEGAN MONTH, DAY, YEAR | 29B. MONTH PRENATAL CARE BEGAN (1ST, 2ND, ...9TH, 9TH) | 29C. NUMBER OF PRENATAL VISITS | 31. PREGNANCY HISTORY (COMPLETE EACH SECTION): LIVE BIRTHS — OTHER TERMINATIONS (EXCLUDE INDUCED ABORTIONS)
29D. PRINCIPAL SOURCE OF PAYMENT FOR PRENATAL CARE — CODE: | 30. FETAL WEIGHT — GRAMS | 32A. METHOD OF DELIVERY — CODE(S): | NOW LIVING (NUMBER) A | NOW DEAD (NUMBER) B | BEFORE 20 WKS (NUMBER) D | AFTER 20 WKS (NUMBER) E
32B. EXPECTED PRINCIPAL SOURCE OF PAYMENT FOR DELIVERY — CODE: | 33. COMPLICATIONS AND PROCEDURES OF PREGNANCY AND CONCURRENT ILLNESSES — CODE(S): | DATE OF LAST LIVE BIRTH MONTH, DAY, YEAR C | DATE OF LAST OTHER TERM. MONTH, YEAR F

SAMPLE

34. COMPLICATIONS AND PROCEDURES OF LABOR AND DELIVERY — CODE(S): | 35. ABNORMAL CONDITIONS AND CLINICAL PROCEDURES RELATING TO THE FETUS — CODE(S):

STATE REGISTRAR: A. | B. | C. | D. | E. | F. | CENSUS TRACT

VS 12 (REV 7/91) PENALTY FOR UNAUTHORIZED RELEASE, $500 FINE OR SIX MONTHS IMPRISONMENT. OSP 00 36252

FIGURE 6.3 Example of a Standard Certificate of Fetal Death for the State of California. (Revision July 1991)

The causes of death entered on the death certificate are those diseases, injuries, and morbid conditions that resulted in or contributed to the death. Circumstances of any accident or violent act that produced death are also recorded. The reported conditions are then translated into medical codes according to the classification structure and the selection and modification rules of the current ICD, published by the World Health Organization.[6] The coding rules established by the applicable revision of the ICD give preference to certain categories, consolidate conditions, and systematically select a single cause of death from a sequence of reported conditions. The selected single cause is called the underlying cause of death. The other reported causes are called the nonunderlying causes of death.

Underlying Cause of Death

Found on the death certificate is a space for the underlying cause of death. This is stated on a death certificate directly after the main cause of death. The underlying cause is any disease or injury that initiated the set of events leading to the death. Any violent act or accident that produced the death would be stated on this section of the death certificate. For example, a tumor, such as malignant melanoma, is often the underlying cause of death because cancer cells can spread to distant parts of the body and disrupt the normal functioning of vital organs (eg, the brain, liver, and lungs).

Death Certificate Data

Data from death certificates and the formal death-reporting system provide a database for studying a variety of epidemiologic issues and events. The main cause of death is entered first on a death certificate. Two additional or contributing causes can also be listed (see Figure 6.2). The existing diseases and conditions at the time of death may hold as much epidemiologic value as the listed cause of death.

TYPES OF MORTALITY RATES

Many different mortality rates are used in epidemiology. Below are definitions of the death rates commonly found in national reports and used in community health assessment.

Mortality Rate

The first and most basic measure of death is the crude mortality rate. The **crude mortality rate** is calculated as follows.

$$\text{Crude Mortality Rate} = \frac{\begin{array}{c}\text{Number of deaths occurring}\\ \text{during a given time period}\end{array}}{\text{Population from which deaths occurred}} \times 100{,}000$$

The denominator is the midpoint of the specified time period. The term *crude* is used because it does not account for differences of age, sex, or other variables in any aspect of death. When deaths from a specific cause are of interest, the **cause-specific mortality rate** is calculated.

$$\text{Cause-Specific Mortality Rate} = \frac{\begin{array}{c}\text{Number of deaths from a specific cause}\\ \text{occurring during a given time period}\end{array}}{\text{Population from which death occurred}} \times 100{,}000$$

When comparisons are made of these rates between populations or across time, age-adjusted rates may be more appropriate because they control for differences in the age distribution (see Chapter 4). Crude and age-adjusted mortality rates in the United States for all causes and for diseases of the heart are shown for the years 1950 through 2002 in Figure 6.4. The age-adjusted rates show much more pronounced improvements in mortality rates across these years than do the crude rates. Also, the decline in all-cause mortality rates is explained primarily by decline in rates of diseases of the heart.

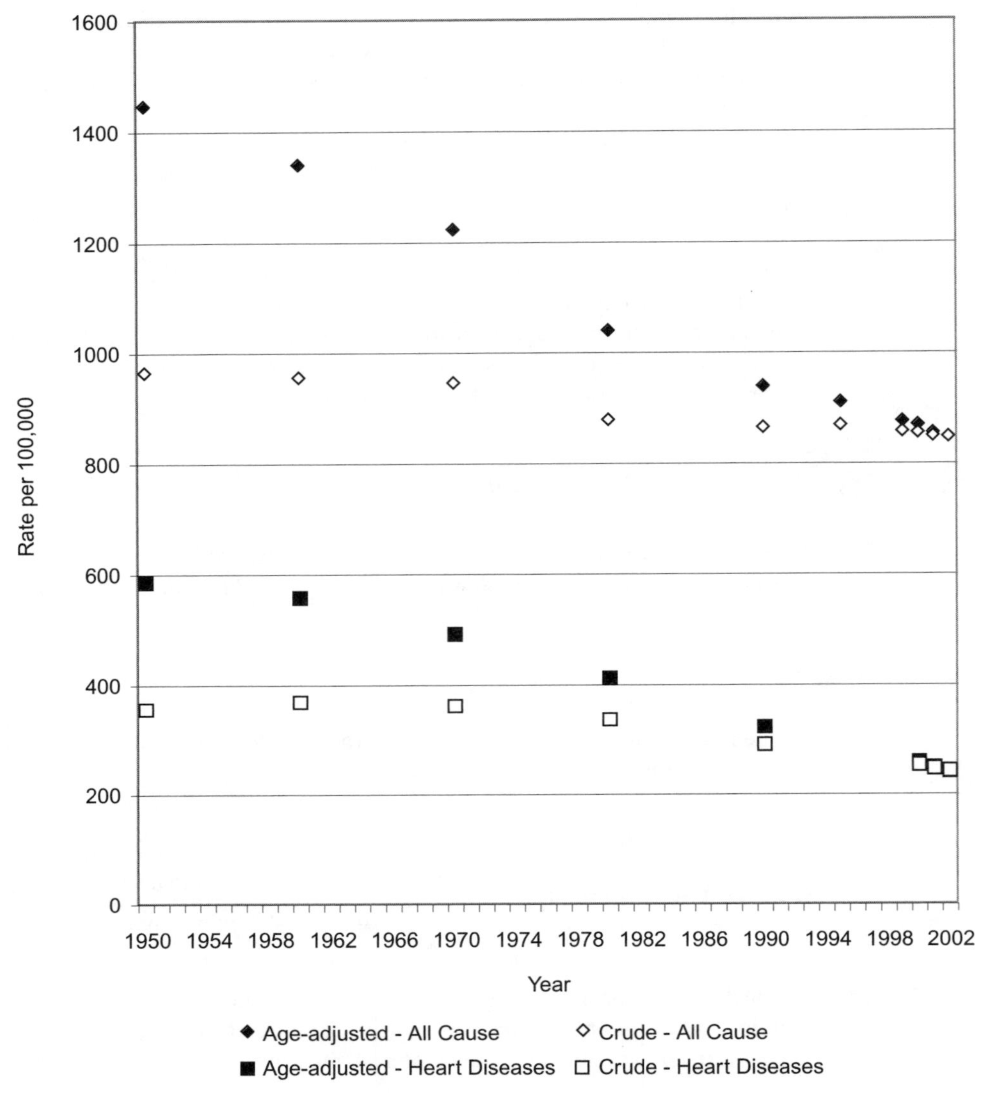

FIGURE 6.4 Crude and Age-adjusted Mortality Rates in the United States for All Causes and Diseases of the Heart. (National Center for Health Statistics. *Health, United States, 2004 with Chartbook on Trends in the Health of Americans.* Hyattsville, MD: NCHS; 2004: Tables 35, 36.)

INFANT MORTALITY

Infant mortality is a major health status indicator of populations and a key measure of the health status of a community or population. Reflected in infant mortality is prenatal and postnatal nutritional care or the lack thereof. If pregnant women have an intake of sufficient calories and nutrients, including appropriate weight gain, this will improve infant birth weight and reduce infant mortality and morbidity. Seeking immediate medical care upon becoming pregnant, along with total abstinence from any drugs, chemicals, alcohol, and smoking, can reduce infant mortality. Declining infant mortality in developing countries has been linked primarily with affordable health services, improvements in the status of women, nutrition standards, universal immunization, and the expansion of prenatal and obstetric services.[7] Breastfeeding has been shown to protect against gastroenteritis and respiratory infections in developing countries.[7]

Infant Mortality Rate

Infant (the period from birth to 1 year) morality rates are often used as an indicator of health in a country. The **infant mortality rate** is calculated as follows.

$$\text{Infant Mortality Rate} = \frac{\text{Number of deaths among infants ages 0–1 year during a specified time period}}{\text{Number of live births in the same time period}} \times 1{,}000$$

Infant mortality varies considerably throughout the world. In Table 6.1, infant mortality rates and life expectancy at birth in 2004 are presented for selected countries. A bivariate scatter plot shows the relationship between infant mortality and life expectancy (Figure 6.5). As the infant mortality rate increases by one, life expectancy decreases on average by 0.3. About 79% of the variability in life expectancy can be explained by the infant mortality rate.

TABLE 6.1 Infant Mortality Rates and Life Expectancy at Birth* in 2004

Country	*Infant Mortality Rate*	*Life Expectancy*
Sweden	2.8	80.3
Japan	3.3	81
Finland	3.6	78.2
Norway	3.7	79.2
Czech Republic	4	75.8
Germany	4.2	78.5
France	4.3	79.4
Switzerland	4.4	80.3
Spain	4.5	79.4
Denmark	4.6	77.4
Austria	4.7	78.9
Australia	4.8	80.3
Canada	4.8	80

(continued)

TABLE 6.1 *(Continued)*

Country	*Infant Mortality Rate*	*Life Expectancy*
Portugal	5.1	77.3
United Kingdom	5.2	78.3
Ireland	5.5	77.4
Greece	5.6	78.9
New Zealand	6	78.5
Italy	6.1	79.5
United States	6.6	77.4
Israel	7.2	79.2
Korea, South	7.2	75.6
Cyprus	7.4	77.5
Slovakia	7.6	74.2
Hungary	8.7	72.2
Poland	8.7	74.2
Chile	9.1	76.4
Costa Rica	10.3	76.6
Sri Lanka	14.8	72.9
Russia	17	66.4
Panama	20.9	72.1
Mexico	21.7	74.9
Albania	22.3	77.1
Venezuela	23	74.1
Ecuador	24.5	76
China	25.3	72
Syria	30.6	69.7
Brazil	30.7	71.4
Peru	33	69.2
Egypt	33.9	70.7
Guatemala	36.9	65.2
Iran	42.9	69.7
India	57.9	64
South Africa	62.2	44.2
Kenya	62.6	44.9
Bangladesh	64.3	61.7
Zimbabwe	67.1	37.8
Nigeria	70.5	50.5
Pakistan	74.4	62.6
Mozambique	137.1	37.1
Angola	192.5	36.8

[*]In years. (Source: US Census Bureau International Database. Available at: http://www.census.gov/ipc/www/idbprint.html. Accessed June 14, 2005.)

NEWS FILE

Infant Mortality Rises in the United States for the First Time in Decades

US life expectancy increased from 77.2 in 2001 to 77.4 in 2002. However, during this same time period the infant mortality rate also increased, from 6.8 deaths per 1,000 live births to 7.0 deaths per 1,000. The last time the nation's infant mortality rate increased was in 1958. The increase in this important public health indicator drew the prompt attention of public health officials in the United States. Potential explanations for the increase posed by health officials include a long trend among American women toward delaying motherhood, with the risk of deadly complications greater in older aged women, and increased use of fertility drugs to get pregnant, which is associated with multiple births and other high-risk pregnancies. The primary explanation for increasing US life expectancy despite the infant mortality increase is the steady decreases in deaths associated with heart disease, stroke, and cancer.

After further investigation, the CDC reported that an increase in the birth of very small infants is the major explanation for the increase in US infant mortality in 2002. The number of babies weighing less than one pound increased by almost 500 births from 2001 to 2002. The increase primarily occurred in women 20–34. Although most of the increase occurred in babies born in single deliveries, about 3% of births were multiple births, which made up about 25% of the overall increase in infant mortality.

[Source: MacDorman MF, Martin JA, Matthews TJ, Hoyert DL, Ventura SJ. Explaining the 2001–2002 infant mortality increase: Data from the linked birth/infant death data set. MMWR. *2005;53(12):1–24.]*

Infant mortality rates in the United States declined by 90% during the 20th century.[8] Nevertheless, the United States ranks 20th among the selected countries shown in Table 6.1. This lower ranking is explained in part by higher infant mortality rates among blacks. Specifically, from 1995 to 1998, the median black infant mortality rate among the 60 largest cities was 13.9 per 1,000 life births. This rate was substantially higher than for either whites or Hispanics (6.4 and 5.9, respectively).[9]

Neonatal Mortality Rate

Neonatal (ie, the period from birth through 28 days of life) mortality rates reflect poor prenatal care, low birth weights, infections, lack of proper medical care, injuries, premature delivery, and congenital defects. A special concern lies in the proper reporting of neonatal deaths. Some deaths in low birth-weight (under 2,500 grams) infants may go unreported, and this may be even more so for very low birth weights under 1,000 grams.[10]

The **neonatal mortality rate** is calculated as follows.

$$\text{Neonatal Mortality Rate} = \frac{\text{Number of deaths among infants less than 28 days during a specified time period}}{\text{Number of live births in the same time period}} \times 1{,}000$$

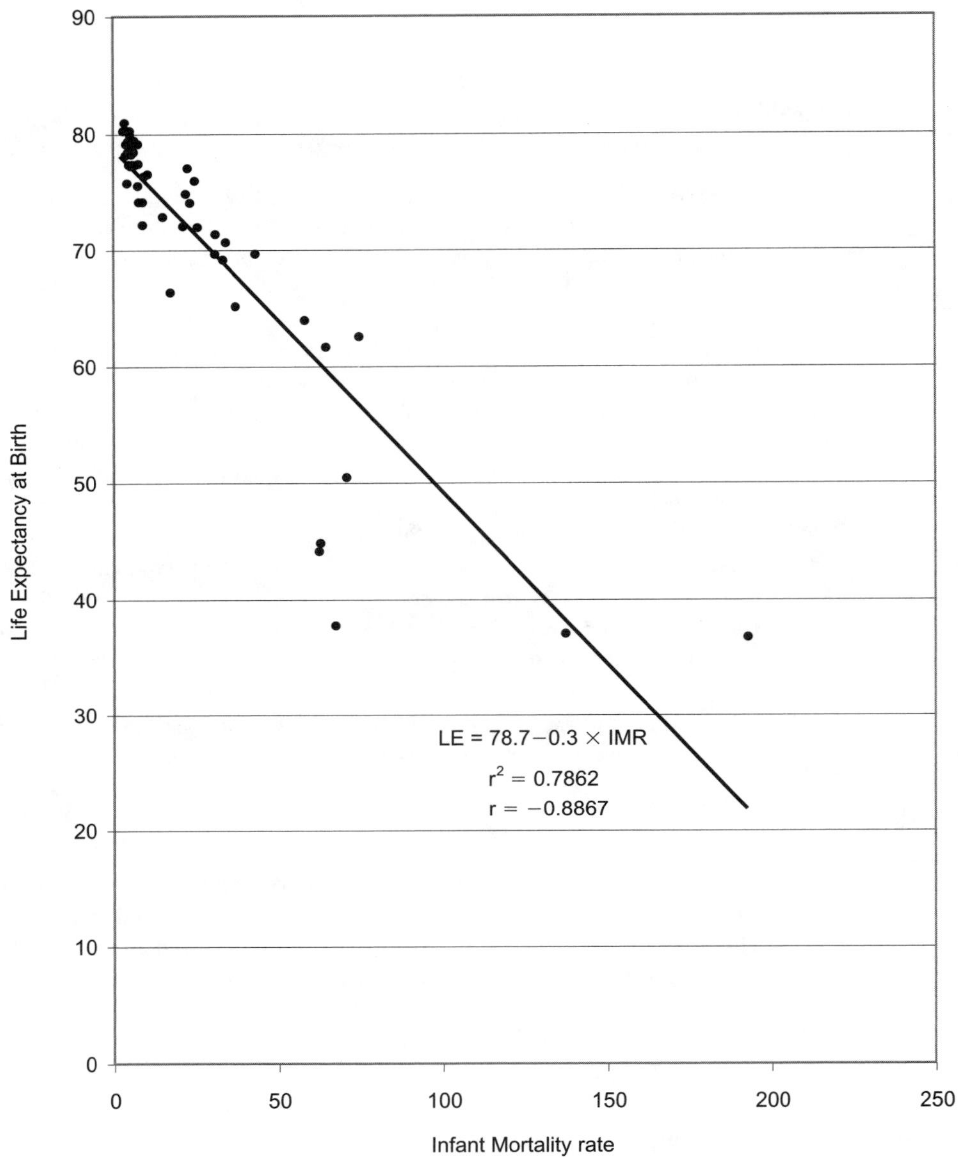

FIGURE 6.5 Correlation Between Infant Mortality Rate and Life Expectancy in 2004 for Selected Countries. (US Census Bureau, International Database. Available at: http://www.census.gov/ipc/www/idbprint.html. Accessed on October 25, 2005.)

Postneonatal Mortality Rate

Postneonatal (ie, from 28 days to 1 year of life) mortality rates are important to track in underdeveloped countries. These rates are influenced primarily by malnutrition and infectious diseases.

The **postneonatal mortality rate** is calculated as follows.

$$\text{Postneonatal Mortality Rate} = \frac{\text{Number of infant deaths between 28 days of age and 1 year of age}}{\text{Number of live births in the same year}} \times 1{,}000$$

Neonatal and postneonatal mortality rates from 1980 to 1994 are shown for whites (Figure 6.6) and blacks (Figure 6.7).

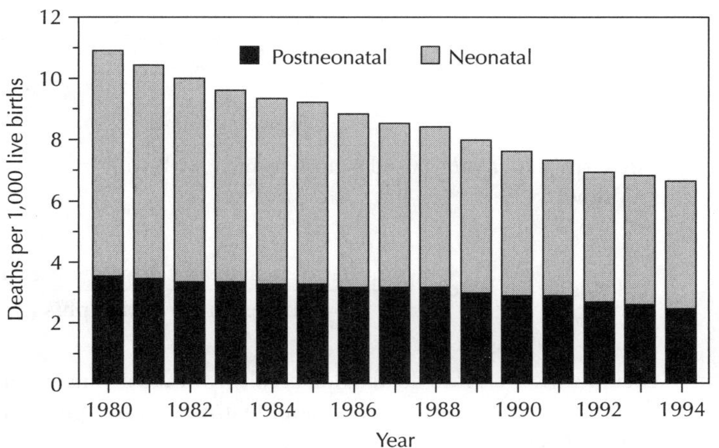

FIGURE 6.6 Infant Mortality Among Whites by Age of Death—United States, 1980–1994. (Centers for Disease Control and Prevention. *MMWR*. 1998;47:SS-2.)

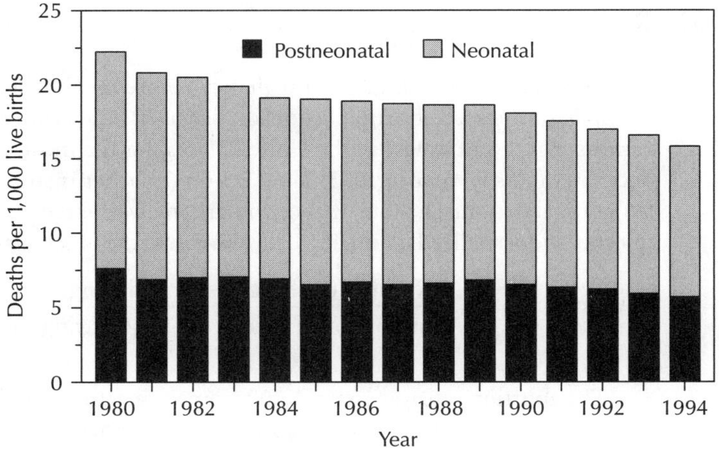

FIGURE 6.7 Infant Mortality Among Blacks by Age of Death—United States, 1980–1994. (Centers for Disease Control and Prevention. *MMWR*. 1998;47:SS-2.)

Perinatal Mortality Rates

The period of greatest risk of death to all populations is the perinatal period (the period around the time of birth) and the period after age 60. The **perinatal mortality rate** is calculated as follows.

$$\text{Perinatal Mortality Rate} = \frac{\text{Number of stillbirths and deaths in infants 6 days of age or younger}}{\text{Number of births (live and still)}} \times 1{,}000$$

Fetal Death Rate

The term *fetal death* is used synonymously with stillbirth. The **fetal death rate** is calculated as follows.

$$\text{Fetal Death Rate} = \frac{\text{Number of fetal deaths after at least 20 weeks gestation}}{\text{Number of live births plus fetal deaths}} \times 1{,}000$$

Fetal deaths are those deaths that result from the expulsion or extraction of the fetus from the womb. When the fetus does not breathe or show signs of life upon leaving the mother's womb, it is dead. Signs of life are usually determined by breathing, a beating heart, pulsating umbilical cord, or voluntary muscle movement. The fetal death rate was developed as a measure of risk of the stages of gestation. The fetal death rate is usually defined by death after the 20th week of gestation.

ABORTION RATE

The deliberate termination of a pregnancy before the fetus is capable of living outside the womb is an induced abortion. Abortion has been legal (with restrictions and limitations in various places and states) in the United States, for the most part, since the Supreme Court decision of *Roe v Wade* in 1973. The Alan Guttmacher Institute and the CDC maintain statistics on abortion. The rate of abortion among women in the United States is greater than in other industrialized countries. The **abortion rate** is calculated as follows.

$$\text{Abortion Rate} = \frac{\text{Number of abortions done during a specified time period}}{\text{Number of women ages 15–44 during the same time period}} \times 1{,}000$$

The abortion rate was 16 per 1,000 women ages 15–44 in the United States in 2001. Surveillance indicates that women most likely to report an abortion are unmarried (82%), white (55%), and younger than 25 years (52%). Among all abortions performed, 88% were performed at less than 13 weeks gestation (59% less than 9 weeks gestation). There were a limited number of abortions performed at later gestational age (4.3% at 16–20 weeks gestation and 1.4% after 20 weeks gestation).[11]

MATERNAL MORTALITY RATES

The **maternal mortality rate** is an important health status indicator of a population. Maternal mortality estimates the proportion of pregnant women who die from causes related to or aggravated by the childbirth process: labor and delivery, poor obstetric care, pregnancy complications, puerperium problems, and poor management. This indicator is influenced by general socioeconomic conditions; unsatisfactory health conditions related to sanitation, nutrition, and care preceding the pregnancy; incidence of the various complications of pregnancy and childbirth; and availability and utilization of health care facilities, including prenatal and obstetric care. Maternal mortality is viewed as a tremendous loss to society because it disrupts the lives of family members, destroys the structure of young families, cuts short the mother's life at an early age, and leaves young children without a mother.

Maternal mortality rate is calculated as follows.

$$\text{Maternal Mortality Rate} = \frac{\text{Number of deaths due to childbirth during a specified time period}}{\text{Number of live births in the same time period}} \times 100{,}000$$

Maternal mortality estimates in 2000 were considerably higher in developing regions of the world than they were in developed regions (Table 6.2). The highest maternal mortality rate is in Africa. In sub-Saharan Africa, the lifetime risk of maternal death is 1 in 16. In contrast, in developed regions, the lifetime risk of maternal death is 1 in 2,800.

TABLE 6.2 World Estimates of Maternal Mortality in 2000

	Maternal Mortality per 100,000 Live Births	*Number of Maternal Deaths*	*Lifetime Risk of Maternal Death: 1 in*
World total	400	529,000	74
Developed regions*	20	2,500	2,800
Developing regions	440	527,000	61
Africa	830	251,000	20
Northern Africa†	130	4,600	210
Sub-Saharan Africa	920	247,000	16
Asia	330	253,000	94
Eastern Asia	55	11,000	840
South central Asia	520	207,000	46
Southeast Asia	210	25,000	140
Western Asia	190	9,800	120
Latin America and the Caribbean	190	22,000	160
Oceania	240	530	83

*Europe, Canada, United States, Japan, Australia, New Zealand.
†Sudan is included in sub-Saharan Africa. (Source: Maternal mortality in 2000: Estimates developed by WHO, UNICEF and UNFPA. Available at: http://www.who.int/reproductive-health/publications/maternal_mortality_2000/index.html. Accessed June 14, 2005.)

PROPORTIONAL MORTALITY RATIO

The **proportional mortality ratio** (PMR) is a ratio of the number of deaths attributed to a specific cause to the total number of deaths occurring in the population during a specified time period. It indicates the burden of a given cause of death relative to all deaths. The PMR is calculated as follows.

$$\text{Proportionate Mortality Ratio (PMR)} = \frac{\text{Number of deaths from a specific cause during a specified time period}}{\text{Number of deaths in the same time period}} \times 100$$

Some epidemiologists suggest caution when using the PMR. If the PMR is used to compare differences between different groups or different time periods, it has some limitations. If different populations have varying causes of disease that lead to death, and if mortality rates are compared with the PMR, it can provide distorted findings. The PMR is not a measure of risk or of probability of dying from a specific cause within a group. Comparing percentages is always risky, and this is true for the PMR. Rates instead of proportions are a more accurate means of comparison.[3,10,12] Here is an example of a PMR.

- Two cities each had a population of 1,000,000.
- Death rate from all causes in Metro City was 400 or 40 per 100,000.
- Death rate from all causes in Suburban City was 900 or 90 per 100,000.
- Cancer deaths in both cities were 4 per 100,000 or 40 deaths per city. Risk of a cancer-caused death for both cities was the same.
- Percentage of all deaths from cancer is the proportionate mortality ratio. For each city the PMR was

$$\text{Metro City} = \frac{40}{400} \times 100 = 10\%$$

$$\text{Suburban City} = \frac{40}{900} \times 100 = 4.4\%$$

The PMR fails to reflect the risk of a cancer death in these two cities, even though the actual numbers are the same. Deaths from all causes are different. PMR can be useful in determining, within a given subgroup or population, the extent to which a specific cause of death contributes to the overall mortality.

CASE FATALITY RATE

The case fatality rate is used to link mortality to morbidity. In this modern era of environmental and occupationally caused diseases, this rate may have wider applications than just its traditional usefulness with infectious diseases. Environmental exposures and injury can cause acute deaths and need to be measured. The **case fatality rate** measures the risk of persons dying from a certain disease within a given time period. One function of the case fatality rate is to measure various aspects or properties of a disease such as its pathogenicity, severity, or virulence.

In the past, the case fatality rate was used more for studying acute infectious diseases. However, it can also be used in poisonings, chemical exposures, or other short-term, non-disease-caused deaths. The case fatality rate has had limited usefulness in the study of chronic diseases because the time of onset may be hard to determine, and the time from diagnosis to death is longer. The number of deaths that occur in a current time period may have little relationship to the number of new cases that occur. Prevention and control measures may already be in place for new cases, but long-term and past exposed cases may still die. Whenever the case fatality rate is used, it is good to make a statement regarding the time element. If the case fatality rate is used for chemical or hazardous waste or occupational health exposures, the time dimension has some limitations and may vary. Occupational or chemical exposures may cause some acute deaths and, at the same time, cause many chronic diseases that bring death years later.

The case fatality rate is calculated as follows.

$$\text{Case Fatality Rate} = \frac{\text{Number of deaths from a specific disease during a specified time period}}{\text{Number of cases of the disease during the same time period}} \times 10^n$$

The rate base is usually $10^2 = 100$.

To illustrate the case fatality rate, consider a study of severe acute respiratory syndrome (SARS) conducted among 1,425 cases reported through April 28, 2003, in Hong Kong. Researchers estimated the case fatality rate to be 13.2% for patients younger than 60 years and 43.4% for patients 60 years and older. Although age was strongly associated with outcome, the time between the onset of symptoms and admission to the hospital did not influence the outcome.[13]

YEARS OF POTENTIAL LIFE LOST

Years of potential life lost (YPLL) is a measure of public health relative to the value of human life and the economic implications of the loss of individuals in a society. Improvements in life expectancy can cause an increase in the available work force, which, in turn, benefits society by increasing productivity. A 20-year-old who dies in an automobile accident that results from drinking and driving could theoretically have lived to an average life expectancy of 75 years of age; thus 55 years of life are lost. When 2,000 deaths like this occur, 110,000 years of potential life are lost.

Some sources calculate YPLL based on the retirement age of 65 because this concept can be seen from a strictly economic point of view. However, the social and humane aspects need to be considered; thus average life expectancy rather than age of retirement may be more appropriate. Questions are often raised such as "What is life worth?" The losses to society in the cost of training, labor, and tax dollars not paid are often considered. The value of human life is an underlying goal of public health, as are economic factors, because both issues have far-reaching societal implications.[14]

YPLL is a measure of premature death in the population. The formula for computation is

$$\text{YPLL} = \Sigma\ (\text{end point} - \text{age at death before end point})$$

where the end point is predetermined at age 65 or the average life expectancy. For grouped data, this formula is modified.

$$\text{YPLL} = \Sigma \text{ for all age groups } (\text{\# deaths in each age group}) \times (\text{end point} - \text{midpoint of the age group})$$

The midpoint is derived as follows.

$$\text{midpoint} = \frac{\text{age group's youngest age in years} + \text{oldest age} + 1}{2}$$

To illustrate, consider the data in Table 6.3. Use an endpoint age of 65 years. Next, calculate the midpoint age for each age group up to the age group just prior to age 65. The years to 65 are obtained by subtracting each midpoint age from 65. This represents the years of life lost on average for a person who dies in the age group. Then multiply the values in this column by the actual number of deaths in that age group to get the age-specific YPLL. The sum of all the age-specific YPLL equals the YPLL across the age groups. The age group representing the highest YPLL because of accidents and adverse effects is 25–29 for white males and 20–24 for black males. The YPLL across all age groups is 1,254,565 for white males and 219,655 for black males.

In order to get a better sense as to whether the burden of death from accidents and adverse effects is different between white and black males, it is useful to calculate the YPLL rate. The **YPLL rate** is calculated as follows.

$$\text{YPLL Rate} = \frac{\text{YPLL}}{\text{Number in the population below the selected endpoint}} \times 10^n$$

The YPLL rate per 100,000 for white males is 1,221.7 (1,254,565/102,690,820 × 100,000). The rate for black males is 1,306.7 (219,655/16,810,259 × 100,000).

The YPLL rate allows meaningful comparisons of the burden of certain diseases or conditions among selected groups. For example, the YPLL through age 89 because of cigarette smoking in Utah, 1994–1998, was estimated to be 22,338 for Latter-Day Saints (LDS or Mormon) men and 21,771 for non-LDS men. Although LDS have a larger burden of smoking-related deaths in Utah, this statistic is misleading because about 70% of the male population in the state are LDS. The YPLL rate gives a much different picture of the burden of smoking-related deaths in Utah: 600.6 for LDS males and 1,676.7 for non-LDS males per 100,000.[15]

A concept related to YPLL is that of quality-adjusted life years. This is an indicator of well-being that measures mental, physical, and social functioning. It combines both mortality and morbidity and is sensitive to changes in health among both the well and the ill. By multiplying the measure of well-being by the number of years of life remaining at each age interval, an estimate of the years of healthy life for a population can be determined. The calculation of years of healthy life uses life tables and the average number of years of life remaining at the beginning of each age interval. Also needed are age-specific estimates of the

TABLE 6.3 Males: Deaths Attributed to Accidents and Adverse Effects by Age Group and Race*

			White				Black			
Age Group (years)	*Midpoint (age)*	*Years to 65*	*No.*	*Population*	*Age-Specific YPLL*	*Cumulative YPLL*	*No.*	*Population*	*Age-Specific YPLL*	*Cumulative YPLL*
0–4	2.5	62.5	1,094	7,812,751	68,375	1,254,565	415	1,619,647	25,938	219,655
5–9	7.5	57.5	497	7,952,436	28,578	1,186,190	185	1,673,129	10,638	193,718
10–14	12.5	52.5	743	8,410,288	39,008	1,157,613	215	1,781,594	11,288	183,080
15–19	17.5	47.5	4,214	8,249,523	200,165	1,118,605	558	1,610,992	26,505	171,793
20–24	22.5	42.5	5,465	8,277,120	232,263	918,440	740	1,500,081	31,450	145,288
25–29	27.5	37.5	3,907	7,656,055	146,513	686,178	677	1,263,507	25,388	113,838
30–34	32.5	32.5	4,079	8,451,370	132,568	539,665	632	1,323,363	20,540	88,450
35–39	37.5	27.5	4,546	8,887,180	125,015	407,098	803	1,359,218	22,083	67,910
40–44	42.5	22.5	5,494	9,427,428	123,615	282,083	789	1,358,995	17,753	45,828
45–49	47.5	17.5	4,949	8,761,339	86,608	158,468	853	1,183,241	14,928	28,075
50–54	52.5	12.5	3,715	7,770,340	46,438	71,860	699	962,180	8,738	13,148
55–59	57.5	7.5	2,681	6,261,800	20,108	25,423	478	670,348	3,585	4,410
60–64	62.5	2.5	2,126	4,773,190	5,315	5,315	330	503,964	825	825
65–69	–	–	1,965	3,860,448			304	400,502		
70–74	–	–	2,351	3,434,848			235	299,667		
75–79	–	–	2,939	2,763,509			256	217,854		
80–84	–	–	3,151	1,818,398			196	130,367		
85+	–	–	4,484	1,244,614			243	92,967		

*Whites and Blacks, United States, 2002.[16]

well-being of a population compared with the population of the life table. As the life span expands, the tradeoffs between quantity and quality of life become more and more critical. Years of healthy life is an important indicator for populations and must be considered in policy and public health administration activities.[17]

EXERCISES

Key Terms

Define the following terms.

Abortion rate
Birth rate
Case fatality rate
Cause-specific mortality rate
Crude mortality rate
Death certificate
Fetal death rate
Infant mortality rate
Maternal mortality rate
Mortality
Neonatal mortality rate
Perinatal mortality rate
Postneonatal mortality rate
Proportional mortality ratio
Years of potential life lost (YPLL)
YPLL rate

Study Questions

6.1 Refer to the following estimated statistics for the United States and Malaysia in 2005.

United States

Crude death rate = 800 per 100,000
Crude birth rate = 14 per 1,000
Life expectancy = 77.7 years

Malaysia

Crude death rate = 500 per 100,000
Crude birth rate = 23 per 1,000
Life expectancy = 72.2 years

Can the lower crude death rate in Malaysia be explained by the fact that the United States has a larger population? What factors could explain differences in birth rates and life expectancy?

6.2 Table 6.4 gives the mortality statistics for a fictitious county in a rural state for the period from July 1 to June 30 (1 year). After reviewing the health status indicators and mortality data, calculate the following mortality rates.

a. crude death rate
b. maternal mortality rate
c. infant mortality rate
d. neonatal mortality rate
e. fetal mortality rate
f. fertility rate
g. age-specific mortality rate for persons ages 55 years or older
h. cause-specific mortality rates for those who died from heart disease
i. cause-specific mortality rates for those who died from stroke
j. *PMR* for cancer among persons ages 55 years or older

TABLE 6.4 Mortality Statistics for a Hypothetical Population, July 1 to June 30

Total one-year population	160,000
Population of women 15–44 years of age	40,000
Population of 55 years of age and older	44,000
Number of live births	3,300
Number of fetal deaths	66
Number of maternal deaths	5
Total deaths	1,444
Number of infant deaths	88
Number of deaths under 28 days old	4
Number of deaths between 20 weeks gestation and 28 days old	8
Number of deaths of persons 55 years and older	848
Number one cause of death in the county is heart disease—deaths from heart disease	133
Number two cause of death in the county is from cancer—deaths from cancer	66
Number three cause of death in the county is from cerebrovascular accident (stroke)	56
Number four cause of death in the county is accidents	45
Number of deaths from cancer age 55 years and older	44
Number of persons diagnosed with heart disease	5,600
Number of deaths from other causes	504
Number of persons diagnosed with high blood pressure, arteriosclerosis, and atherosclerosis (precursors for a stroke)	1,200

6.3 Two cities each had a population of 1,000,000. The death rate from all causes in Desert City was 500 or 50 per 100,000. The death rate from all causes in Sun City was 800 or 80 per 100,000. Cancer deaths in both cities were 4 per 100,000 or 40 deaths per city. Risk of cancer-caused death for both cities was the same. Calculate the *PMR* for cancer in each city.

6.4 Fill out the standard death certificate with the following information: Mr. Captain J. C. Hook was born on October 31, 1790, in Seaside City, Ocean County, Never-Never Land, to Mr. and Mrs. Pegleg Hook. His mother, Lisa, died in childbirth. His first name was John. Captain Hook listed his official occupation as earning his living as a ship's captain. He died in Seaside City, in Ocean View Regional Medical Center; the cause of death was stated as multiple puncture wounds due to crocodile bites, but the autopsy report listed the actual cause of death as drowning. A distinguishing clinical identifying mark on Mr. Hook was that his left hand had been amputated just above the wrist. John Hook had only completed third grade and spent 46 years of his life in Never-Never Land, where he was captain of a ship for 25 years. Mr. Hook was never married but had one survivor, a 22-year-old daughter named Ruby, who lived in Havana, Cuba. The attending physician's name was Sharp E. Blade, DO. The coroner who did the autopsy was Dr. Cutt M. Upp. Captain Hook served in Her

Majesty's Navy from 1808 to 1812. The funeral director who signed the death certificate was Barry M. Deep. Hook was buried on Friday, December 13, 1836, 5 days after his death. Witnesses stated that the crocodile attack occurred at noon during lunch, in a rowboat near the ship.

6.5 Infant mortality and maternal mortality are two of the most commonly used health status indicators. Why?

For questions 6.6 through 6.10 refer to Table 6.5.

6.6 Calculate the crude mortality rate for all causes, all malignant cancers, accidents and adverse events, suicide and self-inflicted injury, and homicide and legal intervention.

6.7 Calculate the YPLL, using age 65 years as the end point, for each of the causes of death listed in the table.

6.8 The number of cancer deaths is about 3.8 times higher than the number of deaths due to accidents and adverse effects, yet the YPLL is about 1.4 times higher for deaths from accidents and adverse effects versus from cancer. Why?

6.9 Calculate the YPLL rate for each of the causes of death listed in Table 6.5.

6.10 If you were interested in comparing the burden of deaths from homicide and legal intervention between white and black males, would you prefer the YPLL rate over YPLL? Why or why not?

TABLE 6.5 Deaths* Attributed to all Causes for Black Males in the United States[16]

	Population	*All Causes*	*All Malignant Cancers*	*Accidents*	*Suicide*	*Homicide and Legal Intervention*
0–4	1,619,647	5,354	38	415	0	148
5–14	3,454,723	998	106	400	29	88
15–24	3,111,073	5,364	140	1,298	351	2,618
25–34	2,586,870	6,848	290	1,309	447	2,157
35–44	2,718,213	11,849	1172	1,592	354	1,084
45–54	2,145,421	21,122	4,240	1,552	219	593
55–64	1,174,312	24,000	7,183	808	99	183
65–74	700,169	28,198	8,931	539	68	75
75–84	348,221	28,478	7,749	452	48	48
85+	92,967	14,584	2,776	243	18	6

*For the year 2002.

REFERENCES

1. US Census Bureau. US and world population clocks—POPClocks. Available at: http://www.census.gov/main/www/popclock.html. Accessed June 12, 2005.
2. Weeks JR. *Population*. 2nd ed. Belmont, CA: Wadsworth; 1981.
3. Mausner J, Bahn A. *Epidemiology, an Introductory Text*. 2nd ed. Philadelphia, PA: Saunders; 1983.
4. Slome C, Brogan D, Eyres S, Lednar W. *Basic Epidemiological Methods and Biostatistics: A Workbook*. Monterey, CA: Wadsworth; 1982.
5. Rothman KJ. *Modern Epidemiology*. Boston, MA: Little, Brown and Company; 1986.
6. World Health Organization. *International Statistical Classification of Diseases and Related Health Problems*, 10th rev., Version for 2003. Available at: http://www3.who.int/icd/vol1htm2003/fr-icd.htm. Accessed September 26, 2005.
7. Golding J, Emmett PM, Rogers IS. Breast feeding and infant mortality. *Early Hum Dev*. 1997;49 (Suppl):S143–S155.
8. Centers for Disease Control and Prevention (CDC). Ten great public health achievements—United States, 1900–1999. *MMWR*. 1999;48:1141–1143.
9. CDC. Racial and ethnic disparities in infant mortality rates—60 largest US cities, 1995–1998. *MMWR*. 2002;51(15):329–332, 343.
10. Fox JP, Hall CE, Elveback LR. *Epidemiology: Man and Disease*. New York, NY: Macmillan; 1970.
11. Strauss LT, Herndon J, Chang J, Parker WY, Bowens SV, Zane SB, et al. Abortion surveillance—United States, 2001. *MMWR*. 2004;53(SS09):1–32.
12. Lilienfeld AM, Lilienfeld DE. *Foundations of Epidemiology*. New York, NY: Oxford University Press; 1980.
13. Donnelly CA, Ghani AC, Leung GM, et al. Epidemiological determinants of spread of causal agent of severe acute respiratory syndrome in Hong Kong. *Lancet*. 2003;361:1761–1766.
14. Pickett G, Hanlon JJ. *Public Health: Administration and Practice*. St. Louis, MO: Times Mirror/Mosby; 1990.
15. Merrill RM, Hilton SC, Daniels M. Impact of the LDS church's health doctrine on deaths from diseases and conditions associated with cigarette smoking. *Ann Epidemiol*. 2003;13:704–711.
16. Surveillance Research Program, National Cancer Institute SEER*Stat software (www.seer.cancer.gov/seerstat) version 6.1.4. Also available at: http://seer.cancer.gov/csr/1975_2002/results_merged/sect_23_prostate.pdf. Accessed May 23, 2005.
17. US Department of Health and Human Services. *Healthy People 2010: Understanding and Improving Health*. 2nd ed. Washington, DC: US Government Printing Office; 2000.

CHAPTER

7

Design Strategies and Statistical Methods in Analytic Epidemiology

OBJECTIVES

After completing this chapter you will be able to

- Define analytic epidemiology.
- Distinguish between observational and experimental analytic epidemiologic studies.
- Define case-control and cohort studies and identify their distinctive features, strengths, and weaknesses.
- Identify appropriate measures of association in case-control and cohort studies.
- Identify common measures used in epidemiology for describing cohort data.
- Identify potential biases in case-control and cohort studies.
- Identify ways to control for biases in case-control and cohort studies at the design and analysis levels.
- Distinguish between effect modification and confounding.

INTRODUCTION

The two general areas of epidemiologic study, descriptive and analytic, have already been introduced. Chapters 4 and 5, "Design Strategies and Statistical Methods in Descriptive Epidemiology" and "Descriptive Epidemiology According to Person, Place, and Time," focused on descriptive study designs. Chapter 6, "General Health and Population Indicators," focused on descriptive health indicators. The focus of this chapter is analytic study designs.

An analytic study attempts to identify causes or risk factors that explain health-related states or events and tests specific *a priori* hypotheses that are often developed in descriptive studies. **Analytic studies** are distinct from descriptive studies in that they make use of a comparison group. Analytic studies have been classified into two general categories: observational and experimental. In analytic observational studies, researchers evaluate the strength of the relationship between an exposure and disease variables. (A **variable** is any characteristic that can be measured or categorized.) The observed variables are beyond the control or influence of the researchers.

On the other hand, in analytic experimental studies, some of the **subjects** (ie, participants in a research study) are assigned an intervention while others are not, or subjects in various groups receive different levels of an intervention. The efficacy of the intervention is then determined. For those interventions that cannot be ethically assigned (eg, subjecting study participants to cigarette smoking, surgery, radiation), potential risk factors can be ethically assessed with observational study designs. When the study is restricted to human subjects who are assigned the intervention on the individual level, it is called a controlled trial. When the intervention is assigned to human subjects on the group level, it is called a community trial. Experimental studies will be discussed further in the next chapter.

OBSERVATIONAL EPIDEMIOLOGIC STUDIES

Observational studies include case-control and cohort (prospective and retrospective) studies. These studies can be exploratory (no specific *a priori* hypothesis) or analytic (specific *a priori* hypothesis). In **exploratory observational studies** a variety of associations are examined. Such studies are useful for identifying clues as to cause-effect relationships. However, the focus of this chapter and the next is on analytic observational and experimental studies, which test specific *a priori* hypotheses.

CASE-CONTROL STUDY DESIGN

Case-control studies originated in the 1920s, and the case-control study design is very common in the literature.[1,2] This study design allows researchers to both evaluate diseases with long latency periods and evaluate one or more exposure variables associated with a given outcome. Other names for case-control studies that appear in the literature are case-comparison studies and case-referent studies. A **case-control study** involves grouping people as cases (persons experiencing a health-related state or event) and controls and investigating whether the cases are more or less likely than controls to have had past experiences, lifestyle behaviors, or exposures. In other words, what is it about their past that made them cases? The outcome is identified before the exposure. Because a case-control study begins with the outcome and looks back at an antecedent variable or variables, it is retrospective in nature. *Retro spicere* means "to look back." Other epidemiologic studies can also be retrospective in nature. These will be discussed later.

Selection of Cases

Establishing the diagnostic criteria and definition of disease is the first step in conducting a case-control study. A strict diagnostic criterion for the disease will ensure that cases reflect as homogeneous a disease entity as possible. Hennekens and Buring[3] refer to the situation before the 1940s when the definition of uterine cancer comprised two diseases (of the corpus uteri and uterine cervix) with very different risk factors. Low numbers of sexual partners and high socioeconomic status has been associated with uterine cancer, and a high number of sexual partners and low socioeconomic status has been associated with cervical cancer. Hence a case-control study attempting to identify the association between number of sexual partners and socioeconomic status with uterine cancer under this old definition might find no association.

Cases may consist of new cases (incidence) that show selected characteristics during a specific time period in a specified population and a particular area. Cases may also consist of existing cases at a point in time (prevalence). With prevalence data it may be more difficult to link a specific cause with a disease outcome because prevalence is influenced by both the development and duration of disease. For example, suppose researchers were interested in assessing whether an association existed between exercise and the prevalence of arthritis. It may be that exercise patterns before the development of arthritis are much different than after the onset of symptoms; thus the timing of when the exposure was evaluated could have a large impact on the association. For this reason, whenever possible, incident cases are preferred to prevalent cases in case-control studies.

Sources for cases can come from records from public health clinics, physician offices, health maintenance organizations, hospitals, and industrial and government sources. Cases should be representative of all persons with the disease. In some situations, all persons with the disease may be included in the study. It is more common, however, that cases come from sampled data. In order for the sampled data to reflect the population of interest, random selection is required. An adequately large random selection of cases from a population of interest ensures that the results of the study can be appropriately generalized. In some situations researchers may use **restriction** (ie, limiting subjects in a study to those with certain characteristics, such as black males in Atlanta aged 40–59 years) in order to reduce potential biases and to increase feasibility. Although restriction may limit generalization, it may be necessary in order to ensure a valid study. Conducting a valid study with definitive results should always be the primary goal of any epidemiologist.

Selection of Controls

To better ensure that a case-control study is valid and reliable, the control subjects should look like the case subjects with the exception of not having the disease. This means, selecting controls from the same population from which the cases were drawn. An epidemiologic assumption is that controls are representative of the general population in terms of probability of exposure and that controls have the same possibility of being selected or exposed as do the cases. Controls drawn from a population of the same area or populace of the cases should reflect the same sex, age groups, and other significant factors. Controls from a general population are assumed to be normal and healthy and to reflect the well population from the area.

Sampling of controls from a general population for large studies is an expensive endeavor and thus is not always realistic or possible. Controls are typically drawn from the same hospital or general population as the cases. They may also be drawn from the family, friends, or relatives of the cases. Some advantages and disadvantages of these types of controls are presented in Table 7.1. In some circumstances it may be useful to select more than one control group to see if the selection of controls influences the measured association between exposure and outcome variables. It may also be useful to collect more controls than cases when only a few cases are available. This increases the power of the study. The ratio of controls to cases should not exceed 4 to 1.[4] Controls can be randomly selected from a larger population when the entire population of eligible controls is known. Selection of controls can also be made systematically (ie, every *n*th person listed), assuming the order of potential controls is not related to factors such as age, sex, education, etc.

Exposure Status

Once the cases and controls have been identified, ascertainment of exposure status is performed. Information about exposure status can be obtained through medical records, in-

TABLE 7.1 Advantages and Disadvantages of Controls From Hospitals, the General Population, and Special Groups[3]

Controls	***Advantages***	***Disadvantages***
Hospital	• Easily identified, sufficient number, low cost • Subjects more likely aware of antecedent events or exposures • Selection factors that influence decision to come to a particular hospital similar to those for cases • More likely to cooperate, thereby minimizing potential bias from nonresponse	• Differ from healthy people such that they do not accurately represent the exposure distribution in the population where cases were obtained
General Population	• Represent the population from which cases were selected	• More costly and time consuming than hospital controls • Population lists might not be available • May be difficult to contact healthy people with busy work and leisure schedules • May have poorer recall than hospital controls • Less motivated to participate than controls from the hospital or special groups
Special Groups (eg, family, relatives, friends)	• Healthier than hospital controls • More likely to cooperate than people in the general population • Provide more control over possible confounding factors	• If the exposure is similar to the one experienced by cases, an underestimation of the true association would result

terviews, questionnaires, or surrogates, such as spouses, siblings, or employers. Information on exposure status should be collected in a similar manner between cases and controls in order to avoid bias. Blinding interviewers as to who the cases are and who the controls are may further minimize bias. It is also preferable to blind those performing the assessment of the hypothesis of the study because such knowledge could influence how they probe or scan records for information.[3]

Because bias can result in studies where the results are based on individual recall, exposure information from medical records is always preferable, when available. For example, researchers interested in assessing the association between chest radiographs during adolescence and female breast cancer should use medical records indicating whether chest radiographs were performed rather than relying on the recall of the study participants, assuming the records exist. It is possible that if the study is based on recall, that women with breast cancer would have better recall of having had chest radiographs than women without breast cancer, thereby biasing the results.

The time window, on which exposure status in relation to the outcome is determined, is critical in case-control studies. This should be influenced by current understanding of the potential causal factors associated with the disease. Is a lifetime duration of smoking (number of years smoked) more important than current smoking for selected disease outcomes? With many forms of smoking-related cancers, the lifetime duration of smoking appears to be more important than current smoking. The level of smoking is also important. Hence, an exposure variable that captures the duration and intensity of smoking is much more informative. On the other hand, current smoking has been associated with myocardial infarction.

When limited information of the mechanisms of disease is available, exploring different combinations of the level and duration of exposure is suggested.

STATISTICAL MEASURES OF ASSOCIATION

A commonly used measure of the relative probabilities of disease in case-control studies is the **odds ratio**, or **relative odds**. Before presenting the odds ratio, however, it is helpful to present the **risk ratio**, or **relative risk**. The odds ratio is appropriate for measuring the strength of the association between exposure and disease variables in case-control studies, whereas the risk ratio is appropriate for measuring the association in cohort studies.

The risk ratio reflects the probability of disease among those exposed relative to the probability of disease among the unexposed. Consider the following 2 × 2 table, a type of table that is commonly used in epidemiology to summarize the relationship between exposure and disease variables (Table 7.2). The letters in the table represent numbers that would actually be present in an epidemiologic study.

TABLE 7.2 2 × 2 Table

	Cases	*Controls*	*Total*
Exposed	a	b	$a + b$
Not Exposed	c	d	$c + d$
Total	$a + c$	$b + d$	$n = a + b + c + d$

The risk ratio (*RR*) is calculated as follows.

$$RR = \frac{P(\text{disease} \mid \text{exposed})}{P(\text{disease} \mid \text{unexposed})} = \frac{a/(a+b)}{c/(c+d)}$$

The numerator of the risk ratio is the cumulative incidence rate (or attack rate) of disease among the exposed. The denominator of the risk ratio is the cumulative incidence rate (or attack rate) of disease among the unexposed. These rates are also referred to as measures of risk. A risk ratio equal to 1 indicates no association between exposure and disease, a risk ratio greater than 1 indicates a positive association between exposure and disease, and a risk ratio less than 1 indicates a negative association between exposure and disease. A risk ratio can range from 0 to infinity.

The risk ratio can be interpreted literally. For example, if a risk ratio equals 2.5 in a study looking at the association between current smoking and myocardial infarction, then current smokers are 2.5 times more likely to develop a myocardial infarction than are nonsmokers. If a risk ratio is equal to 0.5 in a study looking at the association between moderate and/or vigorous weekly exercise and myocardial infarction, then moderate and/or vigorous weekly exercisers are 0.5 times as likely as people with lower levels of exercise to develop myocardial infarction. These risk ratios can also be expressed as *percent change*. The general formulas for expressing risk ratios as percentages are as follows.

$$\%\text{Increase Change} = (RR - 1) \times 100 \quad \text{for } RR > 1$$
$$\%\text{Decrease Change} = (1 - RR) \times 100 \quad \text{for } RR < 1$$

Thus, in the first example it appears that current smokers are 150% more likely to develop myocardial infarction than those who do not currently smoke. In the second example, people who engage in moderate and/or vigorous exercise every week are 50% less likely to develop myocardial infarction than those who do not participate in this level of exercise.

With case-control data, unless data are considered for the entire population, the total number of exposed or unexposed people will not be known. Hence, the incidence rate of disease among exposed and unexposed people in the population cannot be determined. In a case-control study, the number of cases and controls is chosen by the researchers. In this situation, the appropriate measure of the association between exposure and disease is the odds ratio (*OR*). This measure compares the odds of disease among exposed individuals divided by the odds of disease among unexposed individuals.

$$OR = \frac{P(\text{disease} \mid \text{exposed})/[1 - P(\text{disease} \mid \text{exposed})]}{P(\text{disease} \mid \text{unexposed})/[1 - P(\text{disease} \mid \text{unexposed})]} = \frac{a/b}{c/d} = \frac{a \times d}{b \times c}$$

Like the risk ratio, an odds ratio equal to 1 indicates no association between exposure and disease, an odds ratio greater than 1 indicates a positive association between exposure and disease, and an odds ratio less than 1 indicates a negative association between exposure and disease. An odds ratio can range from 0 to infinity. Generally, interpretation of the odds ratio should be limited to saying the association is positive, negative, or does not exist. The odds ratio has nice mathematical properties that make its use attractive to researchers, one of which is the ability to calculate odds ratios with the use of logistic regression.

For diseases that are rare, which is thankfully true of many diseases, $a + b$ can be approximated by b, and $c + d$ can be approximated by d. Under such circumstances

$$\text{OR} = \frac{a / b}{c / d} \approx \text{RR} = \frac{a /(a + b)}{c /(c + d)}$$

and interpreting the odds ratio literally, as one would the risk ratio, is appropriate.

BIAS IN CASE-CONTROL STUDIES

Bias is defined as systematic error in the collection or interpretation of epidemiologic data. Bias results in inaccurate overestimation or underestimation of the association between exposure and disease. Avoiding bias at the design stage of a study is paramount because of the difficulty of identifying and accounting for it thereafter. Certain potential biases that require consideration as possible explanations for deviations of the results from the truth include selection bias, recall bias, and confounding.

Selection Bias

In case-control studies, **selection bias** refers to the selection of cases and controls for a study that is based in some way on the exposure.[3] With selection bias, the relationship between exposure and disease among participants in the study differs from what the relationship would have been among individuals in the population of interest. Recruiting all cases in a population avoids selection bias.

For example, suppose researchers were interested in assessing the association between postmenopausal hormone use and uterine cancer. What if estrogen use was associated with uterine bleeding such that women taking estrogen were more likely to undergo a physician examination? Refer to Table 7.2, the 2 × 2 table, and let uterine cancer cases and hormone use represent those exposed. In this example c would be too small and d would be too big, given the lower examination levels for non–hormone-replacement users. This would cause the odds ratio to be biased upward. The literature does indicate that some, but not all, of the strong positive association observed between hormone use and uterine cancer in case-control studies in the 1970s was explained by selection bias.[5–8]

Hospital-based case-control studies are prone to selection bias. Consider a hospital-based case-control study assessing the strength of the association between smoking and respiratory diseases. Selecting controls from the hospital will likely underestimate the association between smoking and respiratory diseases because patients with nonrespiratory diseases in the hospital are more likely to be smokers than the general population. Considering the formula for the odds ratio, b would be too big and d would be too small, making the odds ratio biased downward. Hospital-patient selection bias has also been called **Berkson's bias**,[9] named after Dr. Joseph Berkson, who described it in the 1940s. Randomization minimizes this potential bias in experimental studies.

Prevalence-incidence bias, also called **Neyman bias**, is a form of selection bias in case-control studies attributed to selective survival among the prevalent cases (ie, mild, clinically resolved, or fatal cases being excluded from the case group).[10,11] This is not a common form of bias in cohort or experimental studies, but it is common in case-control studies based on prevalence data. For example, if cases with coronary artery disease die rapidly, persons available for study are not the more severe cases. The association between serum cholesterol (high vs low) and coronary artery disease will be underestimated.

Observation Bias

Observation bias can result from differential accuracy of recall between cases and controls (**recall bias**) or because of differential accuracy of exposure information because an interviewer probes cases differently than he or she does controls (**interviewer bias**). Recall bias can occur because cases have spent more time pondering why they became cases and consequently have better recall of their exposure status than do individuals who are controls (recall bias). For example, a woman with a child that has neurologic problems may better recall the flu and high temperature she had during pregnancy than would women who do not have a child with a neurologic problem. Similarly, an interviewer who believes there is an association between the flu during pregnancy and having a child with neurologic problems may probe the cases and the controls differently. This is an argument for blinding the interviewer as to which subjects are cases and which are controls. It also supports the use of medical records for data, if they exist, instead of self-reported information. The odds ratio in this example would be too large, because although a and c might be accurate, b might be too small and d too large.

Misclassification occurs when exposure or disease status is inaccurately assigned. In a case-control study, if exposure or disease status is inaccurate for cases but not controls, or for controls but not cases, we refer to this as differential misclassification. Another name for this is nonrandom misclassification. Observation bias resulting from differential recall between cases and controls is an example of **differential** (or **nonrandom**) **misclassification.** If a similar level of inaccurate assignment of exposure status exists between cases and controls, we refer to this as **nondifferential** (or **random**) **misclassification**. Although differential misclassification may result in overestimation or underestimation of the true association, nondifferential misclassification will always result in underestimation of the true association.

Confounding

Confounding occurs when an extrinsic factor is associated with a disease outcome and, independent of that association, is also associated with the exposure. Several variables are routinely considered as potential confounders in epidemiologic research, such as age, sex, educational level, and smoking. Suppose the researcher was interested in the association between exercise and heart disease. Failure to control for age, which is generally lower in those who exercise and higher in those with heart disease, may make exercise appear more protective against heart disease than it really is.

Newman, Browner, and Hulley[12] presented a hypothetical example of confounding involving an assessment of the association between coffee drinking and myocardial infarction. To begin, consider the following data.

	Myocardial Infarction	No Myocardial Infarction
Coffee	90	60
No Coffee	60	90

$$OR = \frac{90 \times 90}{60 \times 60} = 2.25 \text{ for the association between coffee and myocardial infarction.}$$

However, if the data is stratified by smoking status, the data appears differently.

	Smokers		Nonsmokers	
	Myocardial Infarction	No Myocardial Infarction	Myocardial Infarction	No Myocardial Infarction
Coffee	80	40	10	20
No Coffee	20	10	40	80

$$OR = \frac{80 \times 10}{20 \times 40} = 1 \text{ among smokers, and } OR = \frac{10 \times 80}{40 \times 20} = 1 \text{ among nonsmokers.}$$

The difference between the crude odds ratio and the stratified odds ratio quantifies the magnitude of confounding. To verify that smoking is a confounder, it must be associated with both coffee and myocardial infarction. With a little rearranging of numbers and combining the data in this table, it can be shown that smoking is associated with coffee and smoking is associated with myocardial infarction.

CONTROLLING FOR BIAS IN CASE-CONTROL STUDIES

Because the potential for bias is always present in observational epidemiologic studies, researchers should address how they dealt with this in writing up their studies. Selection and observation bias are best controlled for at the design level. Selection bias can be minimized by considering incident cases and general population controls. Observation bias is best controlled for by blinding subjects, interviewers, and persons assessing the data. Confounding can be minimized by restriction and matching. On the analysis level it can also be controlled for through stratification or multiple-regression analysis.

As mentioned previously, a confounder must be associated with the outcome and, independent of that relation, associated with the exposure. To avoid confounding, the level of the potential confounding variable can be restricted such that there is no longer an association between the exposure and the confounding variable. For example, if age and sex are potential confounders of the association between exercise and heart disease, the assessment could be restricted to include only men in their 50s. Although restriction is a simple and convenient way to control for confounding, it reduces the number of subjects eligible for the study, limits the ability to generalize results, and makes it impossible to evaluate whether an association varies across the levels of the confounding factor.

Matching is a strategy for controlling confounding at both the design and analysis levels of a study. In the example assessing the association between exercise and heart disease, for each case, a control of a similar age and sex could be selected to control for the potential confounding effects of these factors. As a result, the distribution of the confounding factors is forced to be similar between the cases and controls.

Matching controls to cases for confounding factors causes these two groups to be more alike with respect to the factors than if the cases and controls were not matched. For matched variables on true confounders, the cases and controls will have similar exposure status than would otherwise be true. Failure to take this into account in the analysis will result in underestimation of the true association. The purpose of the matching is to ensure sufficient statistical power to analyze associations and control for confounding. Specific analysis techniques are then used, such as the McNemar test.[3]

It is possible, if data on the potential confounding factors are collected at the design level of the study, to adjust for confounding at the analysis level of a study. This can be done by stratification and multiple-regression analysis. Stratification eliminates the association between the confounder and exposure within the strata (see the example in the previous subsection). The Mantel–Haenszel method is useful for estimating a pooled odds ratio across homogeneous strata. Multiple logistic regression, another useful technique, computes odds ratios adjusted for other variables (eg, potential confounders) included in the model.

STRENGTHS AND WEAKNESSES OF CASE-CONTROL STUDIES

A number of strengths and weaknesses have been identified in the literature of case-control studies. Some of these are listed in Table 7.3.

COHORT STUDIES

Cohort as a general term means a group, a band, or body of people. As used in the context of epidemiology, it generally refers to a group of persons being studied who were born in the same year or time period. As time passes, the group moves through different and successive time periods of life; as the group ages, changes can be seen in the health and vital statistics of the group. Health factors as well as deaths are tracked in cohorts (Figure 7.1).

A cohort is a group of individuals sharing a statistical factor(s) (often birth year) in common. Cohorts of persons placed in a group can be studied as a group, either forward in time (prospectively) or backward in time (retrospectively). In a **prospective cohort study**, the predictor variable is measured before the outcome has occurred. In a **retrospective cohort study**, a historical cohort is reconstructed with data on the predictor variable (measured in the past) and data on the outcome collected (measured in the past after some follow-up period).

TABLE 7.3 Selected Strengths and Weaknesses of Case-Control Studies[13]

Strengths	*Weaknesses*
• Useful for studying rare outcomes	• Do not establish sequence of events
• Short duration	• Potential bias in measuring exposure variables
• Relatively inexpensive	• Limited to a single outcome variable
• Relatively small	• Do not yield prevalence, incidence, or excess risk
• Yields odds ratio (usually a good approximation of relative risk)	• Prone to selection and observation bias

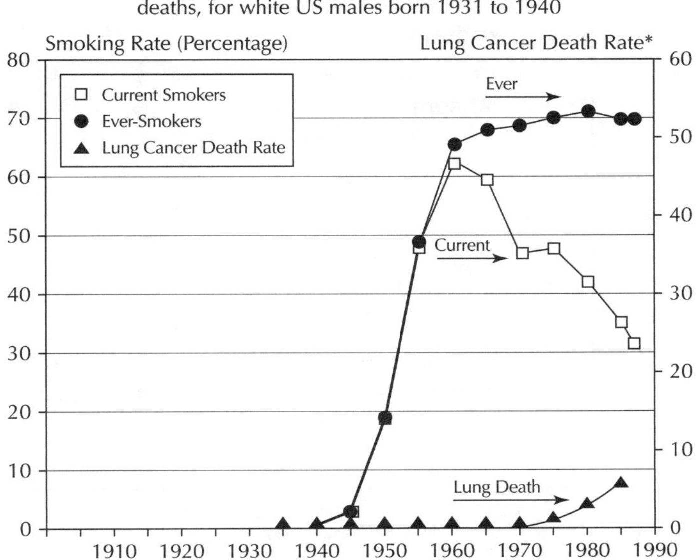

FIGURE 7.1 Smoking Outcomes for Two Different Birth Cohorts. [National Cancer Institute. Strategies to control tobacco use in the United States: a blueprint for public health action in the 1990s. Bethesda, MD: US Department of Health and Human Services, Public Health Service, National Institutes of Health, 1991; DHHS publication no. (NIH) 92-2789.]

Cohorts are divided into exposed and unexposed groups to evaluate whether an association exists between the exposure and the outcome of interest. Figure 7.2 illustrates the interrelationship among exposure status, follow-up time, and outcome for prospective and retrospective cohort studies. The defining distinction between a prospective and retrospective cohort study is the time when the investigator initiates the study, whether before or after the occurrence of the outcome.

Cohort effect, also referred to as generation effect, is the change and variation in the disease or health status of a study population as the study group moves through time. Cohort effects can include any exposure or influence, from environmental factors to societal changes. As each group ages, passes through the phases of the life span, and is exposed to the changes of life, such effects will be seen in each person within a cohort, and this will affect the results of the study.

As the cohort advances through time, the incidence rate of the outcome of interest is tracked and compared between exposed and unexposed groups. An advantage of the cohort study over the case-control study is that the incidence rate of several outcome variables can be determined and associated with the exposure variable. As time passes, an increasing number of outcome variables may be considered.

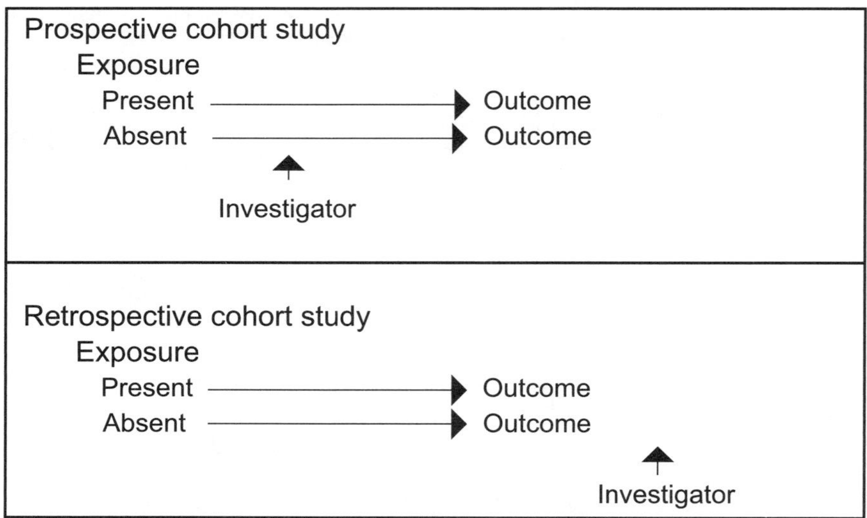

FIGURE 7.2 Time of Prospective and Retrospective.

When the total time that exposed and unexposed subjects are at risk is available rather than the total number of subjects in the two groups, the presentation of the 2 × 2 table is modified (Table 7.4). The cells *a* and *c* still represent the number of exposed and unexposed cases, respectively. However, PT_e now represents the total number of person–time units of follow-up among those exposed and PT_o represents the total number of person–time units of follow-up among those unexposed. Although it may not be possible to derive the values of cells *b* and *d*, it is possible to calculate **person–time rates** for those exposed and not exposed. The ratio of these rates is derived as follows.

$$\text{Rate Ratio} = \frac{P(\text{disease} \mid \text{exposed})}{P(\text{disease} \mid \text{unexposed})} = \frac{a / PT_e}{c / PT_o}$$

When the denominator in a rate calculation is in person–time units, the rate is referred to as an **incidence density rate.** In contrast, when the denominator of the rate calculation reflects the total number of subjects, the rate is called a **cumulative incidence rate** (**attack rate**). The rate ratio is appropriate for measuring the association between exposure and outcome variables in cohort studies when incidence density rates (person–time rates) are in-

TABLE 7.4 Cohort Data with Person-time Denominators

	Disease	*No Disease*	*Total*
Exposed	*a*	—	PT_e
Not Exposed	*c*	—	PT_o
Total	*a* + *c*	—	$PT_e + PT_o$

volved. On the other hand, the risk ratio or relative risk, defined earlier, is appropriate for measuring the association between exposure and outcome variables in cohort studies when cumulative incidence rates (attack rates) are involved.

Although the odds ratio is used to measure associations in case-control studies, it is sometimes used in cohort studies as a matter of convenience when multiple logistic regression is employed to adjust for confounding factors. Also, recall that if the disease outcome is rare, the odds ratio approximates the risk ratio. However, in the strict sense, risk ratio and rate ratios are the appropriate measures for cohort studies.

There are several cohort-based measures that are used in epidemiology for communicating health information. Selected measures are presented in Table 7.5. The formulas for these measures are defined in the context of data in the 2 × 2 table (Table 7.2).

If the numbers of person–time units were available rather than the total numbers of individuals in exposed and unexposed groups, then $a + b$ should be replaced by PT_e and $c + d$ replaced by PT_o in Table 7.5. To illustrate these measures when person-years are involved, refer to Table 7.6 The incidence rate per 100,000 person-years of cardiovascular disease among current smokers is 399 and among noncurrent smokers is 356; overall the rate is 379. The rate ratio (risk ratio) is 1.122, meaning male current smokers are 1.122 times (or 12.2%) more likely than nonsmokers to develop cardiovascular disease.

TABLE 7.5 Commonly Used Epidemiologic Measures for Describing Cohort Data

Cumulative incidence rate in the exposed group:	$I_e = [a/(a + b)] \times 10^n$
Cumulative incidence rate in the unexposed group:	$I_o = [c/(c + d)] \times 10^n$
Cumulative incidence in the total group:	$I_t = [(a + c)/n] \times 10^n$
Risk ratio (or relative risk):	$RR = I_e / I_o$
Attributable risk:	$AR = I_e - I_o$
Attributable risk percent:	$AR\% = (I_e - I_o)/I_e \times 100 = (RR - 1)/RR \times 100$
Population-attributable risk:	$PAR = I_t - I_o$
Population attributable-risk percent:	$PAR\% = (I_t - I_o)/I_t \times 100$

TABLE 7.6 Total Cardiovascular Disease According to Smoking Status*

	Cases	*Controls*	*Person-Years*
Current smoker	882	—	220,965
Nonsmoker	673	—	189,254
Total	1,555	—	410,219

*Study population of 41,782 men aged 40–79 living in 45 communities across Japan from 1988 to 1990 through the end of 1999. (Source: Iso H, Date C, Yamamoto A, et al. Smoking cessation and mortality from cardiovascular disease among Japanese men and women: The JACC study. *Am J Epidemiol.* 2005;161(2):170–179.)

When a causal assumption is made between an exposure and an outcome, the difference in risks is called the **attributable risk**, which is the absolute risk in the exposed group attributable to the exposure. The attributable risk is calculated as the difference in cumulative incidence (risk difference) or incidence densities (rate difference), depending on whether an attack rate or person–time rate is being calculated.[3] The attributable risk is 43 per 100,000 (399–356 per 100,000). Thus the excess occurrence of cardiovascular disease among male smokers that can be attributed to their smoking is 43 per 100,000.

Attributable risk percent can be calculated with the I_e and I_o or the risk ratio. The attributable risk percent equals 10.9% [(1.122 − 1)/1.122 × 100]. This means that if smoking causes cardiovascular disease, nearly 10.9% of cardiovascular disease in males who currently smoke is attributable to their smoking.

Population-attributable risk also assumes a causal association between exposure and disease. The population-attributable risk for the example is 23 per 100,000. This reflects the amount of cardiovascular disease in the population that is attributable to current smoking. This measure says if current smoking were eliminated from the population, the cardiovascular disease incidence rate could be expected to drop by 23 per 100,000.

The **population-attributable risk percent** is perhaps more easily interpretable. In the example, the population-attributable risk percent is 6.2% [(379 − 356)/379 × 100]. This means that if smoking were eliminated from the population, a 6.2% decrease in the incidence rate of cardiovascular disease could be expected.

DOUBLE-COHORT STUDIES

Double-cohort studies are distinct from conventional cohort studies in that two distinct populations are involved with different levels of an exposure of interest. To construct a double-cohort study, samples are taken from each of the two populations, unless the populations are small enough such that they are considered in their entirety. The two cohorts are followed up, and the outcome of interest is measured. Double cohorts are employed when the exposure is rare and a relatively small number of people are affected.

For example, suppose a chemical leak occurred at a manufacturing company. The chemical was suspected of causing neurologic problems. The group of workers exposed to the chemical leak was monitored over time for neurologic disorders. Another group of manufacturing workers at a nearby company served as a comparison group of unexposed persons. This group was also followed into the future, and the level of neurologic disorders was compared with that of the exposed group.

SELECTING THE STUDY COHORT

When selecting the study cohort, the population of study should be reviewed to ascertain those people or groups that are likely to become cases. Individuals who already have a disease outcome of interest (prevalent cases) or who are not at risk (eg, they have had an organ removed such that they cannot become a case) should be excluded from the study. For example, a woman having undergone a total hysterectomy should be excluded from a cohort of women being investigated for uterine cancer. In addition, persons with latent infections or recurring diseases, such as the chronic fatigue immune deficiency syndrome caused by the herpes virus (sometimes implicated in uterine cancer), present a problem because the disease may not be easily diagnosed. It may also be necessary to exclude such individuals. In the interest of saving time and money and avoiding unnecessary testing and effort, appropriate exclusion criteria for a cohort study must be given utmost attention.

Restriction is commonly used in cohort studies. This limits generalization but often improves feasibility and focus. Restriction involves selecting cohorts with limited exposure and a narrow range of behaviors or activities. It can also mean selecting from a limited work environment with restricted exposures or health problems. Heart disease is a health condition often studied among specific working groups, such as mail carriers, longshoremen, and other workers. Cohort studies focusing on respiratory disease may restrict the study to coke workers at steel mills or garment factory workers.

Cohort studies need to come from populations where sampling can be effectively conducted. Adequate sample size is needed to capture the outcome of interest. Hence, researchers may restrict the cohort to high-risk individuals, such as middle aged men, in the study of heart disease. For some rare outcomes, it might not be feasible to conduct a prospective cohort study. In such cases a retrospective cohort or case-control study should be employed.

BIAS IN COHORT STUDIES

Biases related to selection and confounding should be considered in cohort studies. Forms of selection bias common in cohort studies are the healthy worker effect, volunteer bias, and loss to follow-up. Misclassification is also a concern in cohort studies. Confounding can occur in cohort studies, but it is more of a concern in double-cohort studies.

Selection Bias

The **healthy worker effect** occurs in cohort studies when workers represent the exposed group, and a sample from the general population represents the unexposed group. This is because workers tend to be healthier, on average, than the general population. In order to work (eg, some workers must pass a physical examination) and maintain a job, a certain level of health is required. On the other hand, the general population includes persons who are not able to get or keep a job because of health problems.

Suppose the researcher was interested in measuring the association between employment at a steel mill and all-cause mortality. Although the workers may be exposed to certain harmful environmental factors, their jobs are often physically demanding, requiring a relatively high level of physical health. These workers may be in better health than an age-, sex-, and racial/ethnic-matched comparison group of people from the same community where the steel workers reside. Consequently, a positive association between working at the steel mill and all-cause mortality is likely to be negatively biased. To avoid this form of bias, a better comparison group would be workers at another manufacturing plant who are not exposed to the same environmental factors as those in the steel mill.

Loss to follow-up is a circumstance in which researchers lose contact with study participants, resulting in unavailable outcome data on those people. This is a common problem in cohort studies, increasingly so in cohorts with longer follow-up times. Loss of participants eligible for follow-up may arise for a number of reasons. Some subjects may refuse to continue their participation, some cannot be located or are unavailable for interview, and participant death is always a possibility. Loss to follow-up can result in a biased estimate of an association if the extent of loss to follow-up is associated with both exposure and disease. For example, in a study assessing the association between sexual abuse during childhood and psychosocial disorders, sexually abused individuals are more likely to drop out of the study if they develop psychosocial disorders than if a person without a history of sexual abuse develops psychosocial disorders.

As a general rule, the validity of a study requires that loss to follow-up not exceed 20%. Eliminating those not likely to remain in the study, periodic contact with participants, and incentives for participation are approaches frequently used to minimize the problem. The effect of loss to follow-up can be indirectly measured by calculating the risk ratio, assuming that all those lost would have developed the outcome—then recalculating the risk ratio assuming that none of those lost to follow-up would have developed the outcome. This provides a range wherein the true value lies. In some cases, the range of the risk ratio will not overlap 1, such that loss to follow-up would not change the conclusion of there being an association between exposure and disease variables. However, in some cases, loss to follow-up would cause a positive or negative association to become statistically insignificant.

Confounding

Confounding can influence associations in both case-control and cohort studies. Suppose researchers identified a group of men who were bald and a group of men who were not bald. Men with myocardial infarction were excluded from the study. The two groups were then followed into the future in order to see if bald men were more likely to develop myocardial infarction. Age is a possible confounder because it is associated with myocardial infarction and, independent of that relationship, is associated with baldness. Hence, we may find that bald men are more likely to develop myocardial infarction, but that may be explained by the fact that bald men are more likely to be older. In the calculation of the risk ratio, the numerator would be too large and the denominator too small.

Double-cohort studies are particularly susceptible to confounding. In the previous example involving a chemical leak and suspected neurologic disorders, the control group could be different in ways other than just exposure status such that confounding could produce misleading results.

Misclassification

Differential (nonrandom) and nondifferential (random) misclassifications are a primary concern in cohort studies, just as they are in case-control studies. Differential misclassification arises if exposure classification influences differential accuracy in ascertaining outcome information. For example, suppose a group of women were identified as sexually active and not sexually active, and these two groups were then followed into the future to assess whether sexually active women were more likely to develop cervical cancer. If sexually active women are more likely to seek medical attention than those who are not, cervical cancer is likely to be more frequently or accurately diagnosed in the sexually active group. Hence, higher incidence of cervical cancer in sexually active women can be explained, at least in part, by the method of ascertaining the outcome.

Nondifferential misclassification can arise because of inaccuracies in classifying the exposure status of individuals, but these misclassifications occur similarly between exposed and unexposed groups. For example, suppose the researcher was interested in assessing the association between physical activity and myocardial infarction. As a surrogate marker for physical activity, he chose transportation workers who have jobs that are physically demanding (exposed) and workers who have jobs that are not physically demanding (unexposed). Some job switching and time-on-the-job can produce misclassification of some of the subjects, yet this misclassification is likely to be unrelated to myocardial infarction. The effect of nondifferential misclassification is to make the groups more similar, thereby underestimating the association between exposure and disease.

CONTROLLING FOR BIAS IN COHORT STUDIES

Healthy worker bias can be avoided by selecting a comparison group made up of workers, only not exposed to the exposure of interest. Bias resulting from loss to follow-up can be minimized by restricting the study participants to those likely to remain in the study (eg, by excluding those with a highly fatal disease or who are likely to move out of the area), collecting personal identifying information (eg, each participant's telephone number and address as well as those of their employer and a family member) and making periodic contact, and providing incentives (eg, cash or free medical exam). Misclassification can be minimized by refining the definition of the exposed and unexposed groups.

At the study design level, restriction is sometimes used to avoid bias resulting from confounding. In double-cohort studies, confounding can be reduced by choosing comparison groups as similar as possible to the exposed population. Furthermore, collecting data on potential confounders at the beginning of the study makes it possible to adjust for these potential confounders at the analysis level through stratification and multiple-regression techniques.

STRENGTHS AND WEAKNESSES OF COHORT STUDIES

A number of strengths and weaknesses of cohort studies have been identified in the literature. Some of these are listed in Table 7.7.

EFFECT MODIFICATION

When an association between an exposure and disease outcome is modified by the level of an extrinsic risk factor beyond random variation, the extrinsic variable is called an **effect modifier**.[14] Effect modification can occur in either cohort or case-control data. This means effect modification can influence associations measured by either odds ratios or risk ratios. For illustration, this section will focus on odds ratios.

In the example demonstrating confounding in case-control studies, a hypothetical data set showed that the crude odds ratio measuring the association between coffee and heart disease was positive, whereas the stratified odds ratio for smoking showed no association. Confounding was present because the crude odds ratio varied from the stratified odds ratios. When the crude odds ratio is greater than the stratified odds ratios, confounding is positive. When the crude odds ratio is less than the stratified odds ratios, confounding is negative.

TABLE 7.7 Selected Strengths and Weaknesses of Cohort and Double-cohort Studies[13]

Strengths	*Weaknesses*
Cohort	
• Establish sequence of events • Avoid observation (recall, interviewer) bias • Avoid Berkson's bias and prevalence-incidence bias • Several outcomes can be studied • Number of outcomes grows over time • Yield incidence, relative risk, attributable risk	• Often require large sample sizes • Relatively expensive • Not feasible for rare outcomes • Not feasible for long latency periods • Loss to follow-up
Prospective • More control over selection of subjects and outcomes	• More expensive • Longer duration • Limited to one risk factor
Retrospective • Shorter duration • Less expensive • Fewer numbers required • More than one risk factor can be identified in the same data set	• Less control over selection of subjects and outcomes
Double Cohort	
• Useful when distinct cohorts have different or rare exposures	• Potential confounding bias from sampling two populations

In some cases a variable can act as both a confounder and an effect modifier. For example, positive confounding and the presence of effect modification would exist if the crude odds ratio was greater than the stratified odds ratios and if the stratum-specific odds ratio differed beyond random variation. Negative confounding and the presence of effect modification would exist if the crude odds ratio was smaller than the stratified odds ratios, which differed from each other. If the stratum-specific odds ratios differ greatly, to the point that they overlap the crude odds ratio, then effect modification is present, and confounding is not relevant.[15]

Confounding and effect modifying variables are treated differently. On the one hand, a confounder is a nuisance variable that produces a misleading picture of the association between variables. Ways to control for confounding at the study design and analysis levels have been discussed. On the other hand, an effect-modifying variable influences the association between two other variables in an informative way. That is, if the association between two variables differs across the level of a third variable, this is of interest, and this should be described rather than controlled.[3]

EXERCISES

Key Terms

Define the following terms.

Analytic studies
Attributable risk
Attributable risk percent
Berkson's bias
Bias
Case-control study
Cohort effect
Cohort study
Confounding
Cumulative incidence rate (attack rate)
Double-cohort study
Differential (nonrandom) misclassification
Effect modifier
Exploratory observational studies
Healthy worker effect
Incidence density rate
Interviewer bias
Loss to follow-up
Matching
Misclassification
Nondifferential (random) misclassification
Observation bias
Observational studies
Odds ratio (relative odds)
Person–time rate
Population-attributable risk
Population-attributable risk percent
Prevalence-incidence bias (Neyman bias)
Prospective cohort study
Recall bias
Restriction
Retrospective cohort study
Risk ratio (relative risk)
Selection bias
Subjects
Variable

Study Questions

7.1 Discuss the general steps you would take to design a case-control study.

7.2 What are the primary sources of bias in case-control studies?

7.3 What steps would you take to minimize bias and confounding in a case-control study?

7.4 Discuss the advantages and disadvantages of hospital, general population, and special population controls in a case-control study.

7.5 Discuss the strengths and weaknesses of case-control studies.

7.6 Discuss the general steps you would take to design a cohort study.

7.7 What are the primary sources of bias in a cohort study?

7.8 Compare and contrast effect modification with confounding.

7.9 As the hospital epidemiologist, you have been requested by the hospital administration to study the effects of administering antibiotics to patients at different time frames (2-hour intervals up to 24 hours) before they have surgery that involves opening the chest cavity. The study is aimed at reducing infections caused by surgery as well as reducing deaths. The study is to take place over the next 15 years. Design an appropriate study. Explain and justify the study design chosen.

7.10 You have been asked to study the effects of stress across the life span of people who have a close family member with HIV/AIDS. The study is to be from the time of diagnosis until the death of the family member. Design an appropriate study. Explain and justify the study design chosen.

7.11 In the coffee–myocardial infarction example, in which smoking was shown to be a confounder (see the section on confounding under bias in case-control studies), show that there is an association between smoking and coffee and also an association between smoking and myocardial infarction.

REFERENCES

1. Last JM, ed. *A Dictionary of Epidemiology*. New York, NY: Oxford University Press; 1995.
2. Schlesselman JJ. *Case-Control Studies: Design, Conduct, Analysis*. New York, NY: Oxford University Press; 1982.
3. Hennekens CH, Buring JE. *Epidemiology in Medicine*. Boston, MA: Little, Brown and Company; 1987.
4. Gail M, Williams R, Byar DP, et al. How many controls? *J Chron Dis*. 1976;29:723.
5. Smith DC, Prentice R, Thompson DJ, et al. Association of exogenous estrogens and endometrial cancer. *N Engl J Med*. 1975;293:1164.
6. Ziel HK, Finkle WD. Increased risk of endometrial cancer among users of conjugated estrogens. *N Engl J Med*. 1975;293:1167.
7. Horwitz RI, Feinstein AR. Alternative analytic methods for case-control studies of estrogens and endometrial cancer. *N Engl J Med*. 1978;299:1089.
8. Hutchison GB, Rothman KJ. Correcting a bias? *N Engl J Med*. 1978;299:1129.
9. Berkson J. Limitations of the application of fourfold table analysis to hospital data. *Biometrics*. 1946;2:47–53.
10. Reid MC, Lachs MS, Feinstein AR. Use of methodological standards in diagnostic test research. Getting better but still not good. *JAMA*. 1995; 274:645–651.
11. Choi BC, Noseworthy Al. Classification, direction, and prevention of bias in epidemiologic research. *J Occup Med*. 1992;34(3):265–271.
12. Newman TB, Browner WS, Hulley SB. Enhancing causal inference in observational studies. In: Hulley SB, Cummings SR, eds. *Designing Clinical Research: An Epidemiologic Approach*. Baltimore, MD: Williams & Williams; 1988.
13. Newman TB, Browner WS, Cummings SR, Hulley SB. Designing a new study: II. Cross-sectional and case-control studies. In: Hulley SB, Cummings SR, eds. *Designing Clinical Research: An Epidemiologic Approach*. Baltimore, MD: Williams & Williams; 1988.
14. Miettinen OS. Confounding and effect modification. *Am J Epidemiol*. 1974;100:350–353.
15. Kleinbaum DG, Kupper LL, Morgenstern H. *Epidemiologic Research: Principles and Quantitative Methods*. Belmont, CA: Lifetime Learning Publications; 1982.

CHAPTER

8

Experimental Studies in Epidemiology

OBJECTIVES

After completing this chapter you will be able to

- Discuss the role of randomization in controlled trials.
- Discuss the role of blinding in controlled trials.
- Identify the general strengths and weaknesses of controlled trials.
- Identify the advantages to using a run-in design, a factorial design, a randomized matched pair design, or a group-randomized design.
- Discuss some of the ethical issues associated with experimental studies.

INTRODUCTION

Chapter 7, "Design Strategies and Statistical Methods in Analytic Epidemiology," focused on analytic observational studies where study groups were predetermined by variables beyond the control of the epidemiologist. Past experience, lifestyle, personal behaviors, training, immunization levels, exposure to risk factors, and environmental factors all influence the state of health and susceptibility to illness of individuals in groups and are beyond the control of the investigator. Associations are observed, not manipulated by the investigators.

On the other hand, in experimental (or intervention) studies, the investigators intervene in the study by influencing the exposure of the study subjects. Two types of experimental trials are **randomized controlled trials** and **community trials.** In a randomized controlled trial the unit of analysis is the individual. A randomized controlled trial in a clinical setting is referred to as a **clinical trial**. An experimental study where one group of people or one community receives an intervention and another group does not is a community trial. The unit of analysis is the group or community.

In some rare situations in nature, unplanned events produce a natural experiment. A **natural experiment** is an unplanned type of experimental study where the levels of exposure to a presumed cause differ among a population in a way that is relatively unaffected by extraneous factors so that the situation resembles a planned experiment.[1] For example, screening and treatment for prostate cancer in the Seattle–Puget Sound area differed considerably from screening and treatment in Connecticut during the period from 1987 to 1990. Specifically, prostate-specific antigen testing was 5.39 (95% confidence interval: 4.76 to 6.11) times higher in Seattle than in Connecticut, and the prostate biopsy rate was 2.20 (1.81 to 2.68) times higher than in Connecticut. The researchers noted that the ten-year cumulative incidences of radical prostatectomy and external beam radiation up to 1996 were, respectively, 2.7% and 3.9% for those in Seattle compared with 0.5% and 3.1% for those in Connecticut. On this basis, they wanted to assess whether mortality from prostate cancer from 1987 to 1997 differed between Seattle and Connecticut. The adjusted rate ratio of prostate cancer mortality during the study period for Seattle and Connecticut was 1.03 (0.95 to 1.11). In other words, the 11-year follow-up data showed no difference in prostate cancer mortality between the 2 areas, despite much more intensive screening and treatment in Seattle.[2]

Epidemiologic experimental studies resemble controlled experiments performed in scientific research. They are the most useful for establishing cause-effect relationships and for evaluating the efficacy of prevention and therapeutic interventions. When a comparison is made between outcomes observed in 2 or more groups of subjects that receive different levels of the studied intervention, this is called a **between-groups design**. When the outcomes observed in a single group before and after the intervention are compared, it is a **within-group design**.

In Chapter 2, "Historic Developments in Epidemiology," some of the early history of experimental studies in epidemiology was presented, from James Lind's study showing that lemons and oranges were protective against scurvy to Louis Pasteur's demonstration of the effectiveness of his new vaccine against anthrax. One of the first critiques of the therapeutic efficacy of bloodletting was Pierre C. A. Louis. In 1835, he published results on hundreds of patients in Paris hospitals. In his investigation on the efficacy of bloodletting for pneumonia, he showed that bloodletting did not improve the patients' prognosis. Specifically, he revealed that the farther from the onset of symptoms bloodletting occurs, the better the patient survival: 50%, 1–3 days, 65%, 4–6 days, and 84%, 7–9 days.[3] This and other studies likely influenced a decrease from 33 million leeches imported to Paris in 1827 to 7,000 leeches imported to Paris in 1837.

RANDOMIZATION

Once the study group is determined, the subjects are then assigned to the intervention and control groups by **random assignment**. Random assignment makes intervention and control groups look as similar as possible. Chance is the only factor that determines group assignment, thus allowing the application of inferential statistical tests of probability and determination of the levels of significance. Randomized controlled trials are most common in clinical settings.

Subjects can be randomly assigned to more than just 2 study groups when the efficacy of various levels of a treatment or combinations of treatments are being investigated. As with the other research designs, inferential statistical tests of probability are applied and levels of significance determined. An important feature of randomization is that it balances out the effect of confounding. Assuming smoking is a confounding factor, randomization of a sufficiently large number of subjects will produce a similar distribution of smokers (in terms of age started, duration, and intensity of smoking) between the intervention and control groups.

Although it is possible to adjust for confounding factors at the analysis phase of a study, this assumes that data on the suspected confounders was collected at the outset of the study. Nevertheless, although our best thinking might identify many possible confounding factors, there may be some not considered. Randomization has the advantage of controlling for both known and unknown confounders. Thus, randomization of a sufficiently large number of subjects produces groups that are alike on average.

In some situations a physician may strongly believe in an intervention and place patients with more severe health problems in that group. Similarly, patients with more serious health problems may self-select the intervention. Randomization has the advantage of eliminating conscious bias resulting from physician or patient selection and averages out unconscious bias from unknown factors.

BLINDING

Blinding is used in experimental studies to minimize potential bias from a placebo effect. A **placebo** is an inactive substance or treatment given to satisfy a patient's expectation of treatment.[2] In some controlled trials that involve drug treatments, the placebos given to the control group are virtually indistinguishable (to blind the patients and providers, when possible) from the true intervention, providing a comparative basis for determining the effect of the treatment being investigated.[4] A **placebo effect** is defined as the effect on patient outcomes (improved or worsened) that may occur because of the expectation by a patient (or provider) that a particular intervention will have an effect. The placebo effect is independent of the true effect (pharmacologic, surgical, etc.) of a particular intervention. Just as a patient may respond to the intervention itself and not the specific therapeutic benefit of the intervention, an assessing investigator, albeit honest, may believe in a certain intervention, and unconscious bias may arise in the way the researcher evaluates those subjects who receive the intervention.

Blinding patients in controlled clinical trials in order to minimize the placebo effect dates back about 100 years. In 1907, a double-blind placebo-controlled trial was conducted by W. H. R. Rivers to explore the association between alcohol and other substances and fatigue. Harry Gold advanced the double-blind placebo-controlled design in the 1940s and 1950s in several lectures and publications. In the 1950s, Henry Beecher estimated that in over 2 dozen studies he assessed, the placebo effect was responsible for about one third of those who showed improvement. The contributions of these and other researchers led the Food and Drug Administration to initially recommend (in the 1970s) but not require that new drug trials be double-blinded.[5,6]

In a **single-blinded** placebo-controlled study, the subjects are blinded but investigators are aware of who is receiving the active treatment. In a **double-blind study** neither the subjects nor the investigators know who is receiving the active treatment. In a **triple-blind study** not only are the treatment and research approaches kept a secret from the subjects and investigators, but the analyses are completed in a way that is removed from the investigators.[7–11]

In drug studies a placebo is a pill of the same size, color, and shape as the treatment. However, for non-drug studies such as those involving behavior changes or surgery, it may be impossible or unethical to blind. It may also be problematic to blind in drug studies where a treatment has characteristic side effects. Building side effects into a placebo, which has no potential therapeutic advantages, may be unethical.

The need for blinding is related to whether the outcome is subjectively determined. For example, if the outcome measure is pain relief, a placebo would be highly desirable, whereas if the outcome measure was based on a urine sample or blood test, blinding the patient would be unnecessary. In drug studies where placebos are used, compliance and retention in the study may be much better, because patients will think they are benefiting from a given medication.

NONRANDOMIZATION

Several reasons exist for not using random assignment. First, large research populations are not always available, especially in clinical settings. Research is expensive, and funds may not be adequate for the research procedures, follow-up treatments, and testing of large study and control groups. Another restraint is the lack of subjects with the disease or condition or a desire to participate. If a large population is to be treated with a preventive measure such as immunization, the epidemiologist would not purposely have half the population assigned at random to a control group and leave them at risk of getting the disease because they were not immunized.

Randomization cannot be applied if an entire population is to be affected or subjected to the treatment. If fluoride is added to the water supply of a city, there is no way to include or exclude certain individuals. If seat belt laws are implemented, control groups are not selected, and randomization is not used in the enforcement of the law. If randomly selected control groups are available, a comparison group may be selected from individuals with traits similar to those of the subjects in the treatment group. A pretest/posttest approach will allow the treatment group to serve as its own control. The changes from the pretest results to the posttest results often show a statistically significant cause-effect relationship.[7–11]

When randomization is not feasible, a concurrent comparison group in a nonrandom process (convenience sample) may be chosen. If one city has fluoridated water, another city without fluoridated water could serve as a control, and dental outcomes from both groups could be used to evaluate the efficacy of fluoridation. Another example involves seat belt use. If one state requires seat belt use and another does not, the death rate from motor vehicle accidents or some other seat belt-related outcome measure between the 2 states could be compared in order to determine the efficacy of seat belt use. Although convenience samples are common in the literature, they are susceptible to unmeasured confounding factors.

NEWS FILE

Aspirin and Colorectal Cancer

Low-dose aspirin has been shown in several experimental studies to reduce the risk for a second heart attack and certain types of stroke—mainly by preventing blood clots from forming. Aspirin has also been shown to reduce the risk of colon cancer. A study completed in 1991 by American Cancer Society researchers and reported in the *New England Journal of Medicine,* was the first large prospective study to show a link between aspirin use and a reduced risk of colon cancer. The study showed the death rate from colon cancer to be approximately 40% lower in men and women who used aspirin regularly, compared with those who did not. A larger study published in the *New England Journal of Medicine* in 1995, involved 121,701 US nurses between 30 and 55 years of age. The study found that subjects who took 4 to 6 aspirin tablets a week for 20 years were less likely to develop colon cancer, compared with subjects who took less aspirin. However, in a more recent study researchers at Brigham and Women's Hospital found men who took one regular aspirin tablet (325 milligrams) every other day for 5 years in a randomized clinical trial, gained no extra protection against colorectal cancer. The findings were reported in the May 1 issue of *Annals of Internal Medicine* and were based on a nationwide study of 22,000 healthy male physicians between the ages of 40 and 84. The researchers indicated that these results may possibility be explained by the fact that these men made healthy lifestyle choices beyond using aspirin that could have lowered their risk for colorectal cancer. The relatively short duration of time the study participants took aspirin may also explain why there was no reduction in colon cancer risk in those who took aspirin. Dr. Charles Fuchs, Chief of Ambulatory services at the Dana-Farber Cancer Institute in Boston, said: "The longer you take [the aspirin] the more you reduce the risk." Fuchs further said: "It takes about 10 years for epithelial cells in the intestines to turn cancerous, so aspirin use for a decade or more is probably necessary to gain a benefit."

(Source: American Cancer Society News Center. Available at: http://www.cancer.org/docroot/NWS/content/NWS_1_1x_Aspirin_and_Colorectal_Cancer.asp?sitearea=NWS&viewmode=%20print&. Accessed on October 25, 2005.)

DESIGNING A RANDOMIZED CONTROLLED TRIAL

There are several steps involved with designing a randomized controlled trial. Six general steps are presented in this section. These include (1) selecting the intervention, (2) assembling the study cohort, (3) measuring baseline variables, (4) choosing a comparison group, (5) ensuring compliance, and (6) selecting the outcome (also called the **end point**).[12,13]

Selecting the Intervention

Selecting the intervention begins with the research objective, whether it is to treat or prevent disease. In trials aimed at evaluating the efficacy of a treatment, the investigator must establish that the therapy is safe and active against the disease, provide evidence that the therapy is potentially better than another, and provide evidence that the therapy is likely to be implementable in the field.

There are 3 phases of clinical trials that must occur before a drug is granted a license. When laboratory testing shows that a new drug has potential to benefit patients, it is first evaluated as a phase I trial. A **phase I trial** is usually small, typically less than 30 patients. The purpose of phase I trials is to find out the safe dosage, side effects, how the body copes with the drug, and if the treatment is effective in humans. Patients in phase I trials often have advanced disease and have already tried other options. They often undergo intense monitoring. Drugs that show promise advance to phase II trials. These are larger, with up to 50 people. **Phase II trials** assess whether a new treatment is at least as good as existing treatments; if so, it warrants further testing in a phase III trial. Phase II trials also evaluate which types of disease a treatment is effective against, further assess side effects and how they can be managed, and reveal the most effective dosage level. **Phase III trials** are typically much larger and may involve thousands of patients. These trials typically involve random assignment and are used to evaluate the efficacy of a new treatment. Different dosages or methods of administration of the treatment are often part of the evaluation.

Behavioral interventions usually begin with an identified problem. Once a problem, such as relatively high levels of sexually transmitted diseases, is observed in a population through descriptive epidemiologic methods, tailored programs can be developed. Identifying high-risk behaviors for disease, where these risk behaviors are most common, and understanding why these behaviors are more readily adopted by this group and not others is important information for designing the intervention. Behavioral interventions are often developed from behavior theory and refined with focus groups. New interventions are often developed from existing interventions shown to be efficacious in other settings. Evaluation of behavioral interventions often requires pilot testing in order to provide evidence that a larger scale assessment is worth doing.

Assembling the Study Cohort

Before assembling the study cohort, inclusion and exclusion criteria must be established and an appropriate sample size determined. Inclusion and exclusion criteria influence the extent to which the results can be generalized. There is often a compromise between the population most efficient for answering the research question and the population best for generalizing the study findings. If the outcome of interest is rare, it may be necessary to include in your cohort only those at high risk for developing the outcome. For example, a coronary heart disease cohort study may restrict subjects to males who are at least 40 years of age. Generalization of the study results; however, would be limited to a narrower group than the entire population. In a therapeutic trial, only persons with certain clinical criteria may be included. In a prevention trial, only persons at risk of developing an outcome of interest should be included.

Exclusion criteria are employed to help control error. Loss to follow-up is a primary concern in randomized controlled trials. Persons may be excluded from a study if they are likely to be lost to follow-up (eg, alcoholics, psychotic patients, homeless persons, and persons planning on moving out of the country). Exclusion of those with rapidly fatal conditions who are unlikely to be alive at the end of the follow-up period may also be excluded.

Sample size calculations are employed to ensure that the number of participants is adequate to test the specific hypothesis or hypotheses motivating the study. Sample size calculation is based on (1) formulation of the null and 1- or 2-tailed research hypothesis, (2) the search for the appropriate statistical test, (3) effect size (and in some cases, variability), (4) the desired level of statistical significance for a 1- or 2-tailed test and the desired probability of failing to reject the null hypothesis when it is actually false and (5) use of the appropriate table or formula for estimating the sample size. These tables and formulas are available in most introductory biostatistics books.

Measuring Baseline Variables

Measuring baseline variables such as identifying information (name, address, telephone number), demographic information (age, sex, race/ethnicity, marital status, education, income), variables that might be associated with the outcome (eg, cigarette smoking), and clinical features (eg, serum cholesterol, blood pressure, glucose level) allows the researcher to accomplish certain objectives.

Identifying information is necessary for maintaining contact with the study subjects and for minimizing loss to follow-up. Demographic information is also useful for characterizing the study cohort. The first table of reports and papers describing results from randomized controlled trials typically compares baseline characteristics, including demographics, in the study groups. This allows assessment of how well the randomization balances out the effects of these potential confounding factors. In nonrandomized studies, collecting demographic information is particularly important so that potential confounding effects can be adjusted for in the analysis. Measuring variables that might be associated with the outcome, such as smoking habits, allows for statistical adjustment of the potential confounding influence in nonrandomized controlled trials and evaluation of change in risk behaviors between baseline and follow-up. Finally, collecting clinical information serves 3 purposes. It can influence inclusion in or exclusion from the study, it indicates whether randomization balances out clinical features between intervention and control groups, and it provides baseline measures for comparison in within-group designs.

Choice of a Comparison Group

When the efficacy of a new drug for treating a given illness is under investigation and existing drugs are currently available, the new drug is compared with the current treatment. Comparing a new drug with nothing is rarely done, unless there is no efficacious treatment available for the disease. The aim is to identify whether improvements can be made over the status quo. Similarly, in a study assessing the efficacy of a dietary program for recovering heart attack patients, it would be unethical to not allow those who are not randomly assigned the program to assume special diets designed for heart attack patients.

Ensuring Compliance

The power of the study is directly influenced by compliance with the protocol. If study follow-up involves visiting a clinic for medical assessment, adherence can be improved by contacting patients by telephone or mail shortly before their appointments and providing reimbursement for time and travel. If the study involves adhering to the intervention protocol, the investigator should select a drug or behavioral intervention that is well tolerated. Drugs that require several dosages or have severe side effects and behavior interventions that require dramatic lifestyle changes and involve considerable time and effort on the part of the patient will have lower levels of compliance than less complex and intense programs.

Measuring compliance throughout the study will allow the investigators to make changes if needed. Low compliance will require changes to bolster compliance (eg, more regular contact with patients and higher incentives). Compliance can be monitored in drug studies by self-report, pill counts, and urine and blood tests. Compliance in the area of behavioral interventions can be monitored by self-report and direct evaluation.

Selecting the Outcome (End point)

It is not always clear what outcome variable is best. In order to minimize cost and increase feasibility, **surrogate** markers of the actual phenomenon of interest are often used. For example, instead of considering the effect of an HIV/AIDS drug on death, investigators might select a major AIDS-defining event as a surrogate end point for death (eg, parasitic infections, fungal infections, viral infections, HIV dementia, HIV wasting syndrome, a neoplasm). A colon cancer prevention program could use polyps as an end point instead of diagnosis of or death resulting from colon cancer. Surrogate end points become particularly useful in randomized controlled trials when the outcome phenomenon of interest is rare.

The power of a study is greater when the outcome variable is continuous rather than dichotomous (eg, CD4 counts vs the presence or absence of a bacterial infection in HIV/AIDS patients). For dichotomous outcome variables, power is influenced more by the number of occurrences of the outcome than by the number of subjects in the study.[14] However, the decision on an outcome variable should be driven by whichever variable or variables are best for satisfying the research objective.

It is often desirable to consider more than one outcome variable. For example, an intense diet and physical activity modification program, designed to ultimately reduce the risk of chronic health problems, measured change in several health indicators between baseline and 6 weeks. Variables with improved scores included health knowledge, percent body fat, total steps per week, and most nutrition variables measured. Clinical improvements were seen in resting heart rate, total cholesterol, low-density lipoprotein cholesterol, and systolic and diastolic blood pressure.[15]

SELECTED SPECIAL TYPES OF RANDOMIZED STUDY DESIGNS

Under certain conditions variations of the randomized controlled trial may have some advantages. Four of these study designs are presented in this section. They include run-in design, factorial design, randomized matched pairs, and group randomization.

Run-in Design

For placebo-controlled studies the run-in design can be useful for minimizing bias associated with loss to follow-up. In the **run-in design**, all subjects in the cohort are placed on placebo or treatment and followed up for some period of time (usually a week or two). Those who remain in the study are then randomly assigned to either the treatment or placebo arm of the study. A limitation of this design is that the subjects in the cohort at the time of randomization may no longer reflect the population of interest.

In a behavioral intervention, it might be useful to place all subjects on the intervention and then, after a short time period, randomly assign those compliant with the program to the different levels of the intervention. For example, recovering heart attack patients in a selected cohort could all be placed on a new dietary intervention and then, after a run-in period, those who are compliant would be randomly assigned to remain on the program or change to a standard dietary program used for recovering heart attack patients. The efficacy of the new dietary intervention can be assessed, but depending on the extent of initial dropout, it may have limited generalization to the population of heart attack patients as a whole.

Factorial Design

A 2 × 2 factorial design allows investigators to address the efficacy of 2 interventions in a single cohort of subjects. In a **factorial design**, subjects are randomly assigned to one of 4 groups. The groups represent the different combinations of the 2 interventions. In a placebo-controlled drug study, the groups could be (1) drug A and drug B, (2) drug A and placebo B, (3) placebo A and drug B, and (4) placebo A and placebo B. Comparing the outcomes for groups (1) and (2) with groups (3) and (4) allows evaluation of the efficacy of drug A. Comparing the outcomes for groups (1) and (3) with groups (2) and (4) allows evaluation of the efficacy of drug B. Factorial designs also offer an efficient approach for studying combination effects of treatments on an outcome. For example, researchers recently assessed the efficacy of the addition of levamisole or interferon-α to adjuvant chemotherapy with 5-fluorouracil in patients with stage III colon cancer. In one arm of the study, patients received 5-fluorouracil weekly for one year; in arm 2, patients received 5-fluorouracil plus levamisole; in arm 3, patients received 5-fluorouracil plus interferon, and in arm 4, patients received both 5-fluorouracil and both levamisole and interferon. The study found that adding levamisole, interferon, or both levamisole and interferon to the 5-fluorouracil provided no significant benefit over 5-fluorouracil alone.[16]

The factorial design is also useful in primary prevention programs. In one study investigators used the factorial design to evaluate low-dose aspirin (100 mg/day) and vitamin E (300 mg/day) as tools in the prevention of cardiovascular events (cardiovascular death, stroke, or myocardial infarction) in type 2 diabetic patients having at least one cardiovascular risk factor. Although low-dose aspirin was shown to lower the risk of cardiovascular events, no significant reduction in any of the endpoints occurred because of vitamin E.[17]

Randomization of Matched Pairs

Matching is a procedure that aims to make study and comparison groups similar with respect to extraneous (or confounding) factors. **Randomization of matched pairs** improves covariate balance on potential confounding variables. Matched randomization provides more accurate estimates than unmatched randomization and may involve matching on several potential confounders.[18] One subject is randomly assigned the study group (eg, a dietary program, a drug) in each matched pair and the other is assigned to the comparison control group.

Group Randomization

In **group randomization**, instead of individuals being randomly assigned the intervention, groups or naturally forming clusters are randomly assigned the intervention. There are many examples of group randomization where groups may involve practices, schools, hospitals, or communities. Individuals or patients within a cluster are likely to be more similar to each other compared with those in other clusters according to selected variables. For example, the World Health Organization randomly assigned 66 factories in the United Kingdom, Belgium, Italy, and Poland to intervention and control groups. The primary outcome variable was death from coronary heart disease. The intervention significantly reduced coronary heart disease and total deaths.[19] However, sample size calculations and interpretation of the results are more difficult with randomized groups than they are with randomized individuals.[20] The sample size required to maintain adequate statistical power is also larger than with individual level randomization.[21]

STRENGTHS AND WEAKNESSES OF DOUBLE-BLIND RANDOMIZED CLINICAL TRIALS

The best study design for establishing cause-effect relationships is the double-blind randomized clinical trial. This is because blinding minimizes bias and randomization minimizes confounding. In addition, control over exposure status allows investigators to evaluate the influence of precise dosages and amounts on the outcome of interest. However, ethical and practical considerations often make this study design impossible to administer. Beyond drug studies, blinding is often impossible. In addition, many exposures (such as smoking) would be unethical to randomly assign. Some of the strengths and weaknesses of blinded randomized controlled trials are shown in Table 8.1.

TABLE 8.1 Selected Strengths and Weaknesses of Blinded Randomized Controlled Studies[2,12]

Strengths	***Weaknesses***
• Can demonstrate cause-effect relationships with a high level of confidence because of the tightly controlled conditions not possible in observational studies • Sometimes produce a faster and cheaper answer to the research question than observational studies • Only appropriate approach for some research questions • Allow investigators to control the exposure levels as needed	• Often more costly in time and money • Many research questions are not suitable for experimental designs because of ethical barriers and because of rare outcomes • Many research questions are not suitable for blinding • Standardized interventions may be different from common practice (reducing generalizability) • May have limited external validity because of use of volunteers, eligibility criteria, and loss to follow-up

ETHICS IN EXPERIMENTAL RESEARCH

In the United States, the Public Health Service Act of 1985 ratified the establishment of **institutional review boards (IRBs)**. IRBs are charged with the protection of research subjects. The establishment of IRBs in this country was a result, in part, of the moral problems associated with the **Tuskegee syphilis study**, which assessed the natural course of syphilis in untreated black males from Macon County, Alabama.

In the early 1900s the poverty-stricken blacks in the southern United States were referred to as a "syphilis-soaked race." Macon County was one of the worst. This eastern county in Alabama was economically depressed, even though the rich soil made it one of the best agricultural areas in the south, with cotton as its most common crop. In this rural setting much of the agriculture activity was tied to poor black sharecroppers. Medical facilities were meager, and access to physicians and medical care was almost nonexistent. Physicians expected full payment in cash for their services. Blacks only used physicians in extreme emergencies, and conditions like syphilis were simply endured.[22]

Under these conditions, in 1928 the Julius Rosenwald Fund, in collaboration with the Public Health Service, endeavored to identify the prevalence of syphilis in southern rural blacks with the intention of providing treatment to cases. However, the 1929 stock market crash and the Great Depression financially devastated the Rosenwald Fund. Consequently, the treatment phase of the study was not pursued. At this time the Public Health Service decided to conduct a prospective study to evaluate the natural history of syphilis in untreated black men, with the end point being death. Cases and controls were then followed into the future, with the cases falsely led to believe they were receiving free treatment. Beginning in the fall of 1932, the study lasted until 1977, when Peter Buxton, an employee with the Public Health Service, alerted the public of the moral concerns associated with the study.[23]

The Tuskegee study had nothing to do with medical experiments, and no treatment was offered for syphilis. No new drugs were tested, nor were there efforts made to establish the efficacy of older chemical treatments, such as Salvarsan (an arsenic derivative) used to treat syphilis for years. The 3 stages of syphilis were clearly understood as were the incubation periods of each. The mode of transmission of the syphilis spirochete pathogen was also well understood. Still, the Public Health Service never established a formal protocol for this study and withheld treatment. The Wassermann test for syphilis was developed in 1907. Salvarsan was available and moderately successful in treating syphilis. Penicillin was made readily available in 1945, yet no treatment with this antibiotic was attempted (Figure 8.1).[22] There were several ethical problems associated with this study.

1. There was no informed consent; patients were not informed they were subjects in an experiment or that they had a contagious disease.
2. Diagnostic spinal taps (called "back shots") for neurosyphilis were misrepresented as special free treatment when, in actuality, treatment was withheld.
3. The contagious nature of the disease was never made known to families of infected cases, such that transmission to wives and children occurred.
4. Because treatment would eliminate a case from the study, cases were actively prevented from receiving treatment (eg, physicians were told not to treat them, and they were not allowed to be drafted because the pre-induction physical could reveal the condition).

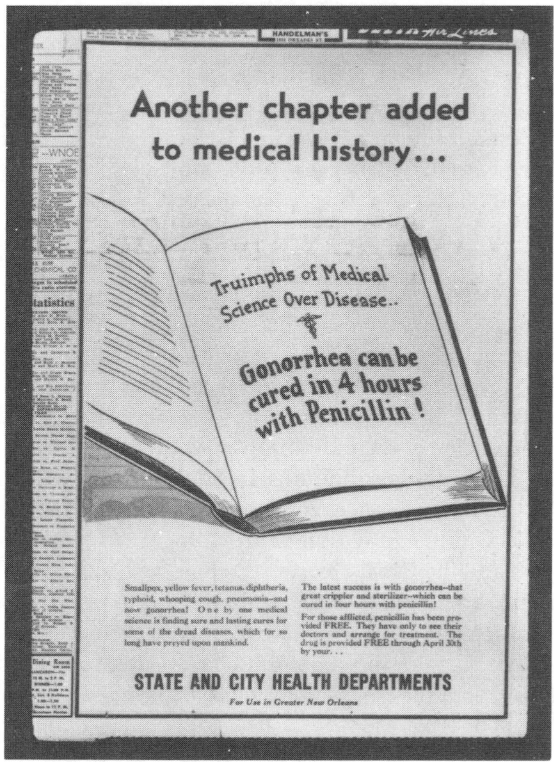

FIGURE 8.1 Penicillin was made widely available in 1945. This antibiotic became known as the "miracle drug," with promises of rapid cures of many infectious diseases, including gonorrhea. (Picture courtesy of Centers for Disease Control and Prevention, Atlanta, Georgia.)

5. Published statistics from the study (eg, that life expectancy was reduced by 20% in patients) were intended to promote fear of the disease in order to encourage further financial support for the study.[23]

Investigators using experimental designs must show respect and do no harm. It is morally required that informed consent be obtained, that subjects be informed that they may or may not be randomly assigned to the treatment group, that subjects be compensated for injury, that vulnerable populations (eg, mentally handicapped, financially destitute) are not taken advantage of, and that controlled clinical trials be stopped when definitive results are available. Subjects should also be protected against poorly designed studies that waste time and resources and that might produce misleading results. For experimental research to be of value, sound scientific methodology and research control methods must be used. Honest reporting and delineation of potential biases are expected.

EXERCISES

Key Terms

Define the following terms.

Between-groups design
Clinical trial
Community trial
Double-blind study
End point
Factorial design
Group randomization
Institutional review boards (IRBs)
Natural experiment
Phase I trial
Phase II trial
Phase III trial
Placebo
Placebo effect
Random assignment
Randomized controlled trial
Randomization matched pairs
Run-in design
Single-blinded study
Surrogate
Triple-blind study
Tuskegee syphilis study
Within-group design

Study Questions

8.1 List some reasons why nonrandomization might be preferred to randomization.

8.2 List some reasons why randomization might be preferred to convenience sampling.

8.3 What is the primary problem that is minimized through randomization?

8.4 What is the primary problem that is minimized through blinding?

8.5 Experimental studies can involve therapeutic or preventive trials. Provide an example for each of these types of trials.

8.6 What study design allows for testing a less mature hypothesis along with a more mature hypothesis?

8.7 What study design allows for answering 2 or more questions in a single study?

8.8 What study design minimizes bias resulting from loss to follow-up?

8.9 Design your own randomized controlled trial using the steps given in the chapter.

8.10 List 5 ethical problems that occurred in the Tuskegee syphilis study.

REFERENCES

1. Oleckno WA. *Essential Epidemiology: Principles and Applications.* Prospect Heights, IL: Waveland Press; 2002.
2. Lu-Yao G, Albertsen PC, Stanford JL, Stukel TA, Walker-Corkery ES, Barry MJ. Natural experiment examining impact of aggressive screening and treatment on prostate cancer mortality in two fixed cohorts from Seattle area and Connecticut. *BMJ.* 2002;325:740.

3. Louis PCA. Recherches sur les effets de la saignée dans quelques maladies inflammatoires, et sur l'action de l'émétique et des vésicatoires dans la pneumonie. Paris: Baillière; 1835.
4. National Library of Medicine. Available at: http://www.nlm.nih.gov/nichsr/hta101/ta101014.html. Accessed June 25, 2005.
5. Shapiro AK, Shapiro E. *The Powerful Placebo: From Ancient Priest to Modern Physician*. Baltimore, MD: Johns Hopkins University Press; 1997: 272.
6. Beecher HK. The Powerful Placebo. *JAMA*. 1955;159(17):1602–1606.
7. Alreck RL, Settle RB. *The Survey Research Handbook*. Homewood, IL: Irwin; 1985.
8. Kerlinger FN. *Foundations of Behavioral Research*. 3rd ed. New York, NY: Holt, Rinehart and Winston; 1986.
9. Neale JM, Liebert RM. *Science and Behavior*. 3rd ed. Englewood Cliffs, NJ: Prentice Hall; 1986.
10. Timmreck TC, Braza G, Mitchell J. Growing older: A study of stress and transition periods. *Occup Health Saf.* 1984;53(9):39–48.
11. Rothman KJ. *Modern Epidemiology*. Boston, MA: Little, Brown and Company; 1986.
12. Hulley SB, Feigal D, Martin M, Cummings SR. Designing a new study: IV. Experiments. In: Hulley SB, Cummings SR, eds. *Designing Clinical Research: An Epidemiologic Approach*. Baltimore, MD: Williams & Williams; 1988.
13. Cancer Research UK. Understanding clinical trials: Types of trials. Available at: http://cancerhelp.org.uk/trials/understanding/default.asp?page=73&order=2848. Accessed June 24, 2005.
14. Yusuf S, Collins R, Peto R. Why do we need some large, simple randomized trials? *Stat Med.* 1984;3:409–420.
15. Aldana SG, Greenlaw RL, Diehl HA, et al. Effects of an intensive diet and physical activity modification program on the health risks of adults. *J Am Diet Assoc.* 2005;105(3):371–381.
16. Lu M, Krams M, Zhang L, Zhang ZG, Chopp M. Assessing combination treatments in acute stroke: Preclinical experiences. *Behav Brain Res.* 2005;162(2):165–172.
17. Sacco M, Pellegrini F, Roncaglioni MC, Avanzini F, Tognoni G, Nicolucci A, PPP Collaborative Group. Primary prevention of cardiovascular events with low-dose aspirin and vitamin E in type 2 diabetic patients: Results of the Primary Prevention Project (PPP) trial. *Diabetes Care.* 2003; 26(12):3264–3272.
18. Greevy R, Lu B, Silber JH, Rosenbaum P. Optimal multivariate matching before randomization. *Biostatistics.* 2004;5(2):263–275.
19. Kornitzer M, Rose G. WHO European collaborative trial of multifactorial prevention of coronary heart disease. *Prev Med.* 1985;14(3):272–278.
20. Cosby RH, Howard M, Kaczorowski J, Willan AR, Sellors JW. Randomizing patients by family practice: Sample size estimation, intracluster correlation and data analysis. *Fam Pract.* 2003;20(1):77–82.
21. Underwood M, Barnett A, Hajioff S. Cluster randomization: a trap for the unwary. *Br J Gen Pract.* 1998;48(428):1089–1090.
22. Jones JH. *Bad Blood: The Tuskegee Syphilis Experiment*. New York, NY: The Free Press; 1993.
23. Fischbach RL. The Tuskegee legacy. *Harv Med Alumni Bull.* 1992;93:24–28.

CHAPTER

9

Statistical and Causal Associations

OBJECTIVES

After completing this chapter you will be able to

- Understand the distinction between statistical association and causal association.
- Know the steps for hypothesis testing and be able to apply hypothesis testing in the search for causal associations.
- Understand the roles of chance, bias, and confounding in statistical associations.
- Know selected criteria for establishing causal associations.
- Understand how webs of causation can be used as tools in epidemiology.
- Understand various aspects of screening and screening tests (including sensitivity, specificity, and predictive value).

INTRODUCTION

A primary role of epidemiology is disease prevention and control. The study of disease causality is a means to this end. Statistics are useful for measuring the strength of associations. Statistical assessment, however, is only part of the process of establishing cause-effect relationships. Epidemiologic study of associations should focus, in general, on learning more about cause-effect relationships so that public health officials can use that knowledge for the protection of the public health through disease prevention and control.

In Chapter 1, "Foundations of Epidemiology," epidemiology was defined as the study of the distribution (frequency and pattern) and determinants of health-related states or events in human populations and the application of this study to the control of health problems.[1] Chapters 4 through 6 introduced descriptive epidemiologic study designs and statistical methods for assessing the distribution of health-related states or events in human populations and emphasized that descriptive epidemiology is useful for formulating etiologic hypotheses. Chapters 7 and 8 introduced analytic epidemiologic study designs and statistical methods for measuring statistical associations. In an effort to identify determinants (causes) of health-related states or events in human populations, a valid statistical association is required. The possibility that chance, bias, or confounding might explain a statistical association should always be considered.

Once a statistical association is deemed valid, then the totality of the evidence needs to be considered before a judgment is made about whether causality exists for a specified hypothesis.[2] The purpose of this chapter is to present an approach for establishing the cause-effect relationships used in epidemiology.

CAUSAL ASSOCIATIONS

It has been shown that when people have particular exposures or characteristics, they are more likely to develop certain diseases than those without those exposures or characteristics. When a person has the disease and the particular exposure or characteristic, then an association exists. Associations have been identified between older age and cancer, less physical activity and heart disease, and a high-fat diet and diabetes. If a person who has smoked for 25 years develops lung cancer, and this is seen over and over again in numerous people, cigarette smoking is the identified exposure associated with the disease. A strong association between the exposure and the disease is observed. If you smoke for 25 years, you might get lung cancer, but if you do not smoke at all, the chance of getting lung cancer is relatively small. When coal miners smoke and are exposed to coal dust, they are more likely to develop lung cancer than coal miners who do not smoke, yet both may get black lung. Thus coal dust is ruled out as the cause of lung cancer, but an association with cigarette smoking and lung cancer is observed.

Although a **statistical association** involves 2 variables that are related, a statistical association does not mean a **causal association.** For example, ice cream consumption and murder are strongly correlated. Does eating ice cream make people want to kill or does killing result in a desire for ice cream? The explanation may be that hot temperatures are related to both ice cream consumption and murder and that it is the heat, not the ice cream that is causally associated with murder. Another example involves coffee drinking and myocardial infarction (see Chapter 7, "Design Strategies and Statistical Methods in Analytic Epidemiology"). A strong association was observed between coffee and myocardial infarction. Does this mean coffee drinking causes myocardial infarction or that myocardial infarction causes coffee drinking? The answer is neither. Cigarette smoking is more common in coffee drinkers and in myocardial infarction such that it is the cigarette smoking that explains the higher incidence of myocardial infarction.

Yet another example involves margarine use and lung cancer. Margarine consumption increased in a fashion similar to that of lung cancer rates in the United States during the 1900s. However, so did smoking prevalence, which is the primary cause of the increase in lung cancer. Smoking is statistically associated with both margarine consumption and lung cancer incidence rates. Associations like these, which involve a third variable jointly associated with the 2 original variables, are spurious, not causal, associations.

Causal associations in disease transmission can be direct or indirect. A **direct causal association** has no intermediate factor and is more obvious. That is, if a person at a picnic eats potato salad that sat in a warm room for a few hours and is contaminated with staphylococcal pathogens, the chance of getting food poisoning directly from the potato salad is quite good. An **indirect causal association** involves one or more intervening factors and is often much more complicated. For example, a high-fat diet is associated with polyps, and polyps are associated with colon cancer. Considerable research has explored mediating variables in the disease process.

Whether direct or indirect causal associations exist, health-related states or events typically have a multifactorial etiology. For example, the formation of cancer usually results from multiple mutations, and the opportunity for mutations to accumulate and for cancer to develop increases with the number of years of life. Cancer of the bladder can result from many causes, from drinking too much coffee and having high levels of chlorine in the drinking water from surface water sources to taking excessive amounts of vitamin C. In paraplegics confined to a wheelchair, the rate for cancer of the bladder is higher than in the nonconfined population. Some urologists suggest that bladder cancer is a result of the person with paraplegia having to hold the urine for long periods of time, causing the urine to become concentrated. The indirect cause of the bladder cancer might be the paraplegia handicap and being confined to a wheelchair. It might also be a combination of excessive coffee drinking and not being able to drain the bladder frequently or the coffee being made too strong or the simple strong concentration of the substance sitting in the bladder for prolonged time periods. The epidemiologist must be careful to assess all variables in the causality of disease, considering both direct and indirect causes.[3–7]

To establish a causal association when one exists, the first step is formulating a testable hypothesis about the proposed causal association. Evaluation of the hypothesis should involve an appropriate research design that allows the researcher to determine valid associations and assess criteria implicit in causal relationships. In 1856, philosopher John Stuart Mill wrote about 3 methods of hypothesis formulation about disease etiology: the method of difference, the method of agreement, and the method of concomitant variation.[8]

1. **Method of difference.** The frequency of disease occurrence is extremely different under different situations or conditions. If a risk factor or event can be identified in one condition and not in a second, it may be that factor, or the absence of it, that causes the disease. For example, Valley Fever (coccidioidomycosis) occurs only in the deserts of the southwestern United States.
2. **Method of agreement.** If events or risk factors are common to a variety of different circumstances and the events or risk factors have been positively associated with a disease, then the probability of that factor being the cause is extremely high. In the United States

cigarette smoking in males and females caused an increased rate of lung cancer in both sexes.

3. **Method of concomitant variation.** The frequency or strength of an event or risk factor varies with the frequency of the disease or condition. Increased numbers of children not immunized against measles causes the incidence rate for measles to go up.

Sir Austin Bradford Hill built on Mill's postulates about causality in 1965 when he outlined specific criteria that could be used to determine whether statistical associations were causal associations.[9] Based on this, the following 6 criteria may serve as a useful guide for establishing causality.

1. **Temporal relationship.** In order for an exposure to cause a disease, the exposure must precede the disease. For example, it has been established that mosquito bites precede malaria. The strength of cohort studies is that they allow researchers to establish a time sequence of events.
2. **Strength of association.** Stronger associations between exposure and outcome variables increase the likelihood of there being a causal association. Stronger associations are less likely explained by chance, bias, or confounding. For example, other factors have failed to explain the strong associations between smoking and lung cancer.
3. **Dose-response relationship.** An increasing amount of exposure increases the risk of disease. Although a dose-response relationship provides strong evidence for causality, the absence of a dose-response relationship does not rule out causality. A threshold may exist such that above that point the risk does not change. Studies have identified a dose-response relationship between pack-years of smoking and age-related macular degeneration, providing evidence that smoking may be causally related to blindness.[10–12]
4. **Consistency of association.** This occurs when associations are replicated by different investigators in different settings with different methods. For example, the 1964 report of the US surgeon general identifying a causal association between cigarette smoking and lung cancer was based on 29 case-control studies and 7 prospective cohort studies.[13]
5. **Biological credibility.** Is the association biologically supported? Biological assessment often involves experiments in controlled laboratory environments. For example, tobacco smoke is known to contain over 60 carcinogens, including formaldehyde and benzoapyrene.
6. **Experimental evidence.** The experimental study design is the best for establishing cause-effect relationships. This is because blinding is effective at controlling bias, and randomization is effective for balancing out the effect of known and unknown confounders. The order in which epidemiologic study designs are effective at establishing causal associations is as follows.

Rank	Study Design
1	Randomized controlled trial
2	Community trial
3	Prospective cohort study
4	Retrospective cohort study
5	Case-control study

6	Cross-sectional study
7	Ecologic study
8	Case report or case series

In addition to controlling for bias and confounding, the ranking is based on an ability to measure a temporal sequence of events, the strength of an association, and the dose-response relationship.

HYPOTHESIS DEVELOPMENT AND TESTING

The first step in determining the causes of a health-related state or event is to formulate a reasonable and testable hypothesis. A **hypothesis** suggests the association of certain variables with other phenomena; a tentative suggestion that certain associations exist in certain activities or in a chain of events. A hypothesis is based on learned and scientific observation from which theories or predictions are made. Hypotheses are used in epidemiology to evaluate suggestions about cause-effect relationships.[14]

Hypothesis Development

Fundamental to the development of hypothesis testing is inductive reasoning. This is the process leading from a set of specific facts to general statements that explain those facts. Inductive reasoning relies on

1. Exact and correct observation.
2. Accurate and correct interpretation of the facts in order to understand findings and their relationship to each other and to causality.
3. Clear, accurate, and rational explanations of findings, information, and facts in reference to causality.
4. Development based on scientific approaches, using facts in the analysis and in a manner that makes sense based on rational scientific knowledge.[14]

Hypothesis Testing

Chapter 7 defined measures of association for case-control (odds ratio, *OR*) and cohort (risk ratio, *RR*) studies and indicated that when the ratios equal 1, there is no association between the exposure and outcome variables. When epidemiologic data represent a sample from the population rather than the entire population, which is almost always the situation, sample data are used to estimate true odds or risk ratios. In hypothesis testing, the aim is to draw a conclusion about a true population value, such as an odds ratio or risk ratio, with the use of sampled data. A hypothesis can be evaluated with either a statistical hypothesis test or a confidence interval. Six steps for hypothesis testing for assessing an association in a case-control study are outlined here.

1. Formulate the null hypothesis (H_o) in statistical terms. The null hypothesis is typically set at no association (eg, $H_o: OR = 1$).

2. Formulate the alternative (or research) hypothesis (H_a) in statistical terms. The investigator may wish to test whether there is an association (eg, $H_a : OR \neq 1$). The null hypothesis is normally assumed correct unless there is strong evidence from the sample data to indicate otherwise.
3. Set the significance level (typically 0.05) and the sample size, n. Sample size formulas are provided in most introductory biostatistics books.
4. Select the appropriate test statistic and identify the degrees of freedom and the critical value. The χ^2-test is useful for evaluating the association between an exposure and outcome in a case-control or cohort study. The shortcut χ^2-formula for 2 × 2 tables (see Table 7.2) is

$$\chi^2 = \frac{n(ad - bc)^2}{(a+b)(c+d)(a+c)(b+d)}$$

Use this formula when no cell in the table has an expected count less than 1, and no more than 20% of the cells have an expected count less than 5.[15] Note that the expected value in each cell is obtained by multiplying the row total by the column total that corresponds with a given cell and dividing by n. When the sample size is small, the Fisher exact test (see a general biostatistics book for details of the test) is more appropriate for evaluating the association between dichotomous variables.[16]

The degrees of freedom (df) for a contingency table with r rows and c columns is $df = (r - 1)(c - 1)$. For the 2 × 2 table, the $df = (2 - 1)(2 - 1) = 1$. The critical value from a χ^2-table that separates the upper 5% of the χ^2-distribution from the remaining 95% is 3.84. A significance level of 0.01 would have given a critical value of 6.63 and so on. The first line of the χ^2-distribution giving the values of the χ^2 for 1 df that cut off specified proportions of the upper tail of the χ^2-distribution is given as follows (Table 9.1).

TABLE 9.1 Values of χ^2 for 1 *df* that Cut Off Specified Proportions of the Upper Tail of the χ^2-Distribution

	Area in Upper Tail			
df	0.10	0.05	0.01	0.001
1	2.71	3.84	6.63	10.83

df, degrees of freedom.

Note that although only the upper tail of the χ^2-distribution is being considered, the test is 2-sided. This is because larger values of the observed χ^2 occur when the association is either positive or negative. It should also be noted that discrete observations are used to estimate the χ^2, which is a continuous distribution. The approximation works better with many degrees of freedom. For the 2 × 2 table that involves 1 *df*, the approximation may be less valid. For this reason a continuity correction can be applied in this situation. The Yates correction (see a general biostatistics book for details of the correction) has been used extensively in the past and is calculated in many statistical software packages. However, some have argued that it is overly conservative.[17]

5. Collect the data and calculate the statistic. Note that a statistic is a measure from a sample, whereas a parameter is a measure from a population.

6. If the observed statistic exceeds the critical value, reject H_o in favor of H_a; else do not reject H_o.

Consider the disease sarcoidosis. This is a systematic granulomatous disease of unknown cause that mostly involves the lungs. It causes fibrosis there, but it also involves the lymph nodes, skin, liver, spleen, eyes, phalangeal bones, and parotid glands.[1] Researchers were interested in exploring the hypothesis that behaviors associated with rural living play some role in the development of sarcoidosis.[18] One of the exposures considered was use of a coal stove. The 2 × 2 table of data on coal stove use and sarcoidosis (Table 9.2) and the steps for hypothesis testing are as follows:

TABLE 9.2 Association between Sarcoidosis and Use of Cole Stoves

	Sarcoidosis		
Use of a Coal Stove	*Yes*	*No*	*Total*
Yes	10	4	14
No	34	84	118
Total	44	88	132

Step 1. Sarcoidosis is not associated with use of a coal stove, expressed in statistical terms as: $H_o : OR = 1$.

Step 2. Sarcoidosis is associated with use of a coal stove, expressed in statistical terms as: $H_a : OR \neq 1$.

Step 3. For this test $\alpha = 0.05$. The sample size was based on an appropriate sample size calculation.

Step 4. The χ^2-test is appropriate for this research question because the observations are nominal data (frequencies).

$$\chi^2 = \frac{132(10 \times 84 - 4 \times 34)^2}{(10 + 4)(34 + 84)(10 + 34)(4 + 84)} = 10.23$$

There is one degree of freedom. The critical value for one degree of freedom and α of 0.05 is 3.841.

Step 5. The odds ratio of sarcoidosis in the group that used a coal stove compared with the group that did not use a coal stove is estimated by

$$OR = \frac{10 \times 84}{34 \times 4} = 6.18$$

Step 6. The estimated $OR = 6.18$ is statistically significant; that is, the null hypothesis is rejected because the observed value of χ^2 is greater than the critical value of 3.841. Had $\alpha = 0.01$ been used, the observed value of χ^2 is still greater than this value such that the results are also statistically significant at the 0.01 level of significance. The observed χ^2 is marginally insignificant at the 0.001 level of significance.

Another way to assess statistical significance is to compare the predetermined significance level α with the p-value. The p-value equals the probability that an effect at least as extreme as that observed in a particular study could have occurred by chance alone, given that there is truly no relationship between the exposure and disease. The p-value is based on the test statistic. To obtain the p-value for the example, go to the row of Table 9.2 that corresponds with one *df* and then go across the row until you get to 10.23 (same table). The observed value does not actually appear on the table but is slightly below 10.83, which is shown. To obtain the corresponding p-value to 10.23, move up a row. The p-value is between 0.01 and 0.001. Because $p < 0.05$, reject H_o. The exact p-value, which in this example is 0.0014, can be determined with the use of a computer package. Computer packages also give the p-value corresponding to the continuity-adjusted χ^2, which in this example is 0.0038.

Role of Chance

Statistical inference involves inference about some characteristic of the population under investigation based on a sample from the population. Generalization requires that the sample be representative of the population, which researchers try to accomplish with random selection. Hypothesis tests allow evaluation of the role of chance.

Most epidemiologic studies rely on sampled data. When samples are involved, however, the characteristics of subjects in a sample may vary from sample to sample. As a result, an association between an exposure and outcome, or a lack thereof, might be the result of **chance**. Sample size is directly related to chance. As the sample size increases, the probability that the results are due to chance decreases. The p-value provides a means for evaluating the role of chance. The p-value ranges from 0 to 1. A small p-value indicates that the result is unlikely to be a product of chance. By convention, a p-value less than or equal to 0.05 indicates that the role of chance is sufficiently small such that the investigators are willing to reject a null hypothesis in favor of the alternative.

Applying a hypothesis test can lead to a wrong conclusion. Two kinds of possible errors are called type I and type II errors. A **type I error** occurs when H_o is rejected but H_o is true. A **type II error** occurs when H_o is not rejected but H_o is false. The probability of committing a type I error is determined by the significance level of the test, represented by the Greek letter α; that is, $\alpha = P$ (type I error). The probability of committing a type II error is denoted by the Greek letter β, where $\beta = P$ (type II error). The **power** of a test of hypothesis is $1 - \beta$, or the probability of rejecting H_o when H_o is false. Power can also be thought of as the chance that a given study will detect a deviation from the null hypothesis when one really exists.

A point estimate, such as the estimated odds ratio above, contains no information about the sample size. Although the p-value is directly influenced by the sample size, it is also influenced by effect size. Consequently, a small p-value may result when there is a strong association between the exposure and outcome but the sample size is moderate or small. On the other hand, a confidence interval reveals more about the sample size because the width of the interval is directly related to the sample size. A **confidence interval** is a range of reasonable values in which a population parameter lies, based on a random sample from the population. A significance level of 0.05 corresponds with a 95% confidence interval. For the odds ratio computed under step 5 in the section titled *Hypothesis Testing*, the 95% confidence interval is 1.81 to 21.05. If each cell is multiplied by 100, the same odds ratio is obtained, but the 95% confidence interval is 2.37 to 2.59.

The confidence interval can also be used to evaluate statistical significance. Recall that $OR = 1$ indicates no association. If the confidence interval for the odds ratio overlaps one, this indicates no statistical association. For the example just mentioned, the 95% confidence interval does not overlap one, indicating statistical significance at the 0.05 level. If a 95% confidence interval overlaps one, the p-value will always be greater than 0.05. On the other hand, if a 95% confidence interval does not overlap one, the p-value will always be less than 0.05. From the example above, $p = 0.0014$ is not statistically significant for $\alpha = 0.001$. Consequently, the 99.9% confidence interval of 0.79 to 48.3 does overlap one.

ROLE OF BIAS

Bias involves deviation of the results from the truth. Like chance and confounding, bias can explain an observed association between exposure and outcome variables. Bias is best controlled for by carefully designing and carrying out the study. Identify likely sources of bias and study their direction and magnitude of effect. Chapters 7 and 8 identified various forms of bias in analytic observational studies (Chapter 7) and experimental studies (Chapter 8, "Experimental Studies in Epidemiology").

ROLE OF CONFOUNDING

Confounding occurs when the relationship between an exposure and a disease outcome is influenced by a third factor, where the factor is related to the exposure and, independent of this relationship, is also a risk factor for the disease. Confounding should always be considered as a possible explanation for an observed association, particularly in descriptive epidemiologic studies (ie, ecologic studies and cross-sectional studies) and nonrandomized analytic epidemiologic studies (ie, observational case-control and cohort studies). Confounding can over- or underestimate a true association. Methods to control for confounding at the design and analysis levels of a study were discussed in Chapters 7 and 8.

FACTORS IN CAUSATION OF DISEASE

Selected factors have been useful in assessing the causation of disease at the community level: predisposing factors, enabling factors, precipitating factors, and reinforcing factors.[19,20]

1. **Predisposing factors.** These are the factors or conditions already present that produce a susceptibility or disposition in a host to a disease or condition without actually causing it. If the host is immunized against the disease or if the host has a natural resistance to the disease, he or she will respond by not getting the disease. If not protected, the host will respond by getting the disease because of exposure to the pathogen or agent. If sensitized to a condition, the host will respond accordingly. For example, if the host has an allergic sensitization to a substance and then is exposed to the substance, an allergic reaction will follow.
2. **Enabling factors.** These factors or conditions allow or assist the disease, condition, injury, disability, or death, letting the process begin and run its course. Some of the factors that can enable a disease to spread can be the lack of public health and medical care

services. Conversely, the availability of and access to public health and medical care services can prevent, control, intervene in, treat, and facilitate recovery from diseases and conditions while improving the health status of the population. The obvious disease causation concern and epidemiologic approach is to enable health services and halt the promotion and production of disease.

3. **Precipitating factors.** These are the factors essential to the development of diseases, conditions, injuries, disability, and death. With regard to causation, the cause of the disease, condition, or injury may be fairly obvious, while in other cases it may not be so obvious. Many times several risk factors may be present in the cause, especially in chronic diseases or those caused by lifestyle and behavior. A communicable disease caused by a single pathogen may have precipitating factors of poor sanitation, lack of immunization, and high levels of susceptibilities in the community.

   In chronic disease or behaviorally related conditions, a multitude of factors can contribute to a condition. Automobile-related and traffic-related deaths have affected the health status of the population of the United States in a detrimental manner. The automobile accident problem was studied. It was found that lack of seat belt use in cars, drinking and driving, and lack of helmet use by motorcycle riders all were precipitating factors in the high levels of traffic deaths. As a result, laws have been passed to prevent deaths by requiring citizens to buckle up, not drink and drive, and wear helmets while riding motorcycles.

4. **Reinforcing factors.** Like enabling factors, reinforcing factors have the ability to support the production of and transmission of disease or conditions, or they have the ability to support and improve a population's health status and help control diseases and conditions. The factors that help aggravate and perpetuate disease, conditions, disability, or death are negative reinforcing factors. Negative reinforcing factors are repetitive patterns of behavior that recur and perpetuate and support a disease that is spreading and running its course in a population. Positive reinforcing factors are those that support, enhance, and improve the control and prevention of the causation of disease.

WEB OF CAUSATION

Epidemiologic investigation of causal association in disease began historically with communicable disease epidemics. Communicable diseases are relatively easy to investigate compared with chronic noncommunicable diseases and conditions because they often have only one cause: a pathogen. Chronic diseases and conditions are often caused by multiple risk factors, often associated with occupation, environment, genetic susceptibility, and behaviors. The variety of factors leading to chronic disease is not easy to investigate. Because of the complexity often involved in noncommunicable diseases and conditions, a method is needed that is effective in the assessment of complex factors of causation.

Webs are graphic, pictorial, or paradigm representations of complex sets of events or conditions caused by an array of activities connected to a common core or common experience or event. In **webs of causation** the core or final outcome is the disease or condition. Webs have many arms, branches, sources, inputs, causes, etc., that are somehow interconnected or interrelated to the core. Webs can also have a chain of events in which some events must occur before others can take place.

One microbe cannot be singled out as the cause of a disease in behaviorally, occupationally, or environmentally caused chronic conditions or disorders. What does occur in lifestyle, work related, and behaviorally induced disease states is that individuals are subject to risk factors in small doses, sometimes in many doses and from many sources, all resulting in a chain of causation. The many risk factors and their various sources make for a complex web of causation for a chronic disease that may involve several organ systems and possibly several sites in a single organ system. A single-line chain of events can be found in parts of or within phases of a web of causation. A single chain of events can be seen in some chronic, behavioral, or environmentally caused diseases or conditions. The complexity of behaviorally or lifestyle-caused conditions or environmentally caused diseases requires that all facets, risk factors, exposures, or contributing causes be understood and shown so that understanding is complete and the investigation is thorough. Cardiovascular disease and heart disease are good examples. Many factors contribute to heart disease; the same factors can also lead to a stroke (cerebrovascular accident). Figure 9.1 is one example of a web of causation for coronary heart disease, and Figure 9.2 is a second web of causation for myocardial infarction. Both webs are slightly different but are also similar and illustrate the complexity of a chronic disease and the multitude of causes that the epidemiologist needs to consider.[3,4]

A web of causation is useful in identifying the risk factors of the disease, the chain of events, and exposures necessary and sufficient to cause the disease. Even though webs of causation are complex, 2 concepts universally apply. First, a complete understanding of the causal factors and mechanisms is not required or necessary for the development of effective prevention and control measures. Second, it is possible to interrupt the production of a disease by cutting the chains of occurrences of the various factors at strategic points that will stop the chain of events in the causation of the disease.

Identifying and ascertaining the specific details of the various factors leading to disease, disability, injury, or death enhance webs of causation. Two approaches to enhancing webs of causation are the use of decision trees and fish bone cause-effect analysis diagrams. The decision tree is a flow chart that visually presents a process through which lines and symbols lead to proper decisions and understanding of the role of certain risk factors in webs of causation. Fish bone diagrams provide a visual display of all possible causes that could potentially contribute to the disease, disorder, or condition under study.

Conditions caused by environmental factors are complex, making it difficult to identify causal factors because an array of sources and risk factors contribute to causation. An example of an environmentally caused disease is lead poisoning, a condition that can be precipitated by a multitude of events and sources. For example, child lead poisoning is a pediatric health problem in the United States that is entirely preventable. Children are particularly susceptible to lead's toxic effects. Lead poisoning, unlike other childhood diseases, produces no symptoms early in the disease; the child has no reaction to the exposure and does not appear ill at first. Thus most cases go undiagnosed and untreated. Over the years, the Centers for Disease Control and Prevention (CDC) have set the safe lead exposure levels lower and lower. Scientific studies and clinical observation in children continue to show that even the smallest amount of lead exposure in children can have detrimental effects. In screening of children to determine levels of lead in the body, the test of choice is now blood lead measurements. The primary control of lead poisoning is prevention measures, especially if these are targeted to high-risk populations. Screening and medical treatment of lead-poisoned children remains important until the sources of lead in the environment are eliminated.[14] Figure 9.3 is an example of the web of causation showing the complexity of environmentally caused diseases, in this case, lead poisoning.

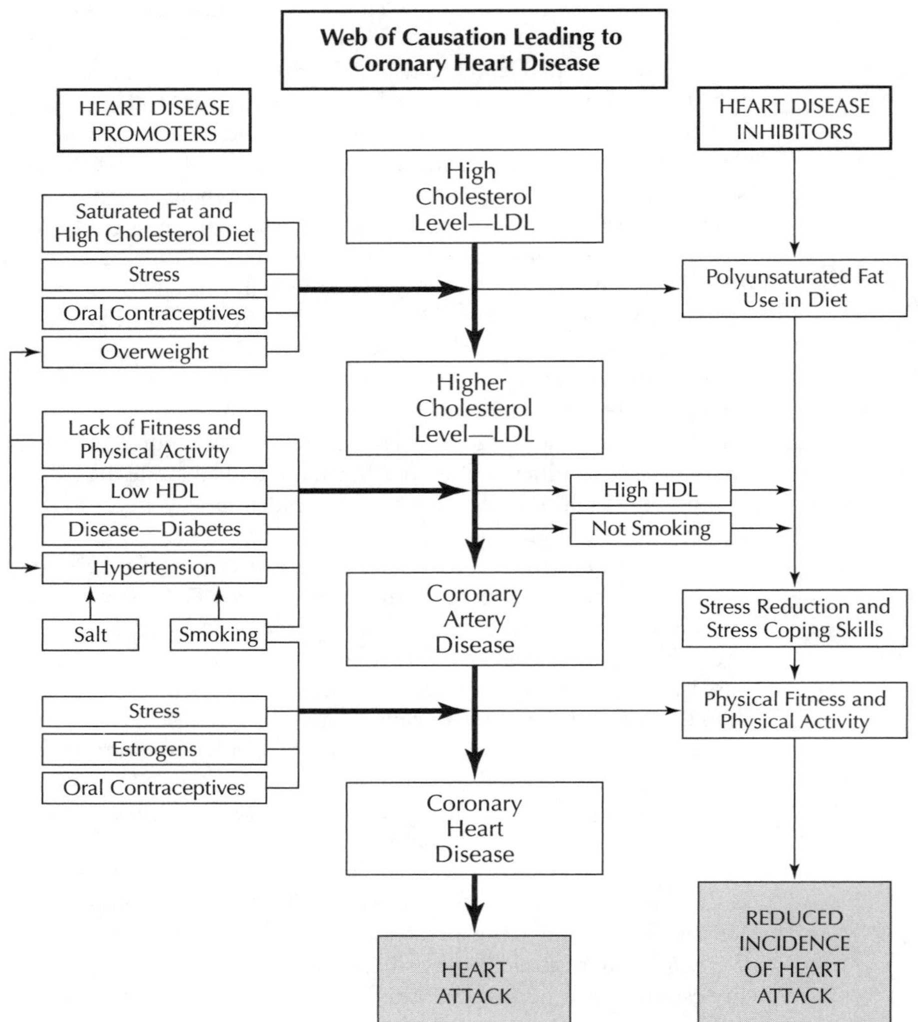

FIGURE 9.1 Example of a web of causation for coronary heart disease. (Adapted from R Sherwin, in Mausner JS, Kramer S. *Epidemiology: An Introductory Text.* Philadelphia, PA: WB Saunders; 1985.)

SCREENING AND DISEASE DETECTION

A primary objective of epidemiology is to identify causal associations so that disease prevention and control programs can be developed and effectively implemented. Screening programs are an important area of secondary prevention. **Screening** is the examination of a group of (usually) asymptomatic people to detect those with a high probability of having a given disease.[1] Persons with a high probability of having a given disease are then encouraged to pursue diagnostic examinations. Thus screening is often a precursor to diagnosis.

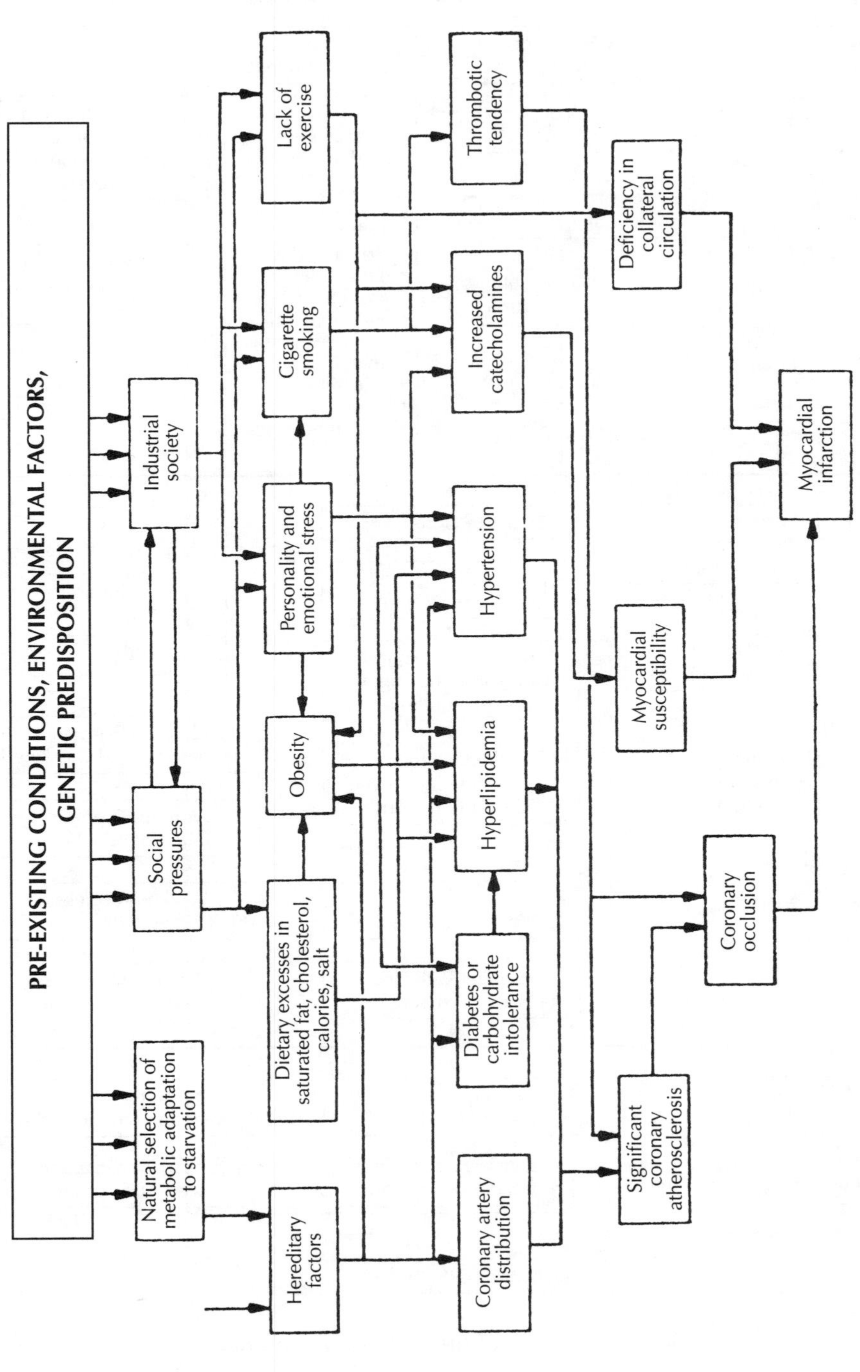

FIGURE 9.2 An example of a web of causation for myocardial infarction used to illustrate complex causation factors of a chronic disease. (Friedman G. *Primer of Epidemiology*. New York, NY: McGraw-Hill; 1974.)

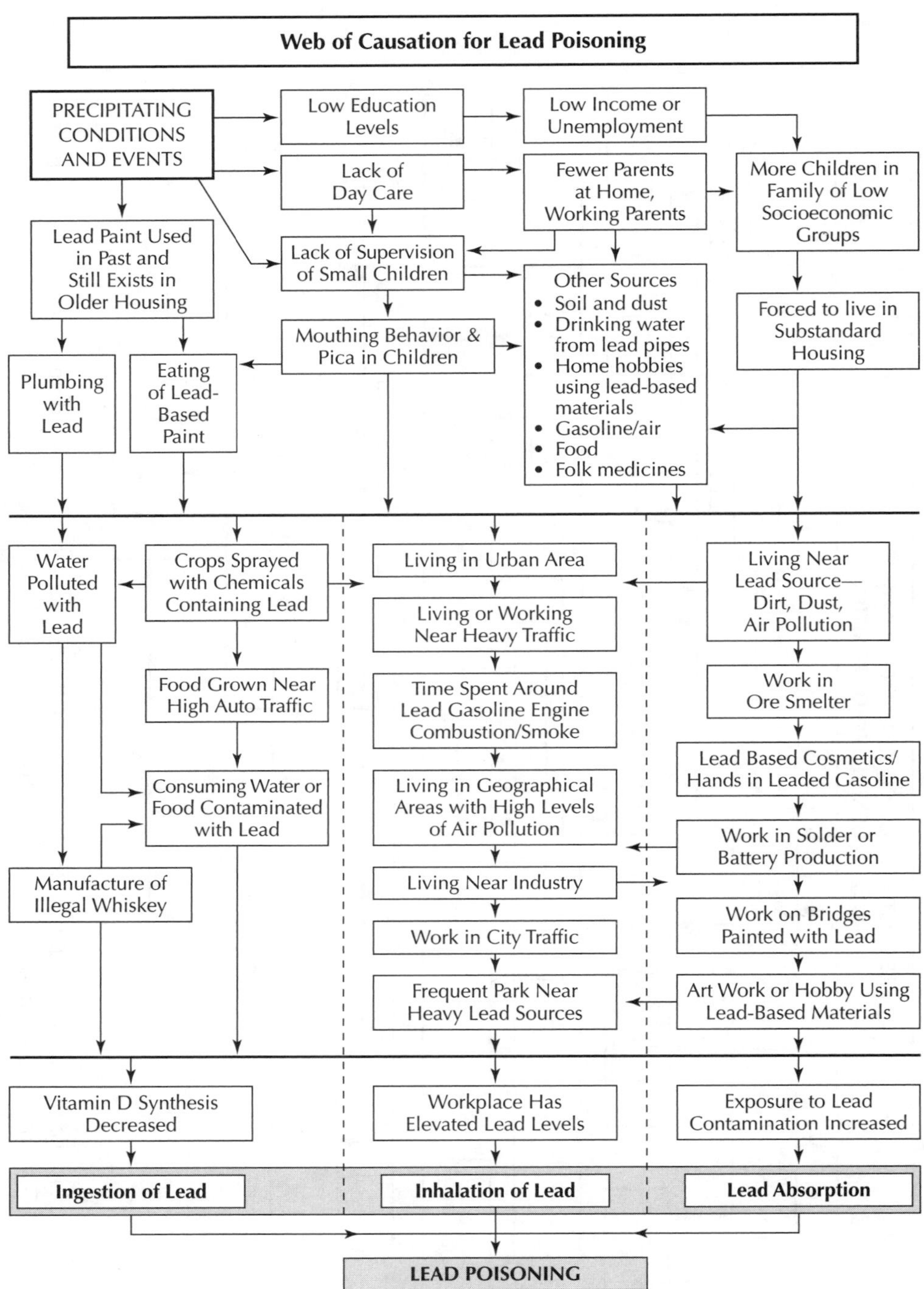

FIGURE 9.3 Example of a web of causation for lead poisoning.

Screening tests have cut points that classify people according to the likelihood of disease. A diagnosis is applied to a patient on a one-on-one basis by a physician or other qualified health care provider in a medical setting. Diagnosis, in addition to using the results of tests, involves the evaluation of signs and symptoms and may involve subjective judgment based on the experience of the physician. Diagnosis is a prerogative of the physician. Screening tests can be conducted by medical technicians under the supervision of a physician. Screening is not meant to compete with diagnosis but is a process used to identify the possibility of a disease state so that it can be referred for diagnosis. Diagnosis cannot only confirm or disprove a screening test, but it can also help establish validity, sensitivity, and specificity of the tests.[3–7,21]

Screening Program Considerations

Wilson and Jungner[22] set forth a list of items that epidemiologists should consider when planning and implementing a screening program. From a public health perspective, screening is most effective when it can reach a large percentage of the population. Ten factors that may be considered when planning a screening program for large population groups are

1. The disease or condition being screened for should be a major medical problem.
2. Acceptable treatment should be available for individuals with diseases discovered in the screening process.
3. Access to health care facilities and services for follow-up diagnosis and treatment for the discovered disease should be available.
4. The disease should have a recognizable course, with identifiable early and latent stages.
5. A suitable and effective test or examination for the disease(s) should be available.
6. The test and the testing process should be acceptable to the general population.
7. The natural history of the disease or condition should be adequately understood, including the regular phases and course of the disease, with an early period identifiable through testing.
8. Policies, procedures, and threshold levels on tests should be determined in advance to establish who should be referred for further testing, diagnostics, and possible treatment.
9. The process should be simple enough to encourage large groups of persons to participate.
10. Screening should not be an occasional activity but should be done as a regular and ongoing process.

Screening Tests

Screening activities are only as effective as the tests and examinations used. Therefore, each screening test needs to have strong validity and reliability. The **validity** of a test is shown by how well the test actually measures what it is supposed to measure. If it is a cholesterol screening test, the question is, can it give accurate enough readings so that the individual actually knows how high or low his or her cholesterol really is? Validity is determined by the sensitivity and specificity of the test. **Reliability** is based on how well the test performs in use over time—-its repeatability. Can the test produce reliable results each time it is used and in different locations or populations? Yield is another term sometimes used in reference to screening tests. **Yield** is the amount of screening the test can accomplish in a time period, that is, how much disease it can detect in the screening process. The validity of a test can be affected by the limitations of the test and the traits of the individuals being tested. The state of the disease, the severity of it, the level and amount of exposure, nutritional health, physical fitness, and other factors influencing the health status of the individual also influence and affect test responses and findings.[3–7,21]

SENSITIVITY AND SPECIFICITY

Table 9.3 shows true disease status as revealed by possible test results. The test results may be (1) **true positive** (TP), (2) **false positive** (FP), (3) **false negative** (FN), or (4) **true negative** (TN). When evaluating a diagnostic test, consider the 4 possible situations shown in the table. Diagnostic tests are preferred if they have few false positives or false negatives. The value of a test is generally determined by its sensitivity and specificity. **Sensitivity** is the proportion of subjects with the disease who have a positive test [TP/(TP + FN)]; that is, sensitivity is the ability of the test to correctly identify those with the disease.[23] **Specificity** is the proportion of subjects without the disease who have a negative test [TN/(FP + TN)].[23] Specificity is the ability to correctly identify those without the disease. An inverse relationship exists between true positives and false positives. Conversely, an inverse relationship exists between false negatives and true negatives.

The proportion of false negatives is the complement of sensitivity. Conversely, the proportion of false positives is the complement of specificity. The epidemiologist wants a sensitive test to identify a high proportion of those who have the disease and a test that will generate few false negatives. The epidemiologist wants the test to be specific enough to detect the disease so that responses are limited to the study group who are truly diseased. Epidemiologists also want a test that produces few false positives. Once a screening process is complete, a diagnosis is needed to establish the disease in those who are suspected of having it and to rule out those persons screened who are suspected of being diseased but are not.[3–7,21]

TABLE 9.3 True Disease Status According to Possible Test Results

	True Disease Status	
Test Result	***Present***	***Not Present***
Positive	True positive (TP)	False positive (FP)
Negative	False negative (FN)	True negative (TN)
	TP + FN	FP + TN

Predictive Value of a Test

The ability of a test to predict the presence or absence of a disease indicates the test's worth. The predictive value of a screening test is influenced by the sensitivity and specificity of the test as well as the prevalence of disease in the population undergoing testing. The higher the prevalence of a disease in a population, the more likely a positive test will represent a true positive. The lower the prevalence of a disease in a population, the more likely a positive test will represent a false positive. Rare diseases require a more specific test in order to be clinically useful.[23]

The prevalence of disease in specific individuals is referred to as the **prior probability**. It is the probability of having a disease prior to the diagnostic test. It is influenced by factors such as age, sex, and clinical characteristics. For example, the prior probability of prostate cancer may be near zero in an Asian man younger than 40 years of age but above 50% in an African-American man over 70 years of age.

The **predictive value** of a positive test (PV+) is equal to the probability that an individual with a positive test actually has the disease. It can be expressed as

$$PV+ = \frac{\text{Sensitivity} \times \text{Prior probability}}{(\text{Sensitivity} \times \text{Prior probability}) + [(1\text{-specificity}) \times (1\text{-Prior probability})]}$$

On the other hand, the predictive value of a negative test (PV−) is the probability that a person who has a negative test does not have the disease. It can be expressed as

$$PV- = \frac{\text{Specificity} \times (1\text{-Prior probability})}{[\text{Specificity} \times (1\text{-Prior probability})] + [(1\text{-sensitvity}) \times \text{Prior probability}]}$$

Because the predictive value is determined after the test results are known, it is sometimes called the **posterior probability**.

To illustrate, consider a screening test for tuberculosis in a small private college. Hypothetical findings of the screening test are as follows.

Diseased and positive on the test	=	50
Diseased and negative on the test	=	15
No disease and positive on the test	=	75
No disease and negative on the test	=	1,710

Sensitivity is 50/(50 + 15) = 0.77 and specificity is 1,710/(75 + 1,710) = 0.96. If the prior probability of tuberculosis was 3.5%, then the probability that a person with a positive test will have tuberculosis (PV+) is 0.41. On the other hand, the probability that a person with a negative test does not have tuberculosis (PV−) is 0.99. If, however, the prior probability of tuberculosis was 20%, then PV+ becomes 0.83 and PV− becomes 0.94.

EXERCISES

Key Terms

Define the following terms.

Bias
Biological credibility
Causal association
Chance
Confidence interval
Confounding
Consistency of association
Direct causal association
Dose-response relationship
Enabling factors
Experimental evidence
False negative
False positive
Hypothesis
Indirect causal association
Method of agreement
Method of concomitant variation
Method of difference
Power
Precipitating factors
Predictive value
Predisposing factors
Prior probability
Reinforcing factors
Reliability
Screening
Sensitivity
Specificity
Statistical association
Strength of association
Temporal relationship
True negative
True positive
Type I error
Type II error
Validity
Webs of causation
Yield

Study Questions

9.1 For each of the following statements, indicate whether the statistical association is likely a result of chance, bias, or confounding.

a. A case-control study showed that a strong association exists between birth order and Down syndrome.

b. A case-control study found a positive association between self-reported chest radiographs during pregnancy and breast cancer.

c. A randomized clinical trial found that drug A versus placebo did not significantly improve 10-year survival ($RR = 0.35$; 95% confidence interval 0.14 – 55.01).

d. A cohort study found no statistical association between smoking and pancreatic cancer ($RR = 1$; p-value = 0.85).

e. A hospital-based case-control study identified a strong association between oral contraceptives and thromboembolism. Many doctors suspected the association and hospitalized some women who used oral contraceptives for evaluation.

9.2 Match the following methods for minimizing chance, bias, and confounding in an experimental study.

__ Chance a. Randomization

__ Bias b. Blind

__ Confounding c. Increase sample size

9.3 Recall the criteria presented by Sir Austin Bradford Hill in 1965 for providing evidence that a valid statistical association is a causal association. Discuss how these criteria relate to smoking and lung cancer.

9.4 Suppose you suspect, based on descriptive epidemiology, that college students who perform better academically are more likely to have an office job and be obese 10 years after graduation. You decide to randomly select 500 graduating seniors and you classify them according to grade point average as high versus low (where the cut point is at the median of the GPAs for these students). The resulting 2 × 2 table is as follows.

	Obese at 10 Years		
GPA	Yes	No	Total
High	60	190	250
Low	40	210	250
Total	100	400	500

Apply this data to the 6 steps of hypothesis.

9.5 A screening test for a newly discovered disease is being evaluated. In order to determine the effectiveness of the new test, it was administered to 880 workers, and 120 of the individuals diagnosed with the disease tested positive. A negative test finding occurred in 50 people who had the disease. A total of 40 persons not diseased tested positive for it. Construct a 2 × 2 table, similar to the one in Table 9.3, and calculate the following:

a. the prevalence of the disease

b. the sensitivity of the test

c. the specificity of the test

d. predictive value of a positive test

e. predictive value of a negative test

9.6 As an occupational health epidemiologist you are required to measure the effect of stress on the workers in your manufacturing plant. Two different tests previously developed to measure stress in industrial workers are selected: stress test alpha and stress test delta. The sensitivity and specificity of each test are shown below.

Stress Test Alpha	*Stress Test Delta*
Sensitivity = 60%	75%
Specificity = 95%	90%

a. Which test generates the greatest proportion of false negatives?

b. Which test generates the greatest proportion of false positives?

c. Which test would you prefer?

9.7 Give specific examples of how a predisposing factor, an enabling factor, and a precipitating factor can influence causal associations.

9.8 Compare a direct causal association with an indirect causal association. Use specific examples.

REFERENCES

1. *Stedman's Medical Dictionary for the Health Professions and Nursing*. 5th ed. New York, NY: Lippincott, Williams & Wilkins; 2005.
2. Hennekens CH, Buring JE. *Epidemiology in Medicine*. Boston, MA: Little, Brown and Company; 1987.
3. MacMahon B, Pugh TF. *Epidemiology: Principles and Methods*. Boston, MA: Little, Brown and Company; 1970.
4. Mausner JS, Kramer S. *Epidemiology: An Introductory Text*. Philadelphia, PA: WB Saunders; 1985.
5. Lilienfeld AM, Lilienfeld DE. *Foundations of Epidemiology*. New York, NY: Oxford University Press; 1980.
6. Friedman GD. *Primer of Epidemiology*. New York, NY: McGraw-Hill; 1974.
7. Kelsey JL, Thompson WD, Evans AS. *Methods in Observational Epidemiology*. New York, NY: Oxford University Press; 1986.
8. Mill JS. *A System of Logic, Ratiocinative and Inductive*. 5th ed. London: Parker, Son and Bowin; 1862.
9. Hill AB. The environment and disease: Association or causation? *Proc R Soc Med*. 1965;58: 295–300.
10. Delcourt C, Diaz JL, Ponton Sanchez A, Papoz L. Smoking and age-related macular degeneration. The POLA study. *Arch Ophthalmol*. 1998;116:1031–1035.
11. Hankinson SE, Willett WC, Colditz GA, et al. A prospective study of cigarette smoking and risk of cataract surgery in women. *JAMA*. 1992;268:994–998.
12. Christen WG, Manson JE, Seddon JM, et al. A prospective study of cigarette smoking and risk of cataract in men. *JAMA*. 1992;268:989–993.
13. US DHEW. Smoking and health: Report of the advisory committee to the Surgeon General of the Public Health Service. PHS Publication No. 1103. Washington, DC: US Government Printing Office; 1964.
14. Shindell S, Salloway JC, Oberembt CM. *A Coursebook in Health Care Delivery*. New York, NY: Appleton-Century-Crofts; 1976.
15. Cochran WE. Some methods for strengthening the common χ^2-test. *Biometrics*. 1954;10: 417–451.
16. Rosner B. *Fundamentals of Biostatistics*. 4th ed. Belmont, CA: Wadsworth Publishing Company; 1995.
17. Grizzle JE. Continuity correction in the χ^2 test for 2×2 tables. *Am Stat*. 1967;21:28–32.
18. Kajdasz DK, Lackland DT, Mohr LC, Judson MA. A current assessment of rurally linked exposures as potential risk factors for sarcoidosis. *Ann Epidemiol*. 2001;11:111–117.
19. Evans AS. Causation and disease: The Henle-Koch postulates revisited. *Yale J Biol Med*. 1976;49:175–195.
20. Green L, Krueter M. *Health Promotion Planning*. 2nd ed. Mountain View, CA: Mayfield Publishing Company; 1991.
21. Fox JP, Hall CE, Elveback LR. *Epidemiology: Man and Disease*. New York, NY: Macmillan; 1970.
22. Wilson JMG, Jungner F. *Principles and Practice of Screening for Disease*. Paper No. 34. Geneva, Switzerland: World Health Organization; 1968.
23. Browner WS, Newman TB, Cummings SR. Designing a new study: III. Diagnostic tests. In: Hulley SB, Cummings SR, eds. *Designing Clinical Research: An Epidemiologic Approach*. Baltimore, MD: Williams & Williams; 1988.

CHAPTER

10

Field Epidemiology

OBJECTIVES

After completing this chapter you will be able to

- Define field epidemiology.
- Discuss the role of the epidemiologist in planning and establishing an epidemiologic study for assessing epidemics.
- Know how to plan and conduct an epidemiologic field study.
- Be familiar with epidemiologic questions that may assist the epidemiologist in an investigation.

INTRODUCTION

An interesting, exciting, and challenging part of epidemiology is to work in the field conducting epidemiologic investigations of epidemics. Epidemiologists have been called disease detectives.[1] Epidemiologic field investigations typically involve disease outbreaks that are limited in scope and are usually communicable diseases or have a common source. The purpose of this chapter is to provide a definition of field epidemiology and discuss specific activities conducted by field epidemiologists.

Field epidemiology has been defined as the application of epidemiology under a set of general conditions:

- The problem is unexpected.
- A timely response may be demanded.
- Travel to and from work in the field is required by epidemiologists to solve the problem.
- The investigation time is likely to be limited because of the need for a timely intervention.[2]

Field investigations involving acute problems may differ from conventional epidemiologic studies in three important ways. First, field investigations often do not start with a clear hypothesis. Gathering descriptive data on person, place, and time may be required before the hypothesis can be formulated and tested. Second, acute problems involve an immediate need to protect the public and resolve the concern. Hence, in addition to data collection and analyses, public health action often occurs. Third, field epidemiologists must decide when the available information is sufficient to take appropriate action.[2]

Field investigations involve several activities. These activities may include abstracting information from a variety of sources, collecting specimens for laboratory tests, conducting clinical exams to confirm cases, identifying the natural course of disease, and producing reports and graphs.[3,4] However, field investigation may pose unique challenges beyond the scientific ideal more closely achieved in many epidemiologic studies. For example, abstracted information may vary considerably in completeness and accuracy, small numbers may greatly restrict statistical power, collecting biologic specimens "after the fact" may be impossible, and cooperation may be low.[2] Nevertheless, the highest scientific quality possible should be sought under such limitations.

CONDUCTING A FIELD INVESTIGATION

Epidemiologic field investigations generally involve disease outbreaks confined to localized areas and traced to a common source, spread from person-to-person, or a combination of the two. Disease outbreaks investigated in field investigations are typically confined to a limited time period. Disease outbreak is a term used synonymously with epidemic and is technically more correct to use if the epidemic is confined to a localized area.[5] Several steps will be described in order (Table 10.1), although some of these steps may be applied simultaneously. The six case studies provided in Appendix I are examples of field investigations.

Establish the Existence of an Epidemic (or Outbreak)

First the epidemiologist must verify a disease outbreak exists. Local health officials will likely know if disease rates are above what are normally expected. However, the presence of a disease

TABLE 10.1 Steps for Conducting a Field Investigation

1	Establish the existence of an epidemic or outbreak
2.	Confirm the diagnosis
3.	Establish criteria for case identification
4.	Search for missing cases
5.	Count cases
6.	Orient the data according to person, place, and time
7.	Classify the epidemic
8.	Determine who is at risk of becoming a case
9.	Formulate a hypotheses
10.	Test hypotheses
11.	Develop reports and inform those who need to know
12.	Execute control and prevention measures
13.	Carry out administration and planning activities

outbreak may be difficult to detect. On the other hand, some perceived outbreaks may not be real. Misdiagnoses by physicians, for example, may give the false impression of an outbreak.

Attack rates are appropriate statistics for investigating disease outbreaks because they describe rapidly occurring new cases of disease in a well-defined population over a limited time period. Attack rates are cumulative incidence rates expressed as a percentage (see Chapter 4 "Design Strategies and Statistical Methods Used in Descriptive Epidemiology"). Attack rates are usually calculated by *person* characteristics (eg, age, sex, race/ethnicity, and occupation) in order to identify high-risk groups.

Confirm the Diagnosis

Clinical diagnosis using laboratory techniques by trained professionals are required to confirm the diagnosis of cases. Assessment of the clinical findings should be done to assure correctness and reliability of the findings. However, in some settings it may not be possible to confirm all cases. If a swift public health response is needed, where several people are confirmed cases, it may be sufficient to identify others as cases if they display the same signs and symptoms. Nevertheless, this should only be done by an appropriately trained individual.

False positive test results may cause considerable concern and give inaccurate information in a disease investigation. Some conditions, injuries, or behaviorally caused occurrences have no laboratory tests that are applicable. It is easier to diagnose a bacteria-caused disease, while an occupational or environmental disorder or condition is not easily diagnosed but still must be verified. On the other hand, some diseases or conditions are only verifiable by laboratory findings and some exotic or unique diseases are determined only by a limited number of specialized labs, including the Centers for Disease Control and Prevention.

Establish Criteria for Case Identification

A case definition involves a set of standard clinical criteria to establish if a person has a particular disease. Applying a standard case definition guarantees that every case is consistently diagnosed when and where the diagnosis occurs. For certain communicable diseases that are rare but very lethal (eg, plague) and a quick response is critical, a loose case definition may be appropriate. On the other hand, in many epidemiologic studies where a quick response is less critical and identifying causal associations is important, it may be more important to be sure people in the study have the disease. In this situation, a stricter set of criteria for establishing the presence of a disease may be in order.

The identifying features (eg, signs, symptoms, disease progression, place and type of exposure, lab findings) will depend upon the condition and disease under investigation.

Search for Missing Cases

The epidemiologist should search for cases that have not been recognized or reported. Physicians, clinics, health maintenance organizations, hospital emergency rooms, public health clinics, migrant health clinics, and related facilities should be canvassed to ascertain if other people might have the disease or condition under investigation. Asymptomatic persons or mild cases and their contacts should be evaluated. Individuals of the group are placed into appropriate categories, initially separating the suspected cases from probable cases.

Count Cases

Exposure status and disease frequency need to be determined and compared with the appropriate at-risk population.

Orient the Data According to Person, Place, and Time

Person—The epidemiologist should quickly become acquainted with the person-related issues and characteristics associated with the disease under investigation. Line listings should include information that characterizes the population and which may be adjusted for in the analysis, including: inherent characteristics or people (age, race/ethnicity, sex), acquired characteristics (immunity or marital status), activities (occupation, leisure, use of medications), and conditions (socioeconomic state, access to health care). The interactions of family, friends, fellow workers, and relatives need to be considered. Certain characteristics of the person will have more relevance to some diseases or conditions than others. For example, if diabetes is discovered to be occurring in epidemic proportions, the epidemiologist should include the characteristics of race in the analysis, because certain races have higher rates of some diseases than others. Specifically, native-Americans have high rates of diabetes; blacks have higher rates of hypertension; Asians have lower rates of cardiovascular diseases.

Place—Concentration of cases needs to be determined with regard to residence, birthplace, place of employment, school district, hospital unit, country, state, county, census tract, street address, map coordinates, etc. This will allow us to understand the geographic extent of disease, gain an understanding of where the agent that causes a disease resides and multiplies, and better understand what may carry or transmit, spread, and cause a disease. A spot map is often an effective way to present this data pictorially. If possible, the epidemiologist might also plot on a map the location of exposures or location of each case at the time of the exposure or when they were identified as being a case.

Time—Presenting each case by time of onset using an epidemic curve can provide important information about the disease outbreak. Recall from Chapter 4 that an **epidemic curve** is a histogram that shows the course of an epidemic by plotting the number of cases by time of onset. It is important to be familiar with the incubation period and how time impacts the modes and vehicles of transmission. Chronological events, step-by-step occurrences, chains of events tied to time, and time distribution of the onset of cases should be determined and plotted on charts and graphs. From the epidemic curve information, determine the nature of the course of the disease and ascertain if the group of people were exposed and infected at about the same time or at different times. Look for clustering of disease by both time and place. Determine and fix the time of the index case and the time of onset of the outbreak. Use the information from incubation periods to determine time factors in the course of the disease peaks and valleys in the epidemic curve.

Classify the Epidemic

The mode of transmission is assessed and a determination made as to whether the disease outbreak arose from a **common source epidemic** (at a specific point, through intermittent or continuous exposure to a source over days, weeks, or years), a **propagated epidemic** (through gradual spread from person-to-person), or resulted from a common source and then by secondary spread from person-to-person. The following questions should be asked when classifying an epidemic:

Common Source or Common Vehicle Epidemic

- Is the outbreak from a single source or a single point exposure?
- Is disease spread from person to person?
- Is there continued exposure to a single source?

Propagated or Progressive Epidemic

- Is the outbreak from multiple sources and/or exposures?
- Is the outbreak airborne, behaviorally or chemically caused, and does it involve multiple events or exposures?
- Are the sources of infection from unapparent sources?
- Is there a vector involved in the transmission?
- Is there an animal reservoir of infection?

Mixed outbreaks involve a combination of both common source and propagated outbreaks. They typically begin with a common source and then are propagated from person-to-person. For example, in September 1973, diarrhea caused by Salmonella typhimurium developed in 32 individuals in a hospital in Maine. The source of the outbreak was raw egg beaten in milk and then drunk as eggnog. However, 14 additional persons developed the illness who had not drunk the eggnog but presumably acquired the infection by person-to-person spread of Salmonella typhimurium.[6]

The shape of the epidemic curve for a point source epidemic typically rises rapidly, peaks, and then gradually declines. With a continuous common source epidemic, the increase may be more gradual and the curve more symmetric, covering a longer period of time. The curve typically contains one primary peak. With a propagated epidemic, the epidemic curve is usually a series of successively larger peaks.

Determine Who is at Risk of Becoming a Case

The epidemiologist must determine and classify the ill people from the well people. Who are the ill persons in the group? Who are the well persons in the group? The people in the group can be classified by their individual disease and exposure histories. Clinical, medical, and lab findings need to be confirmed, evaluated, and analyzed for all cases to substantiate the diagnosis. Asymptomatic individuals or mildly ill persons should be medically evaluated. Search for human and animal sources of infection in those at risk. Those people "exposed" are separated from the "not exposed." The "ill" are separated from the "well." The status of the health of each case needs to be determined by exposure. The 2 × 2 table introduced in Chapter 7, "Design Strategies and Statistical Methods in Analytic Epidemiology," is used to help the epidemiologist classify cases by exposure status.

Analyze the Data

The epidemiologist gathers, compiles, tabulates, analyzes, and interprets the findings. Data analysis and the results of the findings assist in making decisions about hypotheses and those at risk. All the findings and analyses should be consistent across all of the sources and all of the analysis. Findings should support the hypotheses; if not, new hypotheses should be considered.

Formulate Hypotheses

Firmly establish the source and type of epidemic. Is the outbreak from a common source or a propagated one? Identify the most probable source for the epidemic—the event, infection, or exposure source. Establish the mode of transmission. Use and analyze the information acquired earlier in the investigation, including but not limited to case counts, assessing those at risk, the sources of the epidemics, time, place or person, and attack rates. For example, if it is a food-borne epidemic, the source of food must be investigated, as should the food handling, preparation, production, and preservation approaches as well as those ill from the exposure. If the outbreak is environmentally caused, the conditions of the environment in which the individuals spent time must be investigated (eg, the air within the worksite and skin exposure to chemicals). Consider all possible sources from which the disease may be contracted—milk supplies, water supplies, seafood sources, food packing houses, imported foods, and so on.

Animal sources of infection, as well as humans, should be considered. Attack rates for the well/unexposed and the ill/exposed should be studied. All suspected vehicles of transmission should be evaluated. Frequency and levels of exposures should also be assessed. Variations in prevalence and incidence should be evaluated. As information comes in it should be evaluated and data assembled. Pertinent grouping of data based on time, place, and person characteristics and attack rates need to be completed. Findings of collateral investigators and personnel, such as physicians, laboratory personnel, and hospital health care providers, need to be gathered and assessed. Overall, the epidemiologist should develop hypotheses concerning the source of the outbreak as well as the mode of transmission (if an infectious disease).

Hypotheses need to be developed for all aspects of the investigation. For example, in a food-borne outbreak, hypotheses should be developed for the following:

- The source of infection
- The vehicle of infection

- The suspect foods
- The mode of transmission
- The type of pathogen (based on clinical symptoms, incubation periods)
- The time factors in the outbreak and course of the disease
- The place factors in the outbreak
- The person characteristics and factors in the outbreak
- The outside sources of the infection
- The transmission of the disease outside of the study population
- The exposed, unexposed, well and ill cases/individuals

Test the Hypotheses

As data and information are acquired, the various hypotheses need to be evaluated. The various hypotheses need to be tested and established and shown to be consistent or inconsistent with facts. If established facts or information are lacking to substantiate a hypothesis, then more information should be gathered or the research hypothesis should be rejected.

Develop Reports and Inform Those Who Need to Know

The report typically presents a narrative of the investigation and review of the course of the epidemic in the form of a case study. Tables, graphs, charts, or any useful and helpful illustrations are presented as well as any pertinent epidemiologic data, tests, lab reports, information, and characteristics. A good epidemiologic report addresses the information presented under hypotheses ranging from source or mode of transmission and any suggested control and prevention measures.

Communicable diseases pose a more urgent need to inform the public than noncommunicable diseases. When a disease poses a risk or danger to the public, then those who are in a position to intervene and control the epidemic need to be informed first. Public health officials, related government agencies, physicians, hospitals, health maintenance organizations (HMOs), medical clinics, schools, universities, and any group of people who are at risk are among those who need to be informed. Unfortunately, many times public health officials know of a health concern, but fail to inform those who need to know most—the population at risk. Public health officials have a responsibility to warn the public and the population at risk, and should not hesitate to do so. Sometimes officials are fearful that upon informing the population at risk, a panic will occur, but this should not be a reason to not inform the public or at least those who are at risk. Individuals should have a choice to leave the area or take protective measures to protect their families and themselves, and epidemiologists should be supportive of this position.

Execute Control and Prevention Measures

The main purpose of epidemiology and its investigations is to understand disease epidemics so that basic public health morbidity and mortality prevention and control measures can be employed. An epidemiologic investigation not only identifies the source and mode of transmission, but also identifies sources of the outbreak. Once the links to the continuance of the disease are understood, then intervention can occur, the links can be broken and the course of the disease outbreak stopped. The aim of public health disease control programs and epidemiology is to stop the spread of disease, stop epidemics, and prevent them from starting. Immunization programs are the first line of defense in prevention and control of some communicable diseases. Risk factor prevention and health protection programs are the first line of defense in behaviorally caused or environmentally founded chronic diseases. Epidemiologic investigations are conducted if prevention and control measures have failed or were never adequately implemented.

Administration and Planning Activities

Public health measures are accomplished through an organized effort under government assistance and administration. Organization, coordination, communication, planning, and funding assistance is all necessary for epidemiologic activities to occur and be successful. Immunization clinics and programs must be established and implemented. In the case of an epidemic, administrative plans and measures to provide treatment and care for the victims of the epidemic must be considered. Unbiased investigations are best handled by an agency without vested interests. Government agencies often have the experts and professionals carry out appropriate investigations of diseases, conditions, and disorders. Specialized investigations often require assistance from special laboratory facilities, cooperation with private physicians, hospitals, health maintenance organizations and clinics, and individuals, all of which are more likely to cooperate with the administration of a public health department. Financial support to protect the public's health is provided through the administrative activities of government agencies and entities.[3,4,7]

STEPS IN WORKING UP A FOOD-BORNE ILLNESS INVESTIGATION

Food poisoning, food-borne illness, and food-caused epidemics are quite common, but most are not serious and people rarely see their physicians unless it is serious; thus, little public health attention is paid to such occurrences. However, the 1993 Jack-in-the-Box epidemic caused by E. coli, which received national media attention, brought concern for food protection and preparation into the living rooms of families across America. Hamburger meat contaminated in meat processing plants was identified as the possible source of infection.

Even if an epidemic of staphylococcal food poisoning is occurring (eg, being acquired from a fast-food restaurant), most people simply take care of the matter at home, have a bout of diarrhea, take some over-the-counter anti-diarrheal drugs, and feel better the next day. Hundreds of persons could be involved, but the medical and public health community never knows, as the outbreak is short, individuals recover quickly, and the family doctor is rarely seen, let alone the outbreak being reported to the epidemiologist at the public health department. In more serious food-borne and waterborne illnesses such as salmonella, giardia, amoebic dysentery, and shigella, people do not recover so quickly; the symptoms are stronger, last longer, and medical intervention is usually needed. These diseases are serious and sometimes cause death; thus, they are most likely to be reported.

Illnesses arising from consumption of contaminated or spoiled foodstuffs and liquids, that is, solid foods, liquid foods, milk, water, and beverages are classified as **food-borne illnesses**. Food-borne illnesses are usually of three classifications: (1) food infections, (2) food poisoning, and (3) chemical poisoning.

Food infection is a result of the ingestion of disease-causing organisms (pathogens), such as bacteria, and microscopic plants and animals. Examples of food infections are

NEWS FILE

High Rates of Respiratory and Mental Health Problems in World Trade Center Rescue and Recovery Workers

Almost half of over 1,000 screened rescue and recovery workers and volunteers who responded to the World Trade Center attacks have new and persistent respiratory problems. More than half of these people also have persistent psychological symptoms. These results are based on preliminary data from a medical screening program funded by the Centers for Disease Control and Prevention and administered by the Mount Sinai Medical Center, New York City.

The findings reported in the CDC's *Morbidity and Mortality Weekly Report* are based on evaluation of data from 1,138 participants (91% were men and the median age was 41) who voluntarily enrolled in the World Trade Center Worker and Volunteer Medical Screening Program. Through August 2004, the screening program has provided free standardized medical assessments, clinical referrals, and occupational health education to nearly 12,000 workers and volunteers exposed to environmental contaminants, psychological stressors, and physical hazards. Besides respiratory and mental health effects, program participants also reported lower back and upper or lower extremity pain, heartburn, eye irritation, and frequent headache.

Only 21% of the workers and volunteers participating in the screening program had appropriate respiratory protection September 11–14, 2001. Also, 51% met the predetermined criteria for risk of mental health problems. The responses also indicated that the participants' risk for post-traumatic stress disorder (PTSD) was four times the rate of PTSD in the general male population.

The CDC's National Institute for Occupational Safety and Health (NIOSH) has increased efforts to protect emergency responders from health and safety hazards in responding to terrorist incidents. New criteria were established for testing and certifying respirators used by emergency responders against chemical, biological, radiological, and nuclear exposures. NIOSH also is partnering with responders, emergency response agencies, manufacturers, and other federal agencies to improve respirators and other personal protective equipment, improve training and education for responders, and improve safety management at disaster sites.

(Source: Centers for Disease Control and Prevention. Physical health status of world trade center rescue and recovery workers and volunteers—New York City, July 2002–August 2004. MMWR. *2004;53(35):807–812; Centers for Disease Control and Prevention. Mental health status of world trade center rescue and recovery workers and volunteers—New York City, July 2002–August 2004.* MMWR. *2004;53(35):812–815.)*

salomonellosis, giardiasis, amoebiasis, shigellosis, brucellosis, diphtheria, tuberculosis, scarlet fever, typhoid fever, and tularemia.

Food poisoning is the result of preformed toxins in foods prior to consumption, often the waste products of bacteria. The two most common forms are staphylococcus and botulism food poisoning. Staphylococcus food poisoning produces cramps and a short bout of diarrhea about six hours after consumption, being a milder form of food poisoning. The most serious and deadly form of food poisoning is that of botulism. It is said that the amount of botulism that will fit on the head of pin will cause death in humans. Obviously, this toxin is extremely poisonous.

Chemical poisoning from foodstuffs is caused by poisonous chemicals from plants and animals.

Public health and medical personnel, as in any disease investigation, must work together as a team. Personnel involved in a major disease investigation could possibly include epidemiologists, sanitarians, physicians, nurses, and laboratory personnel such as microbiologists, medical technologists, medical lab techs, and chemists.

The epidemiology team interviews, if possible, all persons who were present at the time of the ingestion of suspect foodstuffs. When large groups or populations are involved in an outbreak, it may not be feasible to interview all suspected cases. It has been suggested that in groups of over 50, half be interviewed and in groups over 100, 25% be interviewed. The use of random sampling techniques should be used to select persons to be interviewed and tested. Standardized interviewing procedures should be used. Standardized questions and information should be collected on a standardized form, which all interviewers should use.

Any good epidemiologic investigation should interview both ill and well persons. Half of the study population should come from each category. Tabulation and analysis of the data should be completed as presented in earlier chapters of this book. In food-borne disease outbreaks, certain rates should always be included in the analysis and reports. Those factors necessary to a good investigation will identify and include

- Who ate the food
- Who did not eat the food
- Calculating attack rates for each food
- For each food, calculating the attack rates among those who ate the food
- For each food, calculating the attack rates among those who did not eat the food
- Computing the relative risk (the ratio of the attack rate of those eating the food to those who did not eat the food)

Table 10.2 provides 11 steps in investigating a food-borne disease epidemic.

BASIC EPIDEMIOLOGIC QUESTIONS

Although practicing epidemiologists often ask a set of common questions, they are rarely ever written out, let alone published. This may be because each case or epidemic poses a new and different set of questions. However, some commonality does exist among the many epidemiologic questions that can be asked. Table 10.3 presents some **epidemiologic questions** that the beginning epidemiologist can refer to, if for no other reason than to stimulate thought and possibly stimulate new and different questions about the investigation.

TABLE 10.2 Investigating a Foodborne Disease Epidemic

1. Obtain a diagnosis and make a disease determination.
2. Establish that an outbreak has taken or is taking place.
3. Determine which foods are contaminated and which are suspect.
4. Determine if toxigenic organisms, infectious organisms, or chemical toxins are involved.
5. Ascertain the source of contamination. How did the foodstuff become contaminated? Who contaminated it? Where was it contaminated? Was it contaminated by direct or indirect sources?
6. After determining the source of poison and contamination, ascertain how much growth or the extent of contamination that could occur.
7. Identify foods and people implicated in the contamination and intervene to stop further spread of the disease.
8. Ensure medical treatment.
9. Exercise intervention, prevention, and control measures.
10. Inform those who need to know—private citizens, appropriate leaders, and public officials.
11. Develop and distribute reports.

In short, field epidemiology involves investigative epidemiologic questions. For example, if a disease occurs only in the summer, the epidemiologist searches for the causative factors that would be available only in that time period. Is the increase in the disease due to the exposure of new water sources—for example, drinking from a stream in the mountains, swimming in a contaminated public swimming pool or a lake? Is it a vector-borne disease? What vectors are available for disease transmission in the given time period and are missing at other times of the year or seasons? Are vehicles of transmission present during the time period that is not present during other time periods? Are the cases/subjects exposing themselves during this time period to environments, situations, places, or circumstances not available at other times of the year or in other seasons, such as hiking or camping in the woods in the summer when insects are present that are implicated in vector-borne diseases? Are certain fomites used during a certain time period that might not be used during other seasons, such as shared drinking glasses or containers? Are risk factors only seen in certain locations or places? Do they occur only at work or only at home or at the site of recreation (mountains, beaches, public swimming pool, etc.)?

TABLE 10.3 Some Investigative Epidemiologic Questions to Consider

1. In whom (which groups) is the disease present?
2. In whom (which groups) is the disease absent?
3. What are the sick people doing that the healthy people are not?
4. What are the healthy people doing that the sick people are not?
5. What are the healthy people not doing that the sick people are?
6. What are the sick people not doing that the healthy people are?
7. Can you determine whether certain cause-effect relationships are present in individuals with the condition, disease, or characteristics of interest?
8. Can you determine whether certain cause-effect relationships are blocked or not present in individuals with the condition, disease, or characteristics of interest?

TABLE 10.3 *(Continued)*

9. What are the common experiences among all of the ill persons? Common food? Common water? Common exposure to the disease? Common housing? Common clothing? Common use of fomites? Common exposure to animals/vectors? Frequenting the same places? Common behavior? Common lifestyle?
10. What are the common experiences among the well persons? Common food? Common water? Common immunity to the disease? Common housing? Common use of sanitation? Common control of animals/vectors? Frequenting the same places? Common behavior? Common lifestyle?
11. Does the disease cluster by time and place?
12. What risk factors are present in persons with the condition?
13. Are risk factors present in persons without the condition?
14. What risk factors are absent in persons who do not have the condition (healthy people)?
15. What risk factors are absent in persons with the condition?
16. What exposures to the disease exist in the sick population?
17. What exposures to the disease are lacking in the healthy population?
18. Vehicles of transmission. (Some of the questions above may be useful in reviewing the questions below.)
19. Vectors: What vectors can be implicated in the disease exposure and outbreak?
20. How have the cases been exposed to the vectors?
21. Fomites: What fomites can be implicated in the disease exposure and outbreak?
22. Waterborne transmission: What waterborne activities and exposures are implicated in the disease outbreak?
23. Foodborne transmission: What foodborne activities and exposures are implicated in the disease outbreak?
24. Airborne transmission: What airborne activities and exposures are implicated in the disease outbreak?
25. Risk factors: What risk factor activities and exposures are implicated in the disease outbreak?

EXERCISES

Key Terms

Define the following terms.

Attack rates
Chemical poisoning
Common source epidemic
Epidemic curve
Epidemiologic questions
Field epidemiology
Food-borne illnesses
Food infection
Food poisoning
Mixed outbreaks
Propagated epidemic

Study Questions

10.1 What is the most appropriate type of rate for investigating an outbreak?

10.2 When is it appropriate to refer to an epidemic as an outbreak?

10.3 How would you classify an epidemic if the epidemic curve shows a rapid rise, peak, and gradual decrease?

10.4 A county public health department in a large city received physician reports from five private practices, four clinics, and two health maintenance organizations of a total of 22 cases of tuberculosis in patients 60 years and older in a 30-day period. The city has six senior citizen large housing apartment complexes, where all but two cases were from. Most senior citizens attend a local senior center, which serves a noon meal. List the steps an epidemiologist would have to take and briefly explain key elements of each step in an investigation of this epidemic.

10.5 A fast-food hamburger restaurant chain, Fast-Food Joints of America, has been named as a possible source of a food poisoning outbreak. So far 140 cases of bloody diarrhea have been reported from various clinics and physician offices and the E. coli bacteria is suspected. Cases have been reported from 15 stores in two states. All of the meat was supplied by one supplier and involved two meat processing plants in two counties.

Using the 11 steps to working up an epidemiologic investigation of a food-borne disease epidemic presented in this chapter, outline in detail all of the activities necessary to complete an investigation of the foodborne epidemic in the fast-food restaurant.

REFERENCES

1. Jaret P. Stalking the world's epidemics: the disease detectives. *Natl Geogr Mag*. 1991;179(1): 114–140.
2. Goodman RA, Buehler JW. Field epidemiology defined. In: Gregg MB, ed. *Field Epidemiology*. 2nd ed. New York, NY: Oxford University Press; 2002.
3. Mausner JS, Kramer S. *Epidemiology: An Introductory Text*. Philadelphia, PA: WB Saunders; 1985.
4. Friedman GD. *Primer of Epidemiology*. New York, NY: McGraw-Hill; 1978.
5. Last JM, ed. *A Dictionary of Epidemiology*. 3rd ed. New York, NY: Oxford University Press; 1995.
6. Steere AC, Hall WJ, Wells JG, et al. Person-to-person spread of Salmonella typhimurium after a hospital common-source outbreak. *Lancet*. 1975;1(7902):319–322.
7. Lilienfeld AM, Lilienfeld DE. *Foundations of Epidemiology*. New York, NY: Oxford University Press; 1980.

CHAPTER

11

Chronic Disease Epidemiology

OBJECTIVES

After completing this chapter you will be able to

- Discuss the postulates of chronic disease causation proposed by Robert Koch.
- Define *latency period*, *risk factor*, and other terms frequently used in chronic disease epidemiology.
- Identify multiple risk factors associated with common diseases in the United States.
- Discuss primary prevention and control in chronic disease epidemiology.
- Understand the components and applications of the health belief model.

INTRODUCTION

Historically the main causes of death in the United States and industrialized nations were due to infectious diseases. In its infancy, epidemiology focused on a single pathogen, a single cause of disease. The epidemiologist's challenge was to isolate a single bacteria, virus, or parasite. As improvements were made in the United States and elsewhere in the areas of nutrition, housing conditions, sanitation, water supply, antibiotics, and immunization programs, the emergence of chronic diseases began to parallel the control (and decrease) of infectious disease.

Noninfectious causes of health problems (diseases) can be acute (eg, accidents, suicide, stroke) or chronic (heart disease, cancer, diabetes; see Chapter 3, "Practical Disease Concepts in Epidemiology"). Infectious diseases *can also* be chronic, but the emphasis in this chapter will be primarily on noninfectious chronic diseases. The latency period of chronic disease is the time it takes for the disease to develop once the causes are in place. For cancer the latency period involves initiation of a carcinogen, promotion by one or more agents, and progression as mutated cells multiply at an accelerated rate. When signs and symptoms manifest themselves, the latency period ends. Chronic diseases are characterized by latency periods of 10 to 20 or more years. For example, the latency period for lung cancer is 20 to 25 years. The main causes of chronic diseases are behavioral, environmental, genetic, and social.

CHRONIC DISEASE EPIDEMIOLOGY

William Farr (see Chapter 2, "Historic Developments in Epidemiology") made an important contribution when he promoted the idea that some diseases, especially chronic diseases, have a multifactorial etiology.[1] The idea that many diseases have several interrelated causes has been confirmed through epidemiologic studies in modern times. Given that chronic diseases tend to occur in people of older ages further supports the behavioral connection. Many of the diseases of today are influenced by lifestyles of modern populations: career pressures, sedentary lifestyles, high density population living, poor diet, crime, drugs, gangs, poverty, pollution, fear, stress, and economic struggles.[2,3] The primary objectives set forth by *Healthy People 2010* are to reduce coronary heart disease deaths, cancer deaths (especially lung cancer), mental disorders, work related injuries, and diabetes.[4] The key to achieving these objectives is to promote behavioral, environmental, and social changes.

The list of all chronic diseases known to occur in mankind is quite extensive. The most common noninfectious chronic diseases seen in modern times (and in those over age 65) are listed here.

- Alzheimer's disease
- Arrhythmia
- Atherosclerosis
- Cancer
- Cardiovascular diseases
- Congestive heart failure
- Coronary artery disease
- Depression
- Diabetes

- Glaucoma
- Gout
- Heart attack
- Osteoarthritis
- Osteoporosis
- Parkinson's disease
- Peripheral vascular disease
- Rheumatoid arthritis
- Stroke (cerebral vascular accident)

Figure 11.1 shows (by gender) the percentage of persons 70 years and older who reported selected chronic conditions in the United States in 1995.[5]

Postulates on Chronic Diseases

Robert Koch developed 8 guidelines on chronic disease etiology:

1. The suspected characteristics of a chronic disease must be found more frequently in persons with the diseases in question than in persons without the disease.
2. Individuals possessing the chronic disease characteristic must develop the disease more frequently than do persons not possessing the characteristic.

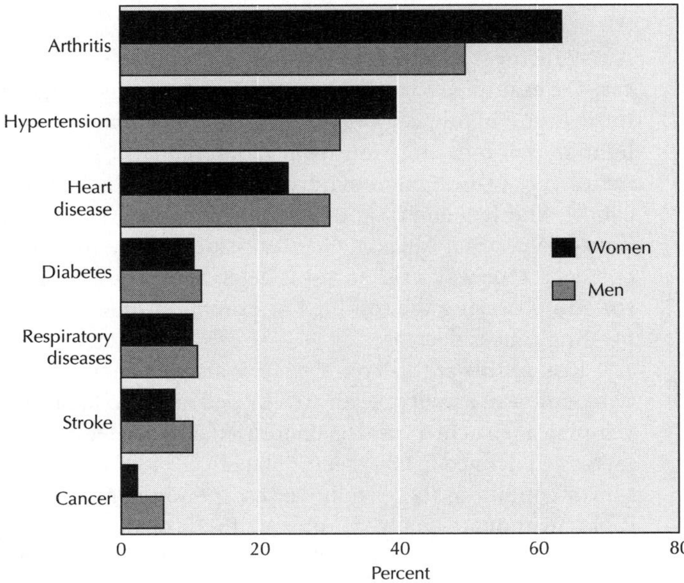

FIGURE 11.1 Percent of persons 70 years and older who reported selected chronic diseases by sex in the United States in 1995. (National Center for Health Statistics. *United States, Health and Aging Chartbook*. Hyattsville, MD: HHS, 1999.

3. If there is any observed association between a risk factor characteristic and the chronic disease, the relationship between the risk factor characteristic and the disease must be tested, as should any similar related risk factor characteristic that could cause the disease under study.
4. The incidence of the chronic disease should increase in relation to the duration and intensity of the risk factor.
5. The distribution of a risk factor should parallel that of the chronic disease in all factors.
6. All facets of a chronic disease illness should be related to the level of exposure to the risk factor.
7. The reduction or removal of the risk factor exposure should reduce or halt the disease.
8. Populations of people exposed to the risk factors in controlled studies should develop the chronic disease more often than those not exposed.[6]

A set of 5 elements relating the association between a suspected cause and the development of a chronic disease has also been developed. These 5 elements follow.

1. Consistency of the cause-effect association.
2. The strength of the cause-effect association.
3. The specificity of the cause-effect association.
4. The time factor aspects of the cause-effect association.
5. The coherence of the cause-effect association.[6]

RISK FACTORS

A **risk factor** is anything that increases a person's chance of developing a disease. In cancer, for example, 4 categories of risk factors have been identified: some chemicals (eg, those found in tobacco smoke, and in diet), radiation (eg, ultraviolet radiation from sunlight and atomic radiation from radiography or those emitted from radioisotopes), genetics (eg, Li-Fraumeni syndrome, which is linked to sarcomas, brain cancer, breast cancer, and leukemia), and some viruses/bacteria (eg, human papillomavirus, which is linked to cervical cancer). Greater risk exposure increases the probability of disease occurrence. One way a risk factor is determined is by modifying the exposure to the risk factor and observing the results. For example, when exposure to smoking is reduced, rates for lung cancer decrease.

Risk factors are also referred to as at-risk behaviors or predisposing factors. An **at-risk behavior** is an activity performed by persons who are healthy, but are at greater risk of developing a particular disease, condition, or disorder because of the behavior. **Predisposing factors**, as defined in Chapter 9, "Statistical and Causal Associations," are those existing factors or conditions that produce a susceptibility or disposition in a host to a disease or condition without actually causing it. Predisposing factors precede the direct cause. For example, the fact that a school-age child's parents smoke is a predisposing factor influencing the possibility of the child also smoking.[7–10]

Table 11.1 presents the top 8 causes of death in the United States and compares risk factors.

TABLE 11.1 Top Eight Leading Causes of Death in the United States According to Selected Risk Factors[7–10]

Risk Factors	*Heart Disease*	*Cancer*	*Stroke*	*Accidents*	*Diabetes*	*Cirrhosis*	*Suicide*	*Homicide*
Behaviorally Related								
Smoking/tobacco use	X	X		X				
Alcohol use/abuse	X	X		X		X	X	X
Nutrition/diet	X	X	X		X	X		
Lack of exercise/fitness	X	X	X		X			
High blood pressure	X		X					
Cholesterol levels	X		X					
Overweight/obesity	X	X			X			
Stress	X		X	X			X	X
Drug use/abuse	X		X	X			X	X
Lack of seat belt use				X				
Environmentally Related								
Worksite risks/exposures		X		X				
Environmental hazards		X		X				
Vehicular hazards				X				
Household hazards				X				
Medical care risks	X	X	X	X	X	X	X	
Radiation exposures		X		X				
Infectious pathogens	X	X						
Engineering/design hazards				X				
Biological/Genetic Related								
Chromosome/genetic defects	X	X	X		X	X	X	
Congenital anomalies	X	X	X		X	X	X	
Developmental defects	X	X	X		X	X	X	
Socially Related								
Poverty	X	X	X	X	X	X	X	X
Low educational level	X	X	X	X	X	X	X	X
Lack of work skills	X	X	X	X	X	X	X	X
Disrupted families	X	X	X	X	X	X	X	X

NONINFECTIOUS DISEASES AND CONDITIONS: WEBS OF CAUSATION

Because behavioral, environmental, genetic, and social factors all contribute to the risk of noninfectious diseases and conditions, a methodology for assessing these factors is needed. Some infectious disease outbreaks have been easy to investigate because sources of causation are based on one agent or pathogen. Even when exposure comes from multiple sources, transmission of the disease is limited.

Some behaviorally founded chronic diseases develop from **multiple exposures** to a single source and a single agent. Cancer of the lip, gums, mouth, and throat from chewing tobacco is a good example. The chewing tobacco is the single agent and the single source to which the user has multiple exposures. The person, place, and time elements are quite limited yet identifiable because smokeless tobacco use is growing in some segments of the population, especially among younger males in certain places in the United States, especially rural areas with the "cowboy" images, trends, and social influences. A **web of causation** for cancer of the mouth with smokeless tobacco would be fairly simple and would include factors such as free samples given to teens from tobacco companies in hopes of hooking the youth, social influences, sex, age, place, parental influences, physiological factors, addiction factors, etc.[9]

When obvious cause-effect associations are seen, as in smokeless tobacco and cancer of the mouth, then investigations are easy to accomplish. However, when a population group comes down with a single disease or several related diseases with a single clear and obviously identifiable source lacking, a web of causation can be of value. For example, if a high rate of pancreatic cancer occurs in a group of children within a limited geographical area, the search for the source and the actual cause is not a simple task. If cancer of the pancreas, kidneys, and liver are seen in the same population group, the investigation becomes even more complicated. Even though all three organs are located within the abdominal cavity, the functions of each and chance for exposure for each vary as each has a totally different physiologic process.

Questions about causation are not easily answered. As for pancreatic cancer, the epidemiologist might ask several questions. What are the sources or types of carcinogen (eg, radiation or chemical)? Is there some genetic predisposition in the population group? When lacking a common and clear source of disease, citizens have looked at all kinds of possibilities. For example, presence of high-tension power lines in the area, such as in a case in Denver, Colorado, has been suspected in certain types of cancer and genetic diseases. When the cause of disease is not clear, other factors must be considered, such as the possible presence of hazardous waste dumps under the homes, problems with food, water, the surface soil; use of pesticides, and herbicides, air pollution, gases; the close proximity to chemical plants or other industries, and other. Thus, a web of causation could be constructed to help solve the mystery of sources and causation.

Webs of Causation and Causation Decision Trees

Webs of causation have limitations in that they may not directly lead the epidemiologic investigator right to the cause. **Decision trees**, used with webs of causation, are the suggested approach. When constructing a web of causation, a separate decision tree would be developed for each aspect, factor, and causation element. The yes–no response of decision trees leads the epidemiologist closer to discovering the cause than a web of causation alone. Decision trees, as used in disease diagnosis, can ask leading questions that are answered either yes or no, thus eliminating possibilities of causation while leading the investigator down the correct path toward discovery, assuming the questions are answered correctly.

Some branches of a web of causation may require second-level assessments as secondary levels of causation or risk factors may have to be taken into account. This may require the development of a second-level set of webs. In some cases a third level of assessment, which includes a third-level set of webs, may be required. The second level and third level of webs feed into the appropriate branches of the main web, accounting for all possible risk factors or factors that contribute to the disease, directly and indirectly.

Web construction approaches have been developed several ways: flow charts starting from the top moving to the disease diagnosis at the bottom in a step-by-step fashion; a central downward flowing core with branches from each side (see Figures 9.1 and 9.3). In the case of lead poisoning, the mode of entry into the body influenced a 3 channel flow toward the cause of the disease (see Figure 9.3). In the spirit of a true web approach, Figure 11.2 presents a spider web configuration to illustrate, in a general fashion, the elements of a web of causation with the disease as the focus.[11] Figure 11.3 presents a second web of causation with a focus on the causes of the disease/risk factors.[11] Figure 11.4 presents an example of a decision tree that must be adapted for each situation and element under consideration in the investigation.[11] In summary, a web of causation is a quasi-flow chart that identifies every remote possible risk factor from every dimension of living, leading eventually to the diagnosed disease. At each step and for each element, a decision tree is established and worked through in order to assure the correct decision is being made leading to causation of the disease.

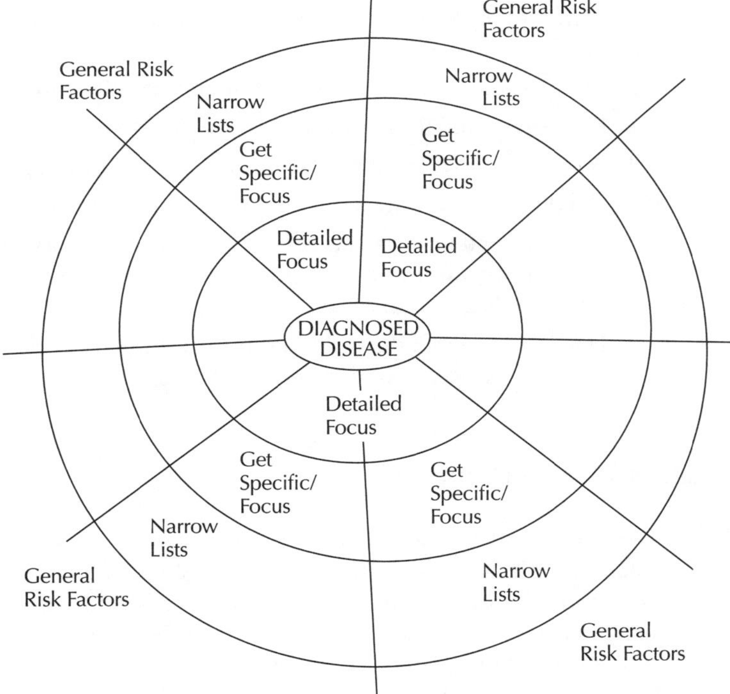

FIGURE 11.2 Basic concepts in the construction of a web of causation with the disease as the focus.

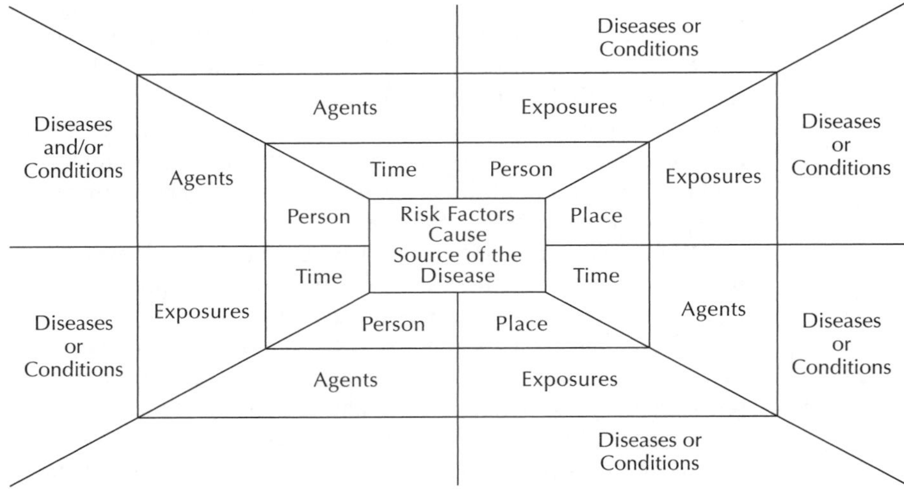

FIGURE 11.3 Web of causation with risk factors, cause, and source of disease as the focus of the investigation.

Construction of a Web of Causation and Decision Trees

1. Identify the problem, affirm the condition, and obtain an accurate diagnosis of the disease.
2. Place the diagnosis at the center or bottom of the web.
3. Brainstorm and list all possible sources for the disease.
4. Brainstorm and list all risk factors and predisposing factors of the disease.
5. Develop sub-webs and tertiary level sub-webs for the various branches of webs if needed.
6. Organize and arrange lists of sources and risk factors from general and most distant from the disease, in steps, being more specific and focused as the steps move closer toward the diagnosis of the disease.
7. Develop and work through causation decision trees for each element under consideration on the way toward the diagnosed disease.

Decision Trees in Webs of Causation

Decision trees have been used as decision-making tools with regard to administration of pharmaceuticals, medical diagnoses, emergency care decision making, health screening, communicable disease investigation, and other related activities. In chronic disease and behaviorally caused diseases and disorder investigations, decision trees are supportive to the web investigation process. In webs of causation, decision trees are not techniques in and of themselves but assist the web investigation method. Multiple decisions may be used in complex disorders with multiple risk factors and multiple exposures and agents, such as found in heart disease, stroke, and cancer.

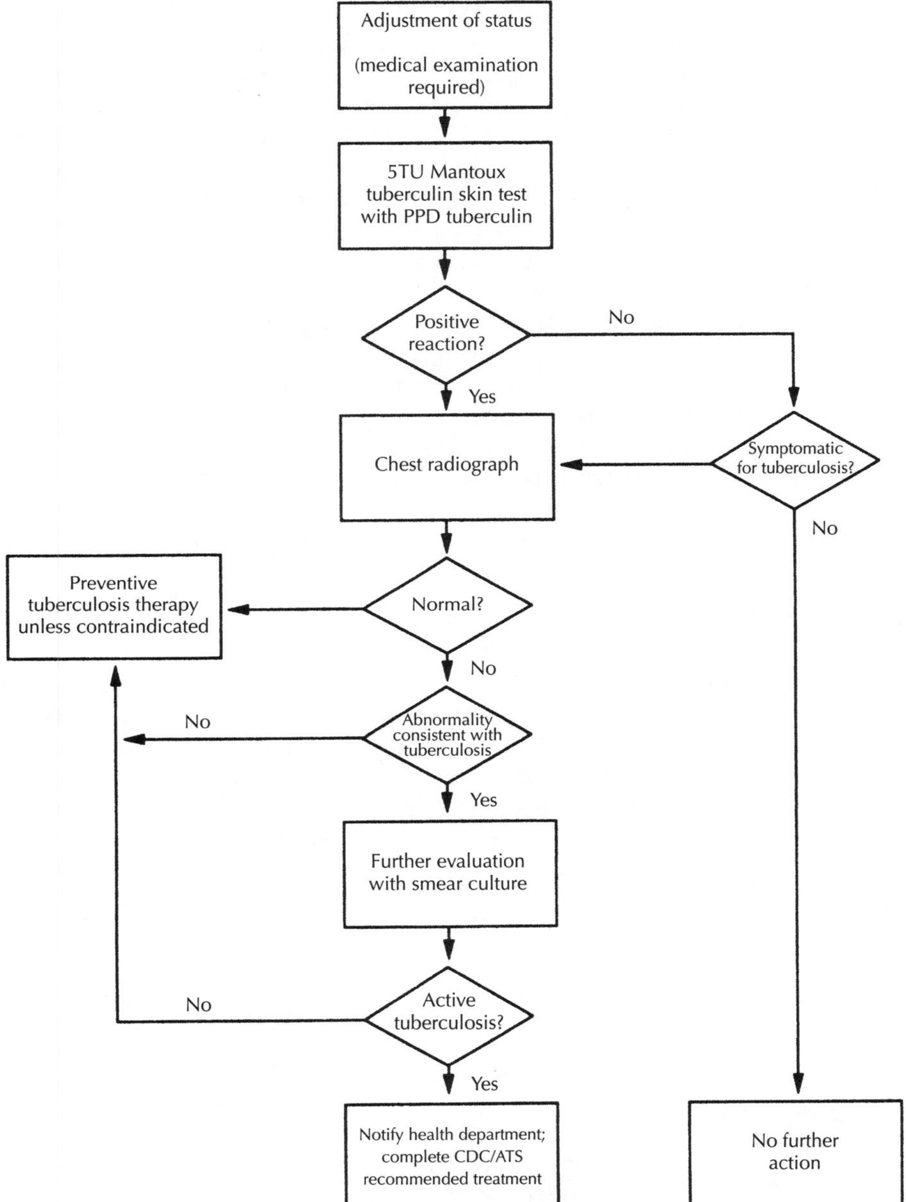

FIGURE 11.4 Example of a decision tree used in epidemiological decision making, showing the decision making activities for tuberculosis screening for non-immigrants in the United States who request permanent residence. (Centers for Disease Control and Prevention. Tuberculosis among foreign-born persons entering the United States. *MMWR.* 1990;39(RR-18):1–13, 18–21.)

Figure 11.4 assists in understanding just how the decision trees work. Diamond-shaped boxes represent decision points. Rectangular boxes represent activities. "Yes" and "No" decision points are indicated while arrows show the direction to the next activity or decision point. Decision trees can reroute activities back toward the beginning if certain criteria are not met or the decision falls short of meeting expectations. Decision trees are followed until the final step is met; in Figure 11.4 "no further action" is the final result.[9]

Using the decision tree technique within the web of causation may be less complex in some cases, and may not require extensive decision trees for all risk factors. On the other hand, certain risk factors may be quite complex and, as a result, the decision trees must also be complex. For example, in a hypothetical case of an outbreak of increased heart attacks in air traffic controllers, all risk factors would be listed. Risk factors considered might be stress, smoking or tobacco use, drug use, illicit drug use, alcohol use, age, hours worked, years in profession, emotional stability, personal problems, social problems, sleep habits, physical fitness, and diet/nutrition.

Decision trees would then be developed for each risk factor or sub-element of the risk factor. Using diet and nutrition as an example, a decision tree could be constructed on eating habits and food selection, vitamin and nutrient intake, fat consumption and cholesterol levels, salt intake, and sugar and caffeine consumption.

Fish Bone Diagrams (Cause-Effect Diagrams)

Fish bone diagrams (Figure 11.5) are also referred to as **cause-effect diagrams** and are developed to provide a visual presentation of all possible factors that could contribute to a disease, disability, or death. **Fish bone diagrams** assist the epidemiologist in defining, determining, uncovering, or eliminating possible causes.

The first step in the fish bone diagram activity is to brainstorm lists of all potential causes or contributing risk factors. The fish bone diagram is then constructed by placing the categories of causes on the "bones" of the diagrams, making it a visual display for easy study and

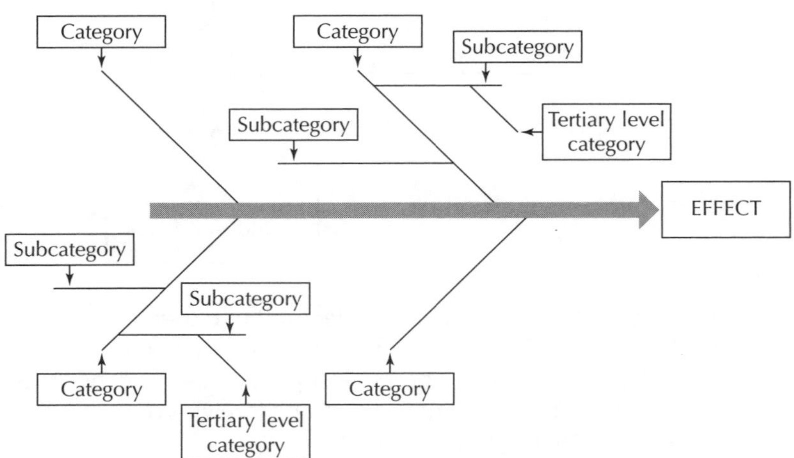

FIGURE 11.5 Example of construction of fish bone diagram.

analysis. The second step is to develop subcategories of all specific causes for each of the major category areas. Each branch of the fish bone is given a label or becomes a category and subcategories are placed on the lines that make up the bones. It is also possible to add a third (tertiary) level of cause to the bones of the diagram. The head of the fish bone is assigned a box that contains the effect or outcome, which is the disease, disability, condition, injury, or death.

The diagram is complete when all possible risk factors or causes have been properly placed within the categories and subcategories of the diagram, on the lines that create the fish bone effect. An outline of the categories, subcategories, and tertiary levels can be developed and presented as well. An assessment of the cause-effect relationship statements of facts of occurrence at the tertiary, subcategory, and category levels should be made for each and every statement. The statements are answered yes or no, or are answered true or not true.

DESCRIPTIVE EXAMPLES OF NONINFECTIOUS DISEASES AND CONDITIONS IN THE UNITED STATES

Cigarette Smoking among Adults in the United States

In 1998 it was estimated that 47.2 million adults, which is 24.1% of the total population, were everyday smokers. Of men, 24.8 million smoke, which is 26.4%, and 22.4 million smokers were women, which is 22.4% of the female population. Of adult smokers, 19.75% are everyday smokers. Smoking was highest for persons in the age range 18–24 years: 27.9%. Historically, persons in the 25–44 age range were the highest percentage of smokers. Prevalence of smoking was highest for American Indian and Alaskan Natives at 40%; the next highest was whites at 25%; next was blacks at 24.7%; next was Hispanics at 19.1%; and the lowest was Asian/Pacific Islanders at 13.7%. Smoking prevalence was highest among those between 9 and 11 years of age and living below the poverty level at 36.8% participating in smoking. It was estimated that 44.8 million adults or 22.9% were former smokers, comprising 25.7 million men and 19.1 million women.

The association between failing and dropping out of high school and smoking is high, with smokers being more likely to fail or drop out of high school. Smokers are encouraged to quit smoking—enroll in smoking cessation programs and use available products such as the nicotine patch, inhaler, or gum—because of the toll that smoking takes on their health. Public health programs are encouraged to continue development of public health education programs, educational commercials, and school health education in order to influence teenagers and preteens to not smoke.[12]

Tobacco use Among Middle and High School Students

Nationally 8.2% of students first smoked a cigarette before age 11. Males were more likely to smoke a cigarette before age 11 than females. The percentage of children smoking a cigarette before age 11 was 9.2% for whites, 10.6% for Hispanics, and 5.3% for blacks. The percent of males who smoked a cigar was 4.9%; the percent for females was 1.4%. Nationally 4.8% of students used smokeless tobacco before age 11. Figure 11.6 shows percentages of middle-school and high-school students who ever used tobacco products.[13]

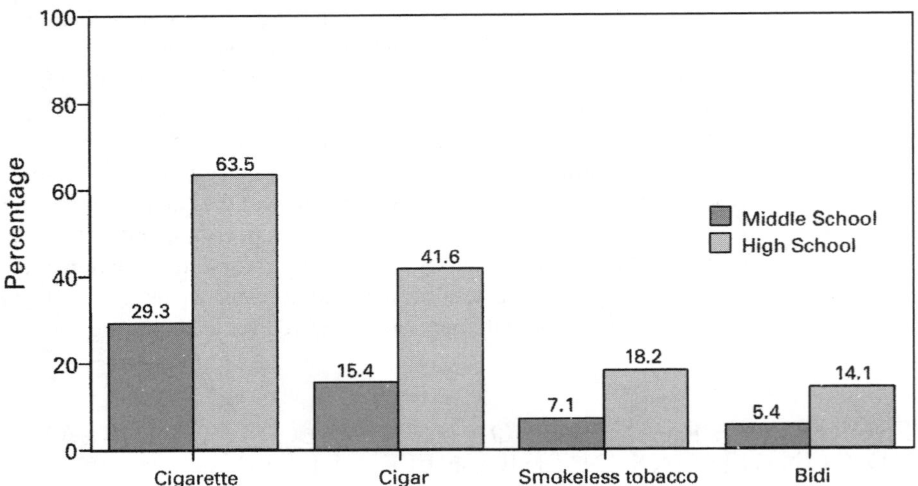

FIGURE 11.6 Percent of middle school and high school students who ever used tobacco products—Nation Youth Tobacco Survey, 1999. (Centers for Disease Control and Prevention. Youth tobacco surveillance United States, 1998–1999. *MMWR.* 2000;49(No. SS-10):9–11.)

Nationally, 96.2% of middle school students who had never smoked cigarettes responded that they would not try a cigarette soon; 85.3% of students responded that they definitely would not smoke in the next year; and 84.2% of students said they would definitely not smoke if a best friend offered them a cigarette. Nationally, 97.6% of high school students who had never smoked cigarettes responded that they would not try a cigarette soon; 82% of students responded that they would definitely not smoke in the next year; and 84.8% of students said they would definitely not smoke if a best friend offered them a cigarette. This is an interesting response because 24% of the people in the United States smoke.

Epidemiology of Hip Fractures

More than 250,000 hip fractures occur each year in the United States. About 20% of people who have a hip fracture are dead within one year, which costs the health care system about $5.4 billion each year, and many of the survivors never regain an acceptable level of function. Women have more hip fractures than men. White men have a 5% lifetime risk of a hip fracture and white women have a 16% lifetime risk. Diet, cigarette smoking, an increasingly sedentary lifestyle, and alcohol use are suggested causes. About 90% of hip fractures are associated with falls. Only 1 to 2% of all falls lead to hip fractures. For the hip to fracture the person must fall so that the point of impact is on or near the hip.

Studies of twins and mother-daughter pairs have shown that bone mass is largely genetically determined. Other studies have shown that replacement estrogen therapy prevents or greatly reduces loss of bone mass in both women who have had their ovaries removed and in women with intact ovaries. Women who had taken estrogen for 7 years before reaching age 75 had a higher bone mass. Women who go through menopause later in life have a reduced risk of hip fracture. Risk factor for hip fractures are: (1) low bone mineral density,

(2) history of falls, (3) direction of fall, (4) neuromuscular impairment, (5) decrease in weight, (6) poor health status, (7) older age, (8) physical inactivity, (9) family history of hip fracture, (10) osteoarthritis, and (11) white race. (The evidence for some of these risk factors is strong and moderate in others.) In nursing home populations it was found that supplemental calcium and vitamin D, plus external hip protectors, can reduce hip fractures by 50%.[14] Figure 11.7 shows the incidence of hip fractures by age, race and sex.

Genetic Epidemiology of Epilepsy

Epilepsy can be defined as unprovoked seizures. Clinically epilepsy is sub-classified according to seizure type. Partial seizures include:

- partial seizures with elementary symptomatology (generally without impairment of consciousness)
- partial seizures with complex symptomatology (generally with impairment of consciousness)
- partial seizures secondarily generalized

Generalized seizures (involves entire brain) are:

- petit mal
- bilateral massive epileptic myoclonus
- infantile spasms
- clonic seizures
- tonic seizures
- tonic–clonic seizures (grand mal)
- atonic seizures
- akinetic seizures

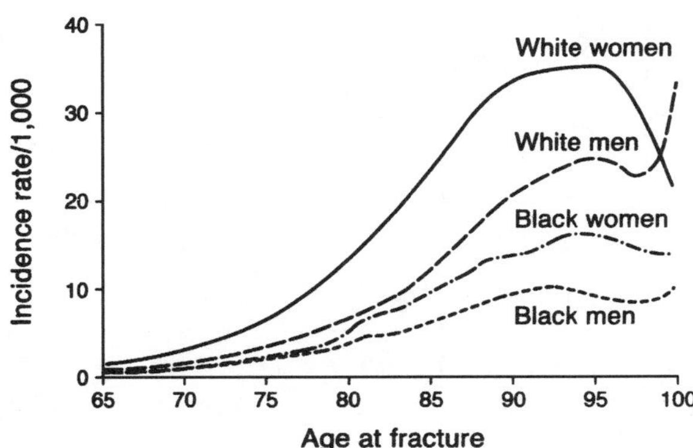

FIGURE 11.7 Age, race, and sex of persons suffering hip fracture in the United States. (Cumming RG, Nevitt MC, Cummings SR. Epidemiology of hip fractures. *Epidemiol Rev*. 1997;19(2):244–253.)

Two additional classifications used are *idiopathic*, which have genetic origins, and *cryptogenic*, which have nongenetic origins, such as head trauma. Epilepsy is the most common neurological disorder, with about 4% of the United States population suffering from this condition. There is strong evidence linking epilepsy to a genetic influence, and two epilepsy genes have been identified. Figure 11.8 shows the risk of unprovoked seizures in offspring of mothers and fathers with epilepsy.[15] Other causes of epilepsy include head trauma, stroke, or brain infection, with 25% of cases resulting from these factors.

Etiology of Brain Tumors in Adults

Brain tumors are among the most lethal. A person with a brain tumor has a 52% chance of surviving one year. Both environmental and genetic factors have been implicated in brain tumors. The list of environmental agents includes physical (radiation), chemical, and biological agents. Very little is known about the cause of brain tumors in adults, but it has been well established that some persons inherit a predisposition to develop them. Exposures to organic solvents, vinyl chloride, pesticides, and polycyclic aromatic hydrocarbons have been implicated as occupational risks.

The main type of brain tumor adults get are gliomas with the main type of glioma being astrocytes (star shaped). It is not uncommon for patients with a glioma to have multiple tumors. It is highly unusual for brain tumors to metastasize outside the central nervous system (CNS); however, there is some seeding within the CNS. The brain is a common place for metastasis from cancers in the lung, breast, rectum, kidney, and stomach. There is a predominance of glioma in men and predominance of meningioma in females. Figure 11.9 shows graphs on the incidence of various types of brain tumors.[16]

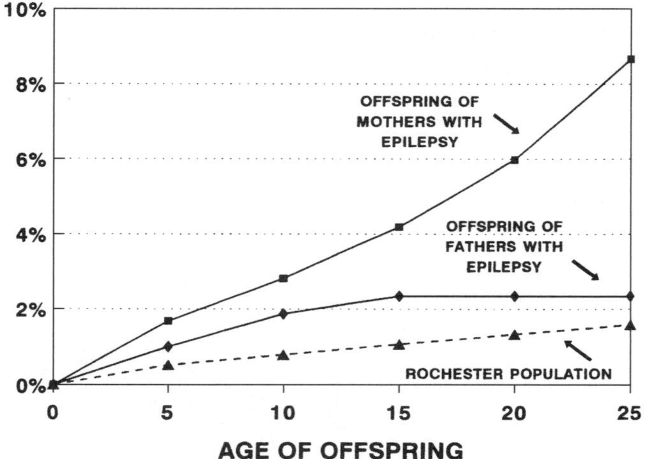

FIGURE 11.8 Risk of unprovoked seizures in offspring of mothers and fathers with epilepsy for the general population of Rochester, Minnesota, 1935–1979. (Ottman R, Genetic epidemiology of epilepsy. *Epidemiol Rev*. 1997;19(1):120–127.)

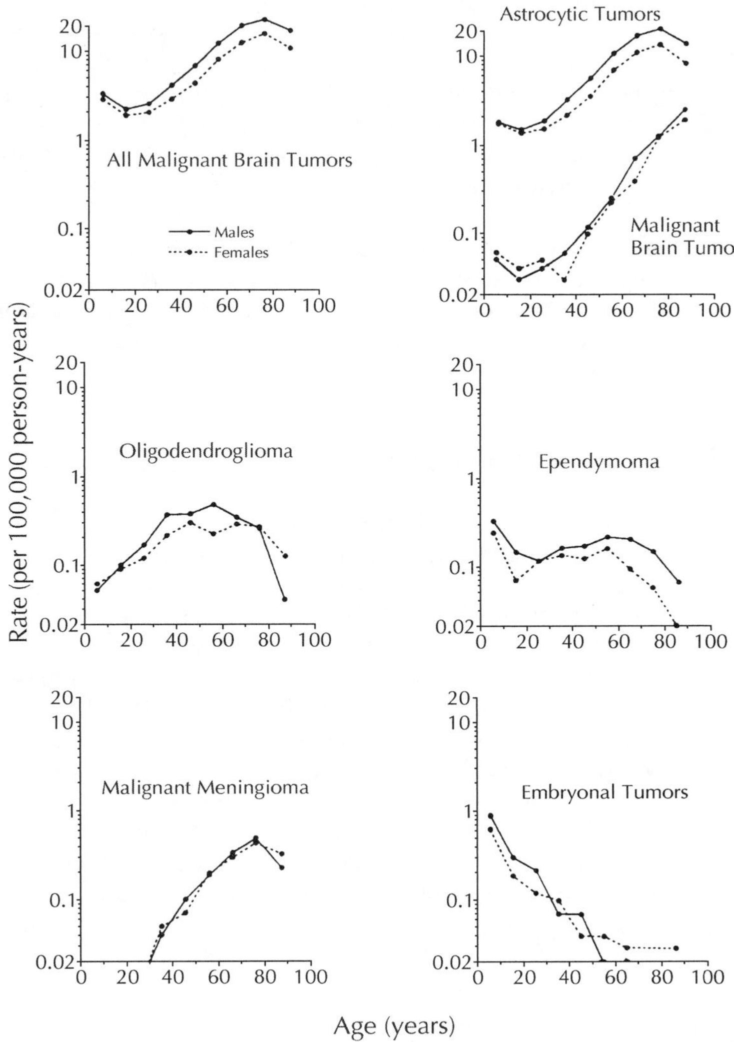

FIGURE 11.9 Age-specific incidence rates for malignant brain tumors. The solid line is for males and the dotted line is for females. (Inskip PD, Linet MS, Heineman EF. Etiology of brain tumors in adults. *Epidemiol Rev.* 1995;17(2):382–404.)

Breast Cancer

Among women in the United States, breast cancer is the most common form of cancer. As a cause of death, it remains second only to lung cancer. The risk for breast cancer increases with advancing age. Risk factors include family history of breast cancer, history of certain benign breast diseases, early age of menarche, late age of menopause, exposure to ionizing radiation, obesity, being Caucasian, having the first child at a late age, not breast feeding, nodular densities on a mammogram, higher socioeconomic status, and living in an urban area in the northeastern United States. The incidence rate of breast cancer among first-generation Japanese-Americans is slightly higher than the rate for their mothers, but the rate among their daughters is considerably higher. The American Cancer Society estimates that 215,990 new cases of female breast cancer and 40,110 deaths from female breast cancer occurred in the United States in 2004.[17] In 2002, female breast cancer incidence rates in the United States (per 100,000) were 138 in whites and 120 in blacks.[18] Corresponding breast cancer mortality rates (per 100,000) were 25 and 34.[18] Mammography is the most effective method of detecting breast cancer in its earliest and most treatable stage. Also it is recommended that women do a breast self-exam on a regular basis. Figure 11.10 shows the incidence and death rates of breast cancer among white and black women in the United States for the years 1975–2002.

Blood Lead Levels in Young Children

Lead exposure adversely affects cognitive development and can cause kidney disease and behavioral problems in young children. Lead poisoning is also chronic and irreversible. Historically older homes and apartment buildings were painted with lead paint, which flakes and forms chips when it gets old. Families below the poverty level cannot afford adequate housing and thus are forced to live in substandard houses and apartment buildings. Children who live in older substandard housing often ingest these peeling paint chips. Also, in some imported ceramic ware, the glaze contains lead. If acidic liquids are put in these containers, the acid will dissolve the ceramic glaze, thus causing the liquid to contain lead. Elevated blood lead levels have decreased by approximately 80% since the late 1970s. High blood lead levels remain among low-income urban dwellers and those living in older housing. A 19-state survey was conducted by the Centers for Disease Control and Prevention to assess the blood lead levels in children. Blood samples were collected from children under six years of age in all of the 19 states. In Figure 11.11, the percentage of children with corresponding blood lead levels is presented.[19]

PREVENTION AND CONTROL

At the beginning of this text, epidemiology was defined. In addition to being the study of the distribution (frequency and pattern) and determinants of health-related states or events in human populations, it involves the application of this study to prevent and control health problems. With the shift from infectious acute diseases to noninfectious chronic diseases in the United States, public health prevention and control efforts have also changed emphasis. As risk factors for disease are identified and the extent of these risk factors made known through epidemiologic study, the potential for effective prevention and control efforts exist. For example, primary prevention of cancer includes the following risk intervention:

- Maintain a healthy weight.
- Eat no more than two or three servings of red meat per week.
- Take a multivitamin with folate every day.

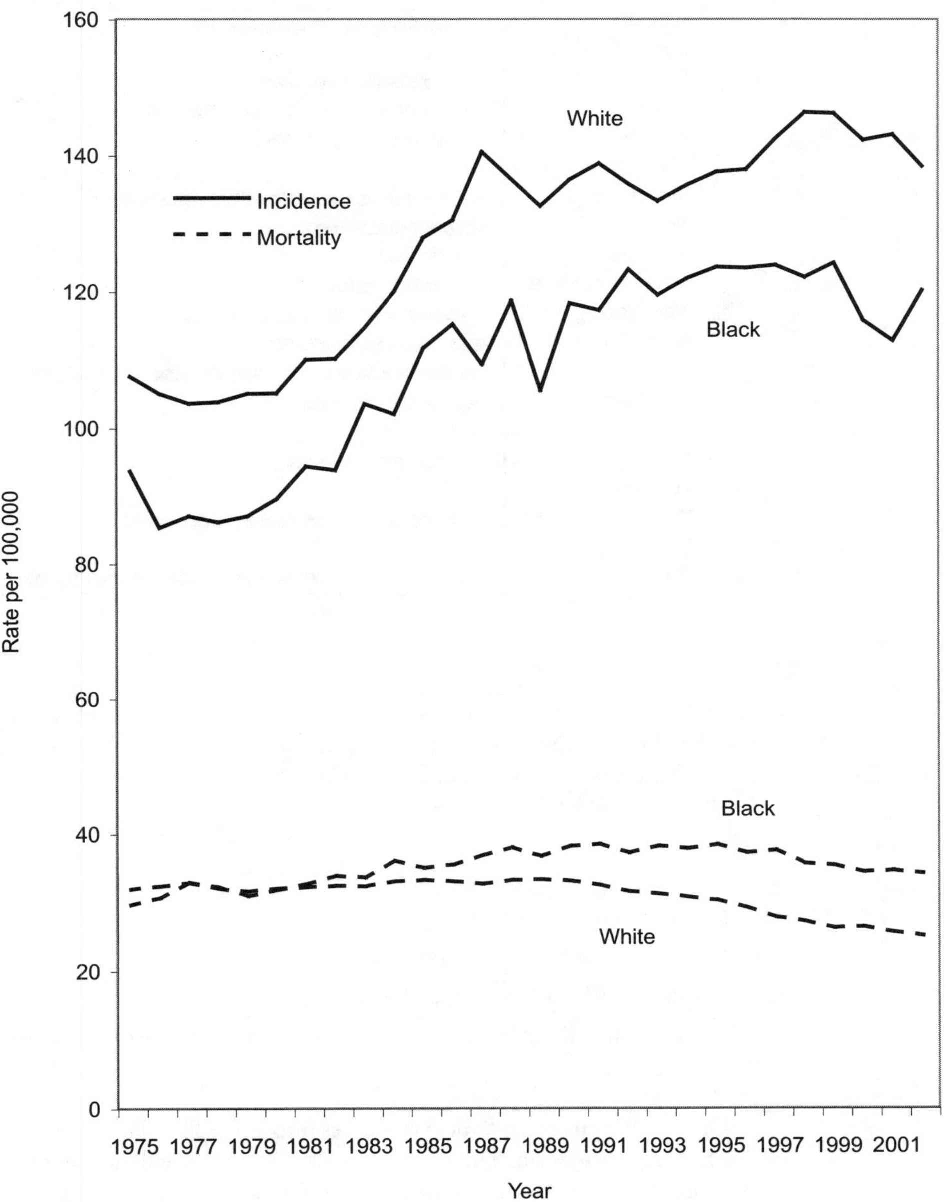

FIGURE 11.10 Age-adjusted (to the 2000 US standard population) incidence death rates of female breast cancer among white and black women in the United States for the years 1975–2002. (Source: Surveillance, Epidemiology, and End Results (SEER).

- Drink less than one alcoholic drink a day.
- Eat five or more servings of fruits and vegetables per day.
- Eat more high fiber foods such as whole grains, wheat cereals, bread, and pasta.
- Include cruciferous vegetables in your diet (such as broccoli, cabbage, etc.).

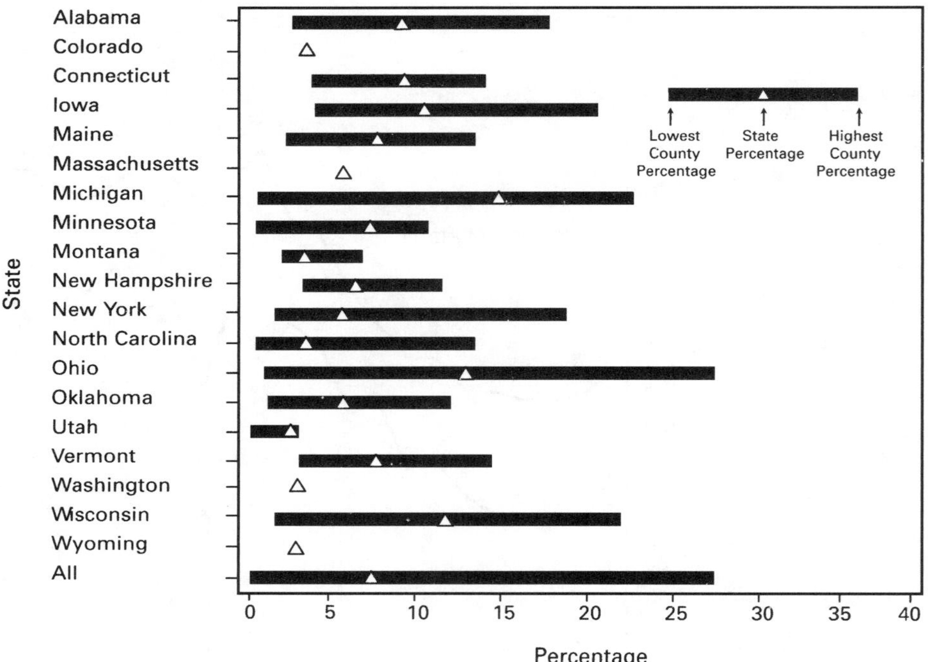

FIGURE 11.11 State-specific percentage of children under the age of 6 who tested positive for elevated blood lead levels. (Centers for Disease Control and Prevention. Blood lead levels in young children—United States and selected states, 1996–1999. *MMWR.* 2000;49(49):1133–1135.)

- Do not smoke.
- Protect yourself from the sun.
- Avoid certain workplace exposures.
- Protect yourself and your partner(s) from sexually transmitted infections.
- Exercise regularly.

The CDC puts considerable resources into annually collecting and disseminating health risk factor information. The Behavior Risk Factor Surveillance System (BRFSS) is a state-level prevalence survey in the United States which monitors actual behavioral risks, rather than information on attitudes or knowledge, associated with premature morbidity and mortality. This information is specifically useful for planning, initiating, supporting, and evaluating prevention programs.[20] It should be emphasized, however, that although BRFSS provides behavior risk factor data, chronic diseases and health-related conditions are often associated with more than just behavior-related risk factors.

The multifactorial etiology of noninfectious conditions was emphasized in Table 11.1. Consequently, prevention and control of noninfectious diseases and conditions is often much more complicated than that of infectious diseases. Health educators often find that effective prevention and control programs require more than just trying to influence be-

NEWS FILE

Climate Conditions Affect Physical Activity among Adults in the United States

A recent study, reported in the *American Journal of Health Behavior,* 2005, quantified the effects of climate on physical activity. The study matched data from 255 weather stations with results from a physical activity survey of people in 355 US counties. Weather measurements—taken four times a day at each weather station—included daily air temperature, dew point temperature, wind speed direction, sea level pressure, and total cloud cover. To gauge physical activity, the researchers took data from an ongoing national telephone survey of adults 18 years and older, a project between the Centers for Disease Control and Prevention and US states and territories. Meeting the recommendation for physical activity was defined as 30 minutes of moderate physical activity five to seven days a week or 20 minutes of vigorous physical activity three to seven days a week. Moderate activity included brisk walking, biking, vacuuming, and gardening; vigorous activity included running, aerobics, and heavy yard work.

The study found that the highest physical activity was linked to moist moderate conditions in winter, dry polar air in spring, dry tropical air in summer, and moist polar air in fall. Moist tropical air is warm and very humid, the researchers say, with cloud cover in winter and partial cloud cover in summer. Muggy conditions "are consistently associated with lowest mean percentages meeting recommendations for physical activity," the researchers found. Dry tropical air is warm and sunny. Polar air, which leads to the coldest conditions, can be either dry with little cloud cover or moist with cloud cover and, often, precipitation. Counties that ranked in the top quarter for physical activity had the highest percentage of dry, moderate days, followed by moist polar days, then dry polar. Counties in the bottom quarter had the highest percentage of days with moist tropical conditions.

After Montana, with 60.9%, the states with the highest percentages of respondents meeting recommended physical activity levels were Utah with 59.2%, Wisconsin with 57.9%, and New Hampshire with 55.9%. On the other hand, after Puerto Rico, at 30.9%, the states with the lowest percentages were Hawaii with 36.4%, North Carolina with 37.4% and Kentucky with 37.6%. Physical activity also varied significantly among seasons, with activity highest in summer at 48.4%, 46.2%, in spring, 45.8%, in fall, and 44.6% in winter.

Source: Merrill RM, Shields EC, White GL Jr, Druce D. Climate conditions and physical activity among adults in the United States. Am J Health Behav. *2005;29(4):371–381.*

haviors. For example, a health education program aimed at reducing risk behaviors associated with heart disease may be ineffective if poverty levels are high such that a nutritious diet is not affordable and the economy promotes feelings of hopelessness. The interaction between behavior, environment, genetic, and social risk factors often make prevention efforts complex and sometimes infeasible. It also emphasizes why prevention programs need to be specifically tailored to given societies and cultures. However, despite the complexities of primary prevention it provides the greatest potential for minimizing public suffering and health care costs.

PRIORITIES IN DISEASE PREVENTION AND CONTROL

The following questions can be used in establishing priorities in disease prevention and health promotion:

1. Which disease, disorder, or condition has the greatest impact on illness, disability, injury, lost work time or school time, unnecessarily using up health resources, rehabilitation costs, causing family disruption, economic impact, and costs?
2. Are special populations or groups of people suffering from exposures to diseases, agents, risk factors, or hazards?
3. Which susceptible populations are most likely to respond to prevention, intervention, and control measures?
4. Which risk factors, diseases, agents, or hazards are most likely to respond to control measures?
5. Are there diseases, disabilities, injuries, disorders, or conditions that need to be investigated, that are being overlooked, or are not being responded to by other organizations or agencies?
6. Of the many risk factors, diseases, agents or hazards, which would yield the greatest improved health status, social impact, and economic benefit to the target population?
7. Of the many risk factors, diseases, agents, or hazards, which are of national, regional, state, or local concern and of major priority for an epidemiological investigation?[10]

HEALTH BELIEF MODEL IN EPIDEMIOLOGY

Many behavior change models are based on the belief that knowledge itself is not a motivating factor in changing problem behaviors. This is a widely accepted premise in health behavior change theory.[21] According to the **health belief model**, a widely used conceptual framework for understanding health behavior, behavior change requires a rational decision-making process that considers perceived susceptibility to illness, perceived consequences or seriousness of the illness, belief that recommended action is appropriate or efficacious to reduce risk, and belief that the benefits of action outweigh the costs.[22–24] For example, an individual may be aware of potential adverse health outcomes associated with smoking, cardiovascular disease and cancer, but unless these health outcomes are perceived to be personally threatening and serious, the potential benefits from not smoking may not outweigh the perceived costs of this behavior.

The health belief model originally involved four concepts representing perceived susceptibility, perceived severity, perceived benefits, and perceived barriers. Two extensions of these concepts in more recent years include cues to action and self-efficacy. The following table in *Theory at a Glance: A Guide for Health Promotion Practice* presents the concepts, along with definitions and applications, of the health belief model (Table 11.2).[25]

Prevention is hard to measure and cannot always be demonstrated by empirical research, but, like quality, it is observable. Common sense dictates that prevention works and must be made the main focus of all health care and public health activity in order to maintain and improve the health status of populations. Fear and pain can be powerful motivational forces in changing behavior. However, to avoid chronic diseases, one must embrace

TABLE 11.2 Concepts, definitions, and applications of the health belief model

Concept Definition	***Application***	
Perceived Susceptibility	One's opinion of chances of getting a condition	Define population(s) at risk, risk levels; personalize risk based on a person's features or behavior; heighten perceived susceptibility if too low
Perceived Severity	One's opinion of how serious a condition and its consequences are	Specify consequences of the risk and the condition
Perceived Benefits	One's belief in the efficacy of the advised action to reduce risk or seriousness of impact	Define action to take; how, where, when; clarify the positive effects to be expected
Perceived Barriers	One's opinion of the tangible and psychological costs of the advised action	Identify and reduce barriers through reassurance, incentives, assistance
Cues to Action	Strategies to activate "readiness"	Provide how-to information, promote awareness, reminders
Self-Efficacy	Confidence in one's ability to take action	Provide training, guidance in performing action

healthy behaviors and lifestyles long before pain or fear occurs. Prevention and control of diseases, disorders, injuries, disabilities, and death in populations remains the primary purpose for the existence of epidemiology.

EXERCISES

Key Terms

Define the following terms.

At-risk behavior
Cause-effect diagram
Decision tree
Fish bone diagram
Health belief model
Multiple exposures
Predisposing factor
Risk factor
Web of causation

Study Questions

11.1 A chronic disease may be which of the following:

a. Infectious, communicable

b. Noninfectious, noncommunicable

c. Neither (a) or (b)

d. Both (a) and (b)

11.2 Chronic diseases are mainly caused by what four general factors?

11.3 Why are primary prevention measures more complex for chronic diseases such as heart disease or cancer than infectious acute conditions like cholera or lyme disease?

11.4 What is the leading cause of cancer in women in the United States? List five known risk factors for this disease.

11.5 Research, develop, and construct a general problem centered web of causation for illicit drug abuse and for alcoholism.

11.6 Based on Figure 11.3 and the supportive concepts of decision trees as a part of a web of causation, develop and explain a decision tree supportive to a web of causation on alcoholism.

11.7 Select a chronic disease example and apply it to the six concepts presented for the health belief model.

REFERENCES

1. Fox JP, Hall CE, Elveback LR. *Epidemiology: Man and Disease*. New York: Macmillan Company; 1970.
2. Program Resources Department. American Association of Retired Persons (AARP) and the Administration on Aging. *A Profile of Older Americans—1989*.
3. Porterfield JD, St. Pierre R. *Healthful Aging*. Guilford, CT: Dushkin Publishing; 1992.
4. US Department of Health and Human Services (DHHS). *Healthy People 2010: Understanding and Improving Health*. 2nd ed. Washington, DC: US Government Printing Office; November 2000.
5. National Center for Health Statistics (NCHS). *United States, Health and Aging Chartbook*. Hyattsville, MD; 1999, p. 89.
6. Evans AS. Causation and disease: The Henle-Koch postulates revisited. *Yale J Biol Med*. 1976;49(2):175–195.
7. Centers for Disease Control and Prevention (CDC). *Chronic Disease and Health Promotion Reprints from MMWR, 1985–1989*. Hyattsville, MD: Public Health Services, US Department of Health and Human Services (DHHS); 1992.
8. National Centers for Health Statistics (NCHS). *Health in the United States—1990*. Hyattsville, MD: Public Health Services, US Department of Health and Human Services (US DHHS); 1991.
9. National Cancer Institute. *Strategies to Control Tobacco Use in the United States*. Hyattsville, MD: Public Health Services, US Department of Health and Human Services (US DHHS); 1992.
10. Green LW, Krueter MW. *Health Promotion Planning: An Educational and Environmental Approach*. Mountain View, CA: Mayfield Publishing; 1991.
11. Centers for Disease Control and Prevention (CDC). Tuberculosis among foreign-born persons entering the United States. *MMWR*. 1990;39(RR-18):1–13, 18–21.
12. Centers for Disease Control and Prevention (CDC). Cigarette smoking among adults—United States. *MMWR*. 1998;49(39):881–884.
13. Centers for Disease Control and Prevention (CDC). Youth tobacco surveillance United States, 1998–1999. *MMWR*. 2000;49(No. SS-10):9–11.
14. Cumming RG, Nevitt MC, Cummings SR. Epidemiology of hip fractures. *Epidemiol Rev*. 1997;19(2):244–253.
15. Ottman R. Genetic epidemiology of epilepsy. *Epidemiol Rev*. 1997;19(1):120–127.
16. Inskip PD, Linet MS, Heineman EF. Etiology of brain tumors in adults. *Epidemiol Rev*. 1995;17(2):382–404.
17. Jemal A, Tiwari RC, Murray T, et al. Cancer statistics, 2004. *CA Cancer J Clin*. 2004;54:8–29.

18. Surveillance Research Program, National Cancer Institute SEER*Stat software (www.seer.cancer.gov/seerstat) version 6.1.4. Also available at: http://seer.cancer.gov/csr/1975_2002/results_merged/sect_23_prostate.pdf. Accessed May 23, 2005.
19. Centers for Disease Control and Prevention (CDC). Blood lead levels in young children—United States and selected states, 1996–1999. *MMWR*. 2000;49(50):1133–1135.
20. Centers for Disease Control and Prevention (CDC). About the BRFSS. National Center for Chronic Disease Prevention and Health Promotion. Behavior Risk Factor Surveillance System. Available at: http://www.cdc.gov/brfss/about.htm. Accessed July 5, 2005.
21. Prochaska JO, DiClemente CC. Stages of change in the modification of problem behaviors. *Prog Behav Modif.* 1992;28:184–218.
22. Rosenstock IM. Why people use health services. *Milbank Mem Fund Q*. 1966;44:94–127.
23. Rosenstock IM. Historical origins of the health belief model. *Health Educ Q*. 1974;2:328–335.
24. Janz NK, Becker MH. The health belief model: A decade later. *Health Educ Q*. 1984;11:1–47.
25. Glanz K, Marcus Lewis F, Rimer BK. *Theory at a Glance: A Guide for Health Promotion Practice.* Bethesda, MD: National Institutes of Health; 1997.

APPENDIX

I

Case Studies

CASE STUDY

I

Snow on Cholera

Snow J. "On the Mode of Communication of Cholera." Excerpted and adapted from the original 1855 edition as found in *Snow on Cholera* by John Snow, Commonwealth Fund: New York, 1936.

Dr. John Snow John Snow was born in 1813 and died in 1858. Dr. Snow was alive at the beginning of the golden era of bacteriology and infectious disease discovery and was actively involved in his professional pursuits at the time of Ignas Semmelweis, MD, Louis Pasteur (1822–1895) of France, and John Koch, MD (1843–1910), of Germany. At the time, these scientists led the world in the discovery of microbes, vaccines, and advanced scientific and biomedical knowledge about communicable diseases. Dr. Snow was a distinguished anesthesiologist in England who, among other accomplishments, administered chloroform to Queen Victoria at the birth of two of her children. Dr. Snow is most famous for his cholera investigations, including the epidemic in the Soho District of London, where he removed the handle from the Broad Street pump as a move to halt the cholera epidemic.

A. OBSERVATIONS ON CHOLERA

Communication of Cholera

There are certain circumstances, connected with the progress of cholera, which may be stated in a general way. Cholera travels along the great tracks more slowly. In extending to fresh inland or continent, it always appears first at a sea-port. It never attacks the crews of ships going from a country free from cholera, to one where the disease is prevailing, till they have entered a port or had intercourse with the shore. Its exact progress from town to town cannot always be traced; but it has never appeared except where there has been ample opportunity for it to be conveyed by human intercourse.

There are also innumerable instances which prove the communication of cholera, by individual cases of the disease, in the most convincing manner. Instances such as the following seem free from every source of fallacy. . . . I called lately to inquire respecting the death of Mrs. Gore, the wife of a labourer, from cholera, at New Leigham Road, Streatham. I found that a son of the deceased had been living and working at Chelsea. He came home ill with a bowel complaint, of which he died in a day or two. His death took place on August 18th. His mother, who attended on him, was taken ill on the next day and died the day following (August 20th). There were no other deaths from cholera registered in any of the metropolitan districts, down to the 26th of August, within 2 or 3 miles of the above place; the nearest being at Brixton, Norwood, or Lower Tooting. . . .

John Barnes, aged 39, an agricultural labourer, became severely indisposed on the 28th of December, 1832; he had been suffering from diarrhoea and cramps for 2 days previously. He was visited by Mr. George Hopps, a respectable surgeon at Redhouse, who, finding him sinking into collapse, requested an interview with his brother, Mr. J. Hopps, of York. This experienced practitioner at once recognized the case as one of Asiatic cholera; immediately enquired for some probable source of contagion, but in vain: no such source could be discovered. When he repeated his visit on the day following, the patient was dead; but Mrs. Barnes (the wife), Matthew Metcalfe, and Benjamin Muscroft, 2 persons who had visited Barnes on the preceding day, were all labouring under the disease, but recovered. John Foster, Ann Dunn, and widow Creyke, all of whom had communicated with the patients above named, were attacked by premonitory indisposition, which was however arrested. Whilst the surgeons were vainly endeavouring to discover whence the disease could possibly have arisen, the mystery was all at once, and most unexpectedly, unravelled by the arrival in the village of the son of the deceased John Barnes. This young man was apprentice to his uncle, a shoemaker, living in Leeds. He informed the surgeons that his uncle's wife (his father's sister) had died of cholera a fortnight (2 weeks/14 days) before that time, and that, as she had no children, her wearing apparel had been sent to Monkton by a common carrier. The clothes had not been washed; Barnes had opened the box in the evening; on the next day he had fallen sick of the disease.

During the illness of Mrs. Barnes, her mother, who was living in Tockwith, a healthy village five miles distant from Moor Monkton, was requested to attend her. She went to Monkton accordingly, remained with her daughter for 2 days, washed her daughter's linen, and set out on her return home, apparently in good health. Whilst in the act of walking home she was seized with the malady, and fell down in collapse on the road. She was conveyed home to her cottage, and placed by the side of her bedridden husband. He, and also the daughter who resided with them, took the malady. All the three died within two days. Only one other case occurred in the village of Tockwith, and it was not a fatal case.

A man came from Hull (where cholera was prevailing), by trade a painter; his name and age are unknown. He lodged at the house of Samuel Wride, at Pocklington; was attacked on his arrival on the 8th of September, and died on the 9th. Samuel Wride himself was attacked on the 11th September, and died shortly afterwards. . . .

Liverpool. (Mr. Henry Taylor, reporter.) A nurse attended a patient in Great Howard Street (at the lower part of the town), and on her return home, near Everton (the higher part of the town), was seized and died. The nurse who attended her was also seized, and died. No other case had occurred previously in that neighborhood, and none followed for about a fortnight. . . .

It would be easy, by going through the medical journal and works which have been published on cholera, to quote as many cases similar to the above as would fill a large volume. But the above instances are quite sufficient to show that cholera can be communicated from the sick to the healthy; for it is quite impossible that even a 10th part of these cases of consecutive illness could have followed each other by coincidence, without being connected as cause and effect.

Besides the facts above mentioned, which prove that cholera is communicated from person to person, there are others which show, first, that being present in the same room with a patient, and attending on him, do not necessarily expose a person to the morbid poison; and, secondly, that it is not always requisite that a person should be very near to a cholera patient in order to take the disease, as the morbid matter producing it may be transmitted to a distance. It used to be generally assumed, that if cholera were a catching or communicable disease it must spread by effluvia given off from the patient into the surrounding air, and inhaled by others into the lungs. This assumption led to very conflicting opinions respecting the disease. A little reflection shows, however, that we have no right thus to limit the way in which a disease may be propagated, for the communicable diseases of which we have a correct knowledge may spread in very different manners. The itch, and certain other diseases of the skin, are propagated in one way; syphilis, in another way; and intestinal worms in a third way, quite distinct from either of the others. . . .

Cholera Propagated by Morbid Material Entering the Alimentary Canal

Diseases which are communicated from person to person are caused by some material which passes from the sick to the healthy, and which has the property of increasing and multiplying in the systems of the persons it attacks. In syphilis, smallpox, and vaccinia, we have physical proof of the increase of the morbid material, and in other communicable diseases the evidence of this increase, derived from the fact of their extension, is equally conclusive. As cholera commences with an affection of the alimentary canal, and as we have seen that the blood is not under the influence of any poison in the early stages of this disease, it follows that the morbid material producing cholera must be introduced into the alimentary canal—must, in fact be swallowed accidentally, for persons would not take it intentionally; and the increase of the morbid material or cholera poison, must take place in the interior of the stomach and bowels. It would seem that the cholera poison, when reproduced in sufficient quantity, acts as an irritant on the surface of the stomach and intestines, or what is still more probable, it withdraws fluid from the blood circulating in the capillaries, by a power analogous to that by which the epithelial cells of the various organs abstract the different secretions in the healthy body. For the morbid matter of cholera having the property of reproducing its own kind, must necessarily have some sort of structure, most likely that of a cell. It is no objection to this view that the structure of the cholera poison cannot be recognized by the microscope, for the matter of smallpox and chancre can only be recognized by their effects, and not by their physical properties.

The period which intervenes between the time when a morbid poison enters the system, and the commencement of the illness which follows, is called the period of incubation. It is, in reality, a period of reproduction, with regards to the morbid matter; and the disease is due to the crop of progeny resulting from the small quantity of poison first introduced. In cholera, this period of incubation or reproduction is much shorter than in most other epidemic or communicable diseases. From the cases previously detailed, it is shown to be in general from 24 to 48 hours. It is owing to this shortness of the period of incubation, and to the quantity of the morbid poison thrown off in the evacuations, that cholera sometimes spreads with a rapidity unknown in other diseases. . . .

The instances in which minute quantities of the ejections and dejections of cholera patients must be swallowed are sufficiently numerous to account for the spread of the disease. Nothing has been found to favour the extension of cholera more than want of personal cleanliness whether arising from habit or scarcity of water. The bed linen nearly always becomes wetted by the cholera evacuations, and as these are devoid of the usual colour and odour, the hands of persons waiting on the patient become soiled without their knowing it; and unless these person are scrupulously clean in their habits and wash their hands before taking food, they must accidentally swallow some of the excretion, and leave some on the food they handle or prepare, which has to be eaten by the rest of the family. The post mortem inspection of bodies of cholera patients has hardly ever been followed by the disease that I am aware, this being a duty that is necessarily followed by careful washing of the hands; and it is not the habit of medical men to be taking food on such occasion. On the other hand, the duties performed about the body, such as laying it out, when done by women of the working class, who make the occasion one of eating and drinking, are often followed by an attack of cholera; and persons who merely attend the funeral, and have no connexion with body frequently contract the disease, in consequence, apparently of partaking of food which has been prepared or handled by those having duties about the cholera patient, or his linen and bedding.

The involuntary passage of the evacuations in most bad cases of cholera, must also aid in spreading the disease. Mr. Baker, of Staines, who attended 260 cases of cholera and diarrhoea in 1849, chiefly among the poor, informed me in a letter with which he favoured me in December of that year, that "when the patients passed their stools involuntarily the disease evidently spread." It is amongst the poor, where a whole family live, sleep, cook, eat and wash in a single room, that cholera has been found to spread once introduced, and still more in those places termed common lodging amongst the vagrant class, who lived in a crowded state, that cholera was most fatal in 1832; but the Act of Parliament for the regulation of common lodging houses, has caused the disease to be much less fatal amongst these people in the late epidemics. When, on the other hand, cholera is introduced into the better kind of houses, as it often is by means that will be afterwards pointed out, it hardly ever spreads from one member of the family to another. The constant use of the hand-basin and towel, and the fact of the apartments for cooking and eating being distinct from the sick room, are the cause for this.

If the cholera had no other means of communication than those we have been considering, it would be constrained to confine itself chiefly to the crowded dwellings of the poor, and would be continually liable to die out accidentally in a place, for want of the opportunity to reach fresh victims; but there is often a way open for it to extend itself more widely and reach well-to-do classes of the community; I allude to the mixture of the cholera evacuations with the water used for drinking and culinary purposes, either by permeating the ground, and getting into the wells, or by running along channels and sewers into the rivers from which entire towns are sometimes supplied with water.

In 1849 there were in Thomas Street, Horsleydown, two courts close together, consisting of a number of small houses or cottages, inhabited by poor people. The houses occupied one side of each court or alley—the south side of Trusscott's Court, and the north side of the other, which was called Surrey Buildings, . . . divided into small back areas in which situated the privies of both courts, communicating with the same drain, and there was an open sewer which passed the further end of both courts. In Surrey Buildings the cholera committed fearful devastation, whilst in the adjoining court there was but one fatal case, and another case that ended in recovery. In the former court, the slops of dirty water, poured down by the inhabitants into a channel in front of the houses, got into the well from which they obtained their water; this being the only difference that Mr. Grant, the Assistant Surveyor for the Commissioners of Sewers, could find between the circumstances of the two courts.

In Manchester, a sudden and violent outbreak of cholera occurred in Hope Street, Salford. The inhabitants used water from a particular pump/well. This well had been repaired, and a sewer which passes within nine inches of the edge of it became accidentally stopped up, and leaked into the well. The inhabitants of 30 houses used the water from this well; among these there occurred 19 cases of diarrhoea, 26 cases of cholera, and 25 deaths. The inhabitants of 60 houses in the same immediate neighbourhood used other water; among these there occurred eleven cases of diarrhoea, but not a single case of cholera, nor one death. It is remarkable, that, in this instance, out of the 26 persons attacked with cholera, the whole perished except one.

Dr. Thomas King Chambers informed me, that at Ilford, in Essex, in the summer of 1849, the cholera prevailed very severely in a row of houses a little way from the main part of town. It had visited every house in the row but one. The refuse which overflowed from the privies and a pigsty could be seen running into the well over the surface of the ground, and the water was very fetid: yet it was used by the people in all the houses except that which had escaped cholera. That house was inhabited by a woman who took linen to wash, and she, finding that the water gave the linen an offensive smell, paid a person to fetch water for her from the pump in the town, and this water she used for culinary purposes as well as for washing.

The following circumstance was related to me, at the time it occurred, by a gentleman well acquainted with all the particulars. The drainage from the cesspools found its way into the well attached to some houses at Locksbrook, near Bath, and the cholera making its appearance there in the autumn of 1849, became very fatal. The people complained of the water to the gentleman belonging to the property, who lived at Weston, in Bath, and he sent a surveyor, who reported that nothing was the matter. The tenants still complaining, the owner went himself, and in looking at the water and smelling it, he said that he could perceive nothing the matter with it. He was asked if he would taste it, and drank a glass of it. This occurred on a Wednesday; he went home, was taken ill with the cholera, and died on the Saturday following, there being no cholera in his own neighbourhood at the time.

Case Study Questions

A.1 Concerning John Barnes, how was cholera communicated? What were the modes of disease transmission? What is the correct epidemiologic term for the modes of transmission that were identified?

A.2 How long is a fortnight?

A.3 In the examples or circumstances presented, what were the various modes of transmission stated or at least alluded to? Which were correct? Which were incorrect and why? What role did personal hygiene and sanitation (including food preparation and hand washing) play in the transmission of the disease and continuation of an outbreak?

A.4 Several instances of causal association were presented or alluded to in the examples presented in the case. List the various instances of association that you can identify from the examples or situations presented in the case. What role did social class, poverty, and housing arrangements play in association? What role did water play in association?

A.5 Describe the disease cholera as presented in the Snow case. Describe cholera as it is known today.

A.6 What hypotheses were developed by John Snow about the cause (etiology), signs and symptoms, spread, and course of the cholera disease? How do the observations and hypotheses of Snow conform with modern understanding and knowledge of cholera?

A.7 What is different about those who develop cholera compared with those who do not?

A.8 What epidemiologic phenomenon can be observed in the Locksbrook, near Bath, example?

B. CHOLERA AND THE BROAD STREET OUTBREAK

The most terrible outbreak of cholera which ever occurred in this kingdom, is probably that which took place in Broad Street, Golden Square, and the adjoining streets, a few weeks ago. Within 250 yards of the spot where Cambridge Street joins Broad Street, there were upwards of 500 fatal attacks of cholera in 10 days. The mortality in this limited area probably equals any that was ever caused in this country, even by the plague; and it was much more sudden, as the greater number of cases terminated in a few hours. The mortality would undoubtedly have been much greater had it not been for the flight of the population. Persons in furnished lodgings left first, then other lodgers went away, leaving their furniture to be sent for when they could meet with a place to put it in. Many houses were closed altogether, owing to the death of the proprietors; and in a great number of instances, the tradesmen who remained had sent away their families: so that in less than six days from the commencement of the outbreak, the most afflicted streets were deserted by more than three-quarters of their inhabitants.

There were a few cases of cholera in the neighbourhood of Broad Street, Golden Square, in the latter part of August and the so-called outbreak, which commenced in the night between the 31st August and the 1st of September, was, as in similar instances, only a violent increase of the malady. As soon as I became acquainted with the situation and extent of this irruption of cholera, I suspected some contamination of the water of the much frequented street-pump in Broad Street, near the end of Cambridge Street; but on examining the water, on the evening of the 3rd of September, I found so little impurity in it of an organic nature, that I hesitated to come to a conclusion. Further inquiry, however, showed me that there was no other circumstance or agent common to the circumscribed locality in which this sudden increase of cholera occurred, and not extending beyond it, except the water of the above mentioned pump. I found, moreover, that the water varied, during the next two days, in the amount of organic impurity, visible to the naked eye, on close inspection, in the form of small white flocculent particles; and I concluded that, at the commencement of the outbreak, it might possibly have been still more impure. I requested permission, therefore, to take a list, at the General Register Office, of the deaths from cholera, registered during the week ending 2nd September, in the subdistricts of Golden Square, Berwick Street, and St. Ann's Soho, which was kindly granted. Eighty-nine deaths from cholera, were registered, during the week, in the three subdistricts (see Figure I.1). Of these, only 6 occurred in the 4 first days of the week. Four (4) occurred on Thursday, the 31st of August; and the remaining 79 on Friday and Saturday. I considered therefore, that the outbreak commenced on the Thursday; and I made inquiry, in detail, respecting the 83 deaths registered as having taken place during the last 3 days of the week.

On proceeding to the spot, I found that nearly all the deaths had taken place within a short distance of the pump. There were only 10 deaths in houses situated decidedly nearer to another street pump. In 5 of these cases the families of the deceased persons informed me that they always went to the pump in Broad Street, as they preferred the water to that of the pump which was nearer. In three other cases, the deceased were children who went to school near the pump in Broad Street. Two of them were known to drink the water; and the parents of the third think it probable that it did so. The other 2 deaths, beyond the district which this pump supplies, represent only the amount of mortality from cholera that was occurring before the irruption took place" (see Figure I.1, map of the Broad Street and Golden Square area of London).

With regard to the deaths occurring in the locality belonging to the pump, there were 61 instances in which I was informed that the deceased persons used to drink the pump-water from Broad Street, either constantly or occasionally. In 6 instances I could get no information, owing to the death or departure of everyone connected with the deceased individuals; and in 6 cases I was informed that the deceased persons did not drink the pump-water before their illness" (see Figure I.1, map of the Broad Street and Golden Square area of London).

The result of the inquiry then was that there had been no particular outbreak or increase of cholera, in this part of London, except among the persons who were in the habit of drinking water of the above mentioned pump-well.

I had an interview with the Board of Guardians of St. James's parish, on the evening of Thursday, 7th September, and represented the above circumstances to them. In consequence of what I said, the handle of the pump was removed on the following day.

The additional facts that I have been able to ascertain are in accordance with those above related; and as regards the small number of those attacked, who were believed not to have drank the water from the Broad Street pump, it must be obvious that there are various ways in which the deceased persons may have taken it without the knowledge of their friends. The water was used for mixing with spirits in all the public houses around. It was used likewise at dining rooms and coffee shops. The keeper of a coffee shop in the neighbourhood which was frequented by mechanics, and where the pump water was supplied at dinner time, informed me (on 6th September) that she was already aware of 9 of her customers who were dead. The pump-water was also sold in various little shops, with a teaspoonful of effervescing powder in it, under the name of sherbet; and it may have been distributed in various other ways with which I am unacquainted. The pump was frequented much more than is usual, even for a London pump in a populous neighbourhood.

There are certain circumstances bearing on the subject of this outbreak of cholera which required to be mentioned. The workhouse in Poland Street is more than three-fourths surrounded by houses in which deaths from cholera occurred, yet out of 535 inmates only 5 died of cholera, the other deaths which took place being those of persons admitted after they were attacked. The workhouse has a pump-well on the premises, in addition to the supply from the Grand Junction Water Works, and the inmates never sent to the Broad Street pump for water. If the mortality in the workhouse had been equal to that in the streets immediately surrounding it on three sides, upwards of 100 persons would have died.

There is a brewery in Broad Street, near to the pump, and on perceiving that no brewer's men were registered as having died of cholera, I called on Mr. Huggins, the proprietor. He informed me that there were above 70 workmen employed in the brewery, and that none of them had suffered from cholera, at least in a severe form, only two having been indisposed, and not that seriously, at the time the disease prevailed. The men are allowed a certain quantity of malt liquor, and Mr. Huggins believes they do not drink water at all; and he is quite certain that the workmen never obtained water from the pump in the street. There is a deep well in the brewery, in addition to the New River water.

A 28-year-old mother in the 8th month of pregnancy, went herself (although they were not usually water drinkers), on Sunday, 3rd September, to Broad Street pump for water. The family removed to Gravesend on the following day; and she was attacked with cholera on Tuesday morning at 7 o'clock, and died of consecutive fever on 15th September, having been delivered. Two of her children drank also of the water, and were attacked on the same day as the mother, but recovered.

In the "Weekly Return of Births and Deaths" of September 9th, the following death is recorded as occurring in Hampstead district: At West End, on 2nd September, the widow of a percussion-cap maker, aged 59 years, diarrhoea two hours, cholera epidemic, 16 hours.

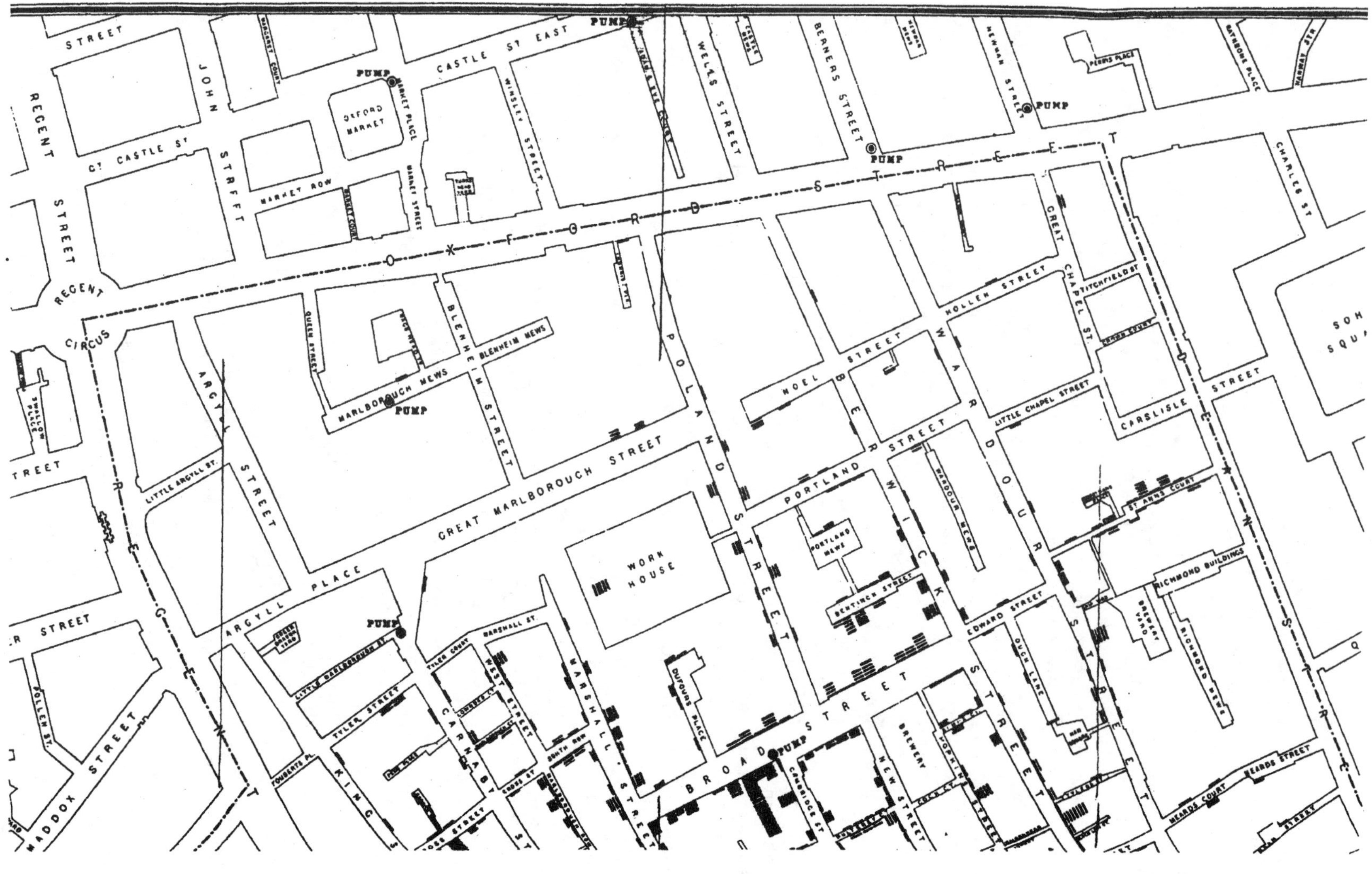

OXFORD STREET
REGENT STREET
REGENT CIRCUS
JOHN STREET
GT CASTLE ST
CASTLE ST EAST
OXFORD MARKET
MARKET PLACE
MARKET ROW
MARKET STREET
WINSLEY STREET
WELLS STREET
BERNERS STREET
NEWMAN STREET
PERRYS PLACE
RATHBONE PLACE
HANWAY STR
CHARLES ST
SOHO SQUA
PUMP
QUEEN STREET
MARLBOROUGH MEWS
BLENHEIM MEWS
BLENHEIM STREET
ARGYLL STREET
LITTLE ARGYLL ST.
ARGYLL PLACE
GREAT MARLBOROUGH STREET
POLAND STREET
WORK HOUSE
DUFOURS PLACE
NOEL STREET
HOLLEN STREET
GREAT CHAPEL ST
TITCHFIELD ST
LITTLE CHAPEL STREET
CARLISLE STREET
PORTLAND STREET
PORTLAND MEWS
BENTINCK STREET
BERWICK STREET
WARDOUR MEWS
WARDOUR STREET
ST ANNS COURT
RICHMOND BUILDINGS
RICHMOND MEWS
BREWERY YARD
EDWARD STREET
DUCK LANE
DEAN STREET
MEARDS COURT
BROAD STREET
CAMBRIDGE ST
NEW STREET
BREWERY
HOPKINS STREET
MARSHALL STREET
MARSHALL ST
WEST STREET
TYLER COURT
TYLER STREET
CARNABY
KING STREET
FOUBERTS PL
POLLEN ST.
MADDOX STREET

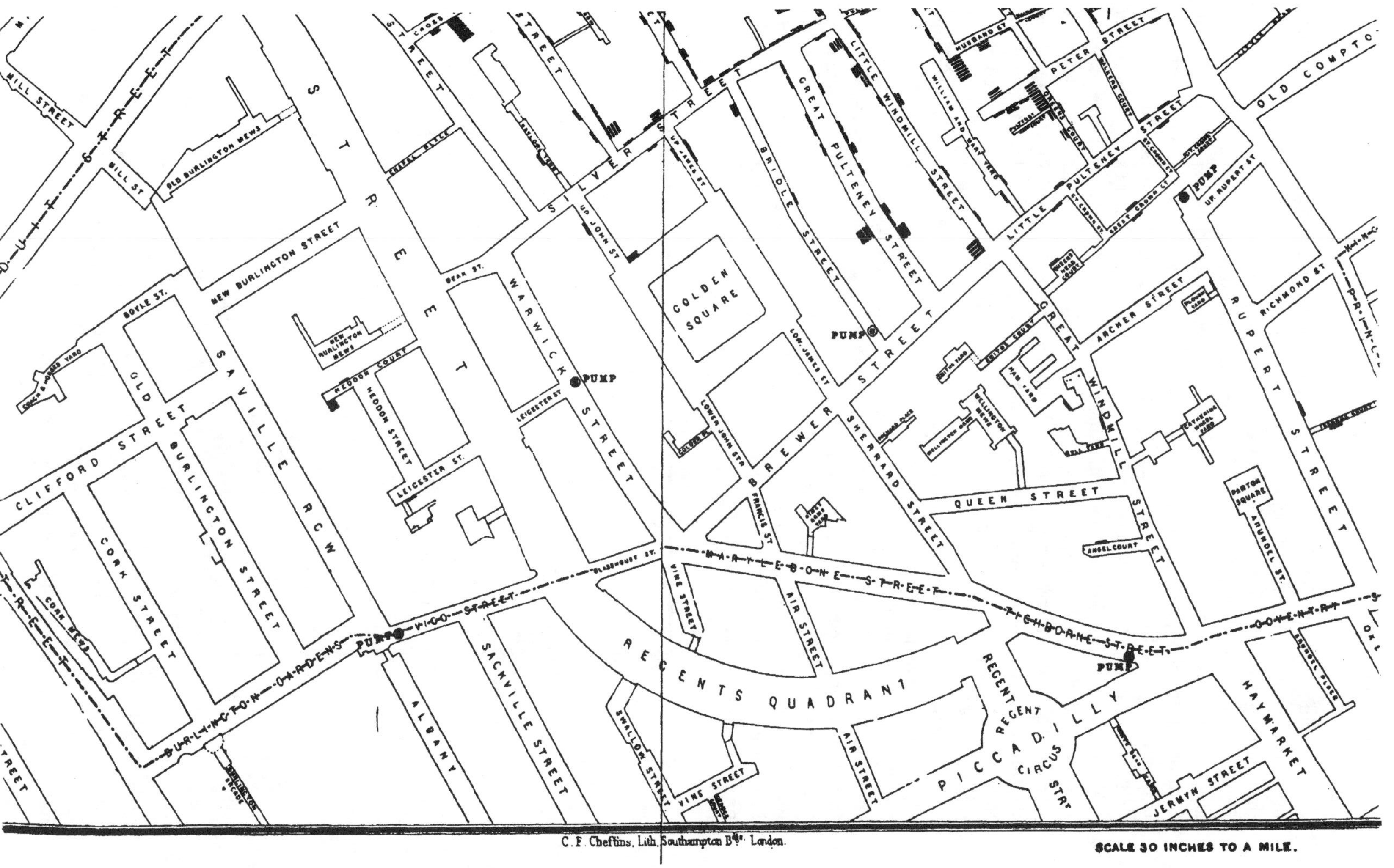

FIGURE I.1 Snow's spot map of the Broad Street and Golden Square area of London. (Snow J. "On the Mode of Communication of Cholera." Excerpted and adapted from the original 1855 edition as found in *Snow on Cholera* by John Snow, Commonweath Fund: New York; 1936.)

I was informed by this lady's son that she had not been in the neighbourhood of Broad Street for many months. A cart went from Broad Street to West End every day, and it was the custom to take out a large bottle of the water from the pump in Broad Street, as she preferred it. The water was taken on Thursday, 31st August, and she drank of it in the evening, and also on Friday. She was seized with cholera on the evening of the latter day, and died on Saturday, as the above quotation from the register shows. A niece, who was on a visit to this lady, also drank of the water; she returned to her residence, in a high and healthy part of Islington, was attacked with cholera, and died also. There was no cholera at the time, either at West End or in the neighborhood where the niece died. Besides these 2 persons, only one servant partook of the water at Hampstead West End, and she did not suffer, or at least not severely. There were many persons who drank the water from the Broad Street pump about the time of the outbreak, without being attacked with cholera; but this does not diminish the evidence respecting the influence of the water, for reasons that will be fully stated in another part of this work.

(These activities are shown in Figure I.2, which presents the dates/chronological events of the Broad Street pump cholera epidemic.)

It is pretty certain that very few of the 56 attacks placed in the table to 31st August occurred till late in the evening of that day. The irruption was extremely sudden, as I learned from the medical men living in the midst of the district, and commenced in the night between the 31st August and 1st September (see Figure I.2.) There was hardly any premonitory diarrhoea in the cases which occurred during the first three days of the outbreak; and I have been informed by several medical men, that very few of the cases which they attended on those days ended in recovery.

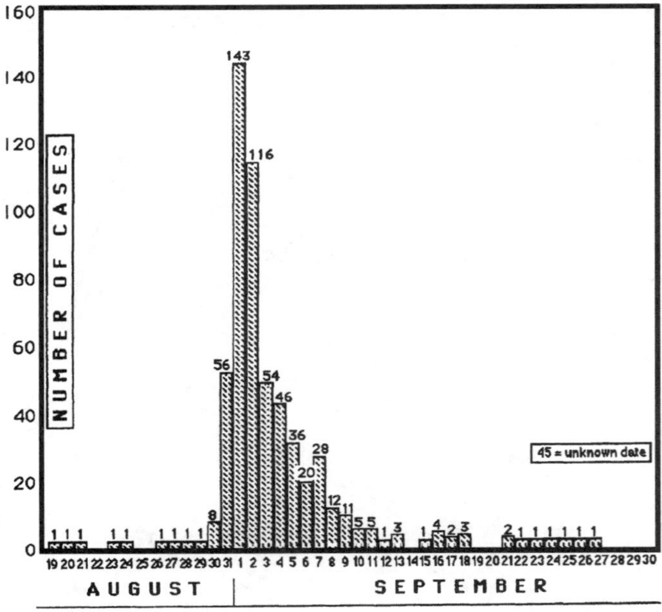

FIGURE I.2 The dates and numbers of attacks of cholera in the Broad Street pump cholera epidemic, London. (Snow J. "On the Mode of Communication of Cholera." Excerpted and adapted from the original 1855 edition as found in *Snow on Cholera* by John Snow, Commonweath Fund: New York; 1936.)

The greatest number of attacks in any one day occurred on the 1st day of September, immediately after the outbreak commenced. The following day the attacks fell from 143 to 116 and the day afterwards to 54. A glance at Figure I.2 and Figure I.3 shows that the fresh attacks and deaths continued to become less numerous every day after 1st and 2nd of September. On September 8th—the day when the handle of the pump was removed—there were 12 attacks; on the 9th, 11 attacks; on the 10th and 11th 5 attacks and on the 12th only 1; after this time, there were never more than 4 attacks on one day. During the decline of the epidemic the deaths were more numerous than the attacks (compare Figure I.2 with Figure I.3.), owing to the decease of many persons who had lingered for several days in consecutive fever.

There is no doubt the mortality was much diminished, by the flight of the population, which commenced soon after the outbreak; but the attacks had so far diminished before the use of the water was stopped, that it is impossible to decide whether the well still contained the cholera poison in an active state or whether, from some cause, the water had become free from it. The pump-well has been opened, and I was informed by Mr. Farrell, the superintendent of the works, that there was no hole or crevice in the brickwork of the well, by which any impurity might enter; consequently in this respect the contamination of the water is not made out of the kind of physical evidence detailed in some of the instances previously related. I understand that the well is from 28 to 30 feet in depth, and goes through the gravel to the surface of the clay beneath. The sewer, which passes within a few yards of the well, is 22 feet below the surface. The water at the time of the cholera contained impurities of an organic nature, in the form of minute whitish flocculi visible on close inspection to the naked eye. Dr. Hassall, who was good enough to examine some of this water with a microscope, informed me that these particles

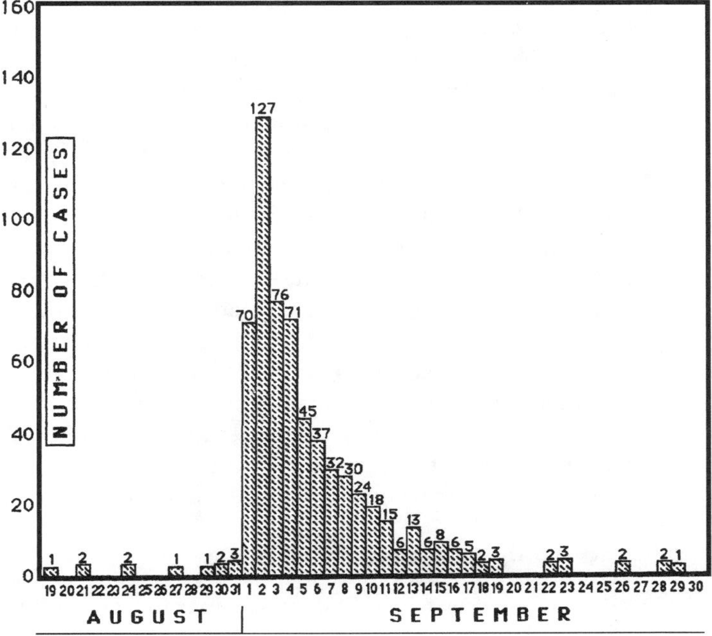

FIGURE I.3 The dates and numbers of deaths from cholera in the Broad Street pump cholera epidemic, London. (Snow J. "On the Mode of Communication of Cholera." Excerpted and adapted from the original 1855 edition as found in *Snow on Cholera* by John Snow, Commonweath Fund: New York; 1936.)

had no organised structure, and he thought they probably resulted from decomposition of other matter. He found a great number of very minute oval animalcules in the water, which are of no importance except as an additional proof that the water contained organic matter on which they lived. The water also contained a large quantity of chlorides, indicating no doubt, the impure sources from which the spring is supplied. Mr. Eley, the percussion-cap manufacturer of 37 Broad street, informed me that he had long noticed that the water became offensive, both to the smell and taste, after it had been kept about two days. This, as I noticed before, is the character of water contaminated with sewage. Another person had noticed for months that a film formed on the surface of the water when it had been kept a few hours.

I inquired of many persons whether they had observed any change in the character of the water, about the time of the outbreak of cholera, and was answered in the negative. I afterwards, however, met with the following important information on this point. Mr. Gould, the eminent ornithologist, lives near the pump in Broad Street, and was in the habit of drinking the water. He was out of town at the commencement of the outbreak of cholera, but came home on Saturday morning, 2nd September, and sent for some of the water almost immediately, when he was much surprised to find that it had an offensive smell, although perfectly transparent and fresh from the pump. He did not drink any of it. Mr. Gould's assistant, Mr. Prince, had his attention drawn to the water and perceived its offensive smell. A servant of Mr. Gould who drank the pump water daily, and drank a good deal of it on August 31st, was seized with cholera at an early hour on September 1st. She ultimately recovered.

Whether the impurities of the water were derived from the sewers, the drains, or the cesspools, of which latter there are a number in the neighbourhood, I cannot tell. I have been informed by an eminent engineer, that whilst a cesspool in a clay soil requires to be emptied every six or eight months, one sunk in the gravel will often go for 20 years without being emptied, owing to the soluble matters passing away into the land-springs by percolation. As there had been deaths from cholera just before the great outbreak not far from this pump-well, and in a situation elevated a few feet above it, the evacuations from the patients might as a matter of course be amongst the impurities finding their way into the water, and judging the matter by the light derived from other facts and considerations previously detailed, we must conclude that such was the case. A very important point in respect to this pump-well is that the water passed with almost everybody as being perfectly pure, and it did in fact contain a less quantity of impurity than the water of some other pumps in the same parish, which had no share in the propagation of cholera. We must conclude from this outbreak that the quantity of morbid matter which is sufficient to produce cholera is inconceivably small, and that the shallow pump-wells in a town cannot be looked on with too much suspicion, whatever their local reputation may be.

Whilst the presumed contamination of the water of the Broad Street pump with evacuations of cholera patients affords an exact explanation of the fearful outbreak of cholera in St. James's parish, there is no other circumstance which offers any explanation at all, whatever hypothesis of the nature and cause of the malady be adopted.

Case Study Questions

B.1 What are the time factors and implications for this case? Explain the time lag from attacks in Figure I.2 to deaths in Figure I.3.

B.2 What are the place factors and implications for this case? Compare the workhouse to the brewery to the pub. Discuss migration and its effect on the epidemic. What *place* issues are important to this case?

B.3 What did the well persons do differently than the ill—those who got the disease (e.g., the inmates in the workhouse)?

B.4 From Figure I.2, what is the index case? What date is the beginning of the epidemic? What other time factors are discerned from this chart? How did Snow establish the time of onset?

B.5 What accurate observations were made about wells, cesspools, ground water, the purity of the water, and its contamination? What inaccurate and misunderstood observations were made about the water, its flow, and its contamination?

B.6 What evidence did Snow use to establish the fact that a cholera epidemic was occurring? Did Snow clearly demonstrate the cause and source of the outbreak of cholera in the Golden Square area? Explain.

B.7 What were Snow's initial and basic hypotheses concerning the epidemic? What processes and procedures did Snow use to establish his hypotheses (prove or disprove them) about the outbreak?

B.8 The obvious control measure applied was the removal of the handle from the Broad Street pump. What role did the removal of the pump handle play in the decline of the epidemic? Did the removal of the pump handle have an effect on the control epidemic? What other social and political roles did removing the handle from the pump play?

C. CHOLERA EPIDEMIC OF 1853 AND TWO LONDON WATER COMPANIES

London was without cholera from the latter part of 1849 to August 1853. During this interval an important change had taken place in the water supply of several of the south districts of London. The Lambeth Company removed their water works, in 1852, from opposite of Hungerford Market to Thames Ditton: thus obtaining a supply of water quite free from the sewage of London. The districts supplied by the Lambeth Company are, however, also supplied, to a certain extent by the Southwark and Vauxhall Co., the pipes of both companies going down every street, in the places where the supply is mixed (different houses getting water from one or the other water companies). Due to this intermixing of the sources of water, the effect of the alteration made by the Lambeth Co. on the progress of cholera was not so evident, to a cursory observer, as it would otherwise have been. It attracted the attention, however, of the Registrar-General, who published a table in the "Weekly Return of Births and Deaths," for 26th November 1853, of which the following is an abstract, containing as much as applies to the south districts of London.

It thus appears that the districts partially supplied with the improved water suffered much less than the others, although, in 1849, when the Lambeth Company obtained their new supply, these same districts suffered quite as much as those supplied entirely by the Southwark and Vauxhall Co. The Lambeth water extends to only a small portion of some of the districts necessarily included in the groups supplied by the companies and when the division is made in a little more detail, by taking subdistricts, the effect of the new water supply is shown to be greater than appears in the Table I.1.

As the Registrar-General published a list of all the deaths from cholera which occurred in London in 1853, from the commencement of the epidemic in August to its conclusion in January, 1854, I have been able to add up the numbers which occurred in the various

TABLE I.1

Water Companies	*Sources of Supply*	*Population*	*Deaths by Cholera in 13 Weeks Ending Nov. 19*	*Deaths in 100,000 Inhabitants*
(1) Lambeth and (2) Southwark & Vauxhall	Thames, at Thames Ditton and at Battersea	346,363	211	61
Southwark & Vauxhall	Thames, at Battersea	118,267	111	94
(1) Southwark & Vauxhall (2) Kent	Thames, at Battersea; the Ravensbourne, in Kent, & ditches and wells	17,805	19	107

subdistricts on the south side of the Thames, to which the water supply of the Southwark and Vauxhall Co. and the Lambeth Companies, extends.

Although the facts shown in the Table I.2 afford very strong evidence of the powerful influence which the drinking of water containing the sewage of the town exerts over the spread of cholera, when that disease is present, yet the question does not end here; for the intermixing of the water supply of the Southwark and Vauxhall Company with that of the Lambeth Company, over an extensive part of London, admitted of the subject being sifted in such a way as to yield the most incontrovertible proof on one side or the other. In the subdistricts enumerated in the above table as being supplied by both companies, the mixing of the supply is of the most intimate kind. The pipes of each company go down all the streets, and into nearly all the courts and alleys. A few houses are supplied by one company and a few by the other, according to the decision of the owner or occupier at that time when the water companies were in active competition. In many cases a single house has a supply different from that on either side. Each company supplies both rich and poor, both large houses and small; there is no difference either in the condition or occupation of the persons receiving the waters of the different companies. Now it must be evident that, if the diminution of cholera, in the districts partly supplied with improved water, depended on this supply, the houses receiving it would be the houses enjoying the whole benefit of the

TABLE I.2

Subdistricts	*Population in 1851*	*Deaths from Cholera—1853*	*Deaths by Cholera in Each 100,000 Living*	*Water Supply*
First 12 subdistricts	167,654	192	114	South & Vauxhall
Next 16 subdistricts	301,149	182	60	Both
Last 3 subdistricts	14,632	0	0	Lambeth Company

diminution of the malady, whilst the houses supplied with the water from Battersea Fields would suffer the same mortality as they would if the improved supply did not exist at all. As there is no difference whatever, either in the houses or the people receiving the supply of the two water companies, or in any of the physical conditions with which they are surrounded. It is obvious that no experiment could have been devised which would more thoroughly test the effect of water supply on the progress of cholera than this, which circumstances placed ready made before the observer.

The experiment, too, was on the grandest scale. No fewer than 300,000 people of both sexes, of every age and occupation, and of every rank and station, from gentlefolks down to the very poor, were divided into two groups without their choice, and in most cases, without their knowledge, one group being supplied with water containing the sewage of London, and amongst it, whatever might have come from the cholera patients, the other group having water quite free from such impurity.

To turn this grand experiment to account, all that was required was to learn the supply of water to each individual house where a fatal attack of cholera might occur. I regret that, in the short days at the latter part of last year, I could not spare the time to make the inquiry; and indeed, I was not fully aware at that time, of the intimate mixture of the supply of the two water companies, and the consequently important nature of the desired inquiry.

Cholera Epidemic of 1854

When the cholera returned to London in July of the present year, however, I resolved to spare no exertion which might be necessary to ascertain the exact effect of the water supply on the progress of the epidemic, in the places where all the circumstances were so happily adapted for the inquiry. I was desirous of making the investigation myself, in order that I might have the most satisfactory proof of the truth or fallacy of the doctrine which I had been advocating for five years. I had no reason to doubt the correctness of the conclusions I had drawn from the great number of facts already in my possession, but I felt that the circumstance of the cholera poison passing down the sewers into a great river, and being distributed through miles of pipes, and yet producing its specific effects, was a fact of so startling a nature, and so vast importance to the community, that it could not be too rigidly examined, or established on too firm a basis.

I accordingly asked permission at the General Register Office to be supplied with the addresses of persons dying of cholera, in those districts where the supply of the two companies is intermingled in the manner I have stated above. Some of these addresses were published in the "Weekly Returns," and I was kindly permitted to take a copy of others. I commenced my inquiry about the middle of August with two subdistricts of Lambeth, called Kennington, first part and Kennington, second part. There were 44 deaths in these subdistricts down to 12th August, and I found that 38 of the houses in which these deaths occurred were supplied by the Southwark and Vauxhall Company, four houses were supplied by the Lambeth Company, and 2 had pump-wells on the premises and no supply from either of the companies.

As soon as I had ascertained these particulars, I communicated them to Dr. Farr, who was much struck with the result, and at his suggestion the Registrars of all the South districts of London were requested to make a return of the water supply of the house in which the attack took place, in all cases of death from cholera. This order was to take place after the 26th August, and I resolved to carry my inquiry down to that date, so that the facts might be ascertained for the whole course of the epidemic.

The inquiry was necessarily attended with a good deal of trouble. There were very few instances in which I could at once get information I required. Even when the water-rates are paid by the residents, they can seldom remember the name of the water company till they have looked for the receipt. In the case of working people who pay weekly rents, the rates are invariably paid by the landlord or his agent, who often live at a distance, and the residents know nothing of the matter. It would, indeed, have been almost impossible for me to complete the inquiry, if I had not found that I could distinguish the water of the two companies with perfect certainty by a chemical test. The test I employed was founded on the great difference in the quantity of chloride of sodium (salt) contained in the two kinds of water, at the time I made the inquiry. On adding solution of nitrate of silver to a gallon of the water of the Lambeth company, obtained at Thames Ditton, beyond the reach of the sewage of London, only 2.28 grains of chloride of silver were obtained, indicating the presence of .95 grains of chloride of sodium in the water. On treating the water of the Southwark and Vauxhall Company in the same manner, 91 grains of chloride silver were obtained, showing the presence of 37.9 grains of common salt per gallon. Indeed, the difference in appearance on adding nitrate of silver to the two kinds of water was so great, that they could be at once distinguished without any further trouble. Therefore when the resident could not find clear and conclusive evidence about the water company, I obtained some of the water in a small phial, wrote the address on the cover, when I could examine it after coming home. The mere appearance of the water generally afforded a very good indication of its source, especially if it was observed as it came in before it had entered the water-butt or cistern; and the time of its coming in also afforded some evidence of the kind of water, after I had ascertained the hours when the turncocks of both companies visited any street. These points were, however, not relied on, except as corroborating more decisive proof, such as the chemical test, or the company's receipt for the rates.

According to a return which was made to Parliament, the Southwark and Vauxhall Company supplied 40,046 houses from January 1st to December 31st 1853, and the Lambeth Company supplied 26,107 houses during the same period; consequently, as 286 fatal attacks of cholera took place, in the first 4 weeks of the epidemic, in houses supplied by the former company, and only 14 in houses supplied by the latter, the proportion of fatal attacks to each 10,000 houses was as follows. Southwark and Vauxhall 71. Lambeth 5. The cholera was therefore 14 times as fatal at this period, amongst persons having the impure water of the Southwark and Vauxhall Company, as amongst those having the purer water from Thames Ditton.

As the epidemic advanced, the disproportion between the number of cases in houses supplied by the Southwark and Vauxhall Company and those supplied by the Lambeth Company, became not quite so great, although it continued very striking. Table I.3 is the proportion of deaths to 10,000 houses, during the first 7 weeks of the epidemic, in the pop-

Table I.3

	Number of Houses	*Deaths from Cholera*	*Deaths in Each 10,000 Houses*
Southwark and Vauxhall Company	40,046	1,263	315
Lambeth Company	26,107	98	37
Rest of London	256,423	1,422	59

ulation supplied by the Southwark and Vauxhall Company, in that supplied by the Lambeth Company and in the rest of London (see Figure I.4, map of River Thames area).

The mortality in the houses supplied by the Southwark and Vauxhall Company was therefore between 8 and 9 times as great as in the houses supplied by the Lambeth Company. See Figure I.4, map of River Thames area.

Case Study Questions

C.1 What are the various aspects of the person presented in the above water company case concerning the epidemic of cholera, especially as the person concept relates to the households that were recipients of the supplies of the water as compared with those who used different water supplies?

C.2 Concerning the water supply system and structure from the two different water companies, explain the soundness of the research approach. Is this a descriptive or analytic epidemiologic research design?

C.3 What were some of the practical problems and barriers that Snow faced that slowed his inquiry of the cholera epidemic of 1854? How would this relate to modern day epidemiologic investigations?

C.4 "As the epidemic advanced, the disproportion between the number of cases in houses supplied by the Southwark and Vauxhall Company and those supplied by the Lambeth Company, became not quite so great. . . ." From an epidemiologic point of view, why was this so? Give detailed epidemiologic reasoning and discussion addressing person, place, and time issues.

D. EPIDEMIOLOGIC ISSUES

John Snow's Answers to Objections

All the evidence proving the communication of cholera through the medium of water, confirms that with which I set out, of its communication in the crowded habitations of the poor, in coal-mines and other places, by the hands getting soiled with evacuations of the patients, and by small quantities of these evacuations being swallowed with the food, as paint is swallowed by house painters of uncleanly habits, who contact lead-colic in this way.

There are 1 or 2 objections to the mode of communications of cholera which I am endeavouring to establish, that deserve to be noticed. Messrs. Pearse and Marston state, in their account of the cases of cholera treated at the Newcastle Dispensary in 1853, that one of the dispensers drank by mistake some rice-water evacuation without any effect whatever. In rejoinder to this negative incident, it may be remarked, that several conditions may be requisite to the communication of cholera with which we are as yet unacquainted. Certain conditions we know to be requisite to the communication of other diseases. Syphilis we know is only communicable in its primary state, and vaccine lymph must be removed at a particular time to produce its proper effects. In the incident above mentioned, the large quantity of the evacuation taken might even prevent its action. It must be remembered that the effects of a morbid poison are never due to what first enters the system, but to the crop of progeny produced from this during a period of reproduction, termed the period of

MAP 2.

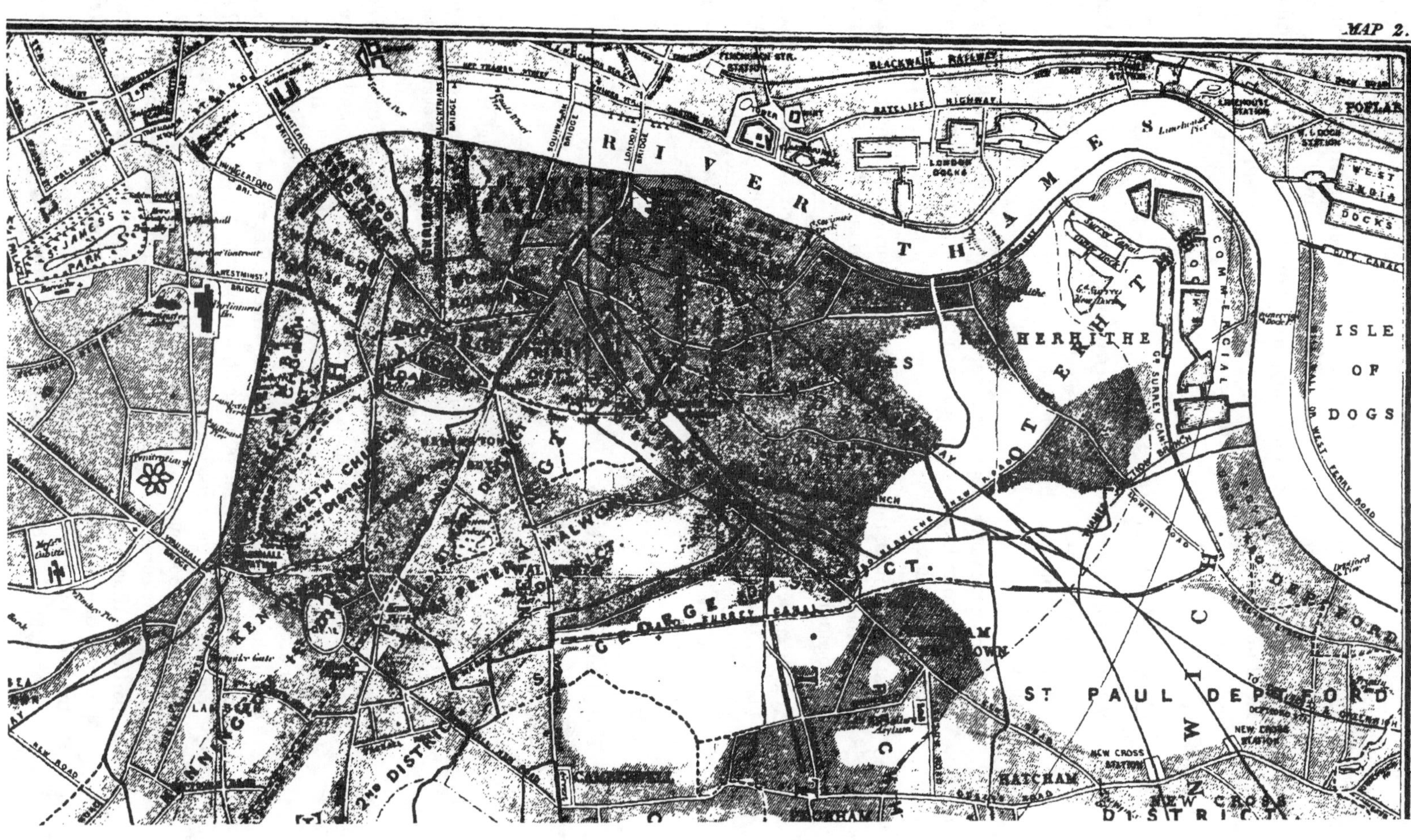
RIVER THAMES
ISLE OF DOGS
COMMERCIAL DOCKS
WEST INDIA DOCKS
LONDON DOCKS
POPLAR
BLACKWALL RAILWAY
HIGHWAY
RATCLIFF
FENCHURCH STR. STATION
LONDON BRIDGE
SOUTHWARK BRIDGE
BLACKFRIARS BRIDGE
WATERLOO BRIDGE
HUNGERFORD BRI.
WESTMINST. BRIDGE
VAUXHALL BRIDGE
ST JAMES'S PARK
ST PAUL DEPTFORD
NEW CROSS STATION
NEW CROSS DISTRICT
HATCHAM
GEORGE
GR SURREY CANAL
WALWORTH
LAMBETH
KENNINGTON
2ND DISTRICT
CAMBERWELL
PECKHAM
DEPTFORD
NEW ROAD
LOWER ROAD

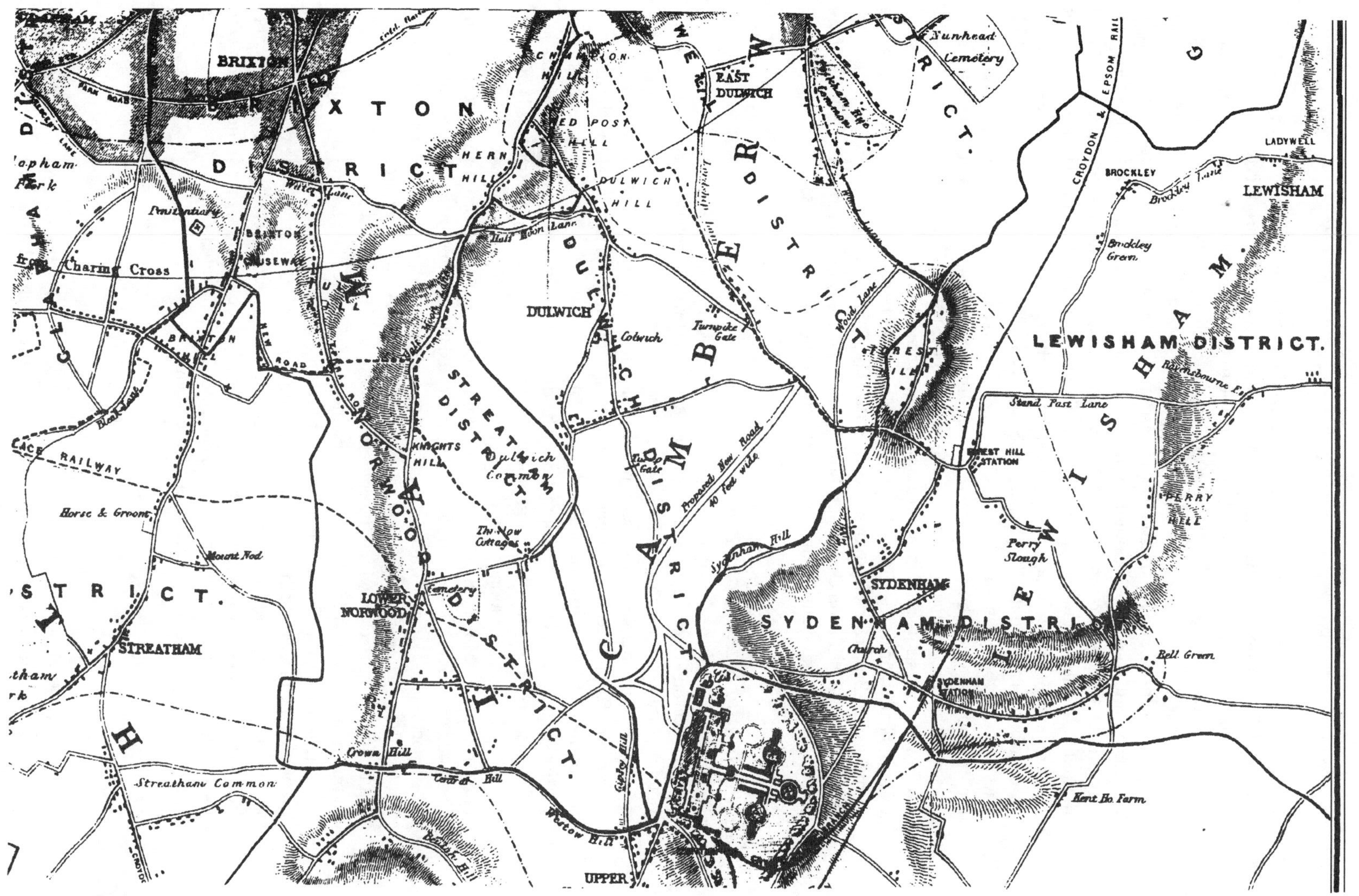

FIGURE I.4 River Thames area of London (shaded parts are the areas served by the two different water companies). (Snow J. "On the Mode of Communication of Cholera." Excerpted and adapted from the original 1855 edition as found in *Snow on Cholera* by John Snow, Commonweath Fund: New York; 1936.)

incubation; and if a whole sack of grain, or seed of any kind, were put into a hole in the ground, it is very doubtful whether any crop whatever would be produced.

An objection that has repeatedly been made to the propagation of cholera through the medium of water, is, that every one who drinks of the water ought to have the disease at once. This objection arises from mistaking the department of science to which the communication of cholera belongs, and looking on it as a question of chemistry, instead of one of natural history, as it undoubtedly is. It cannot be supposed that a morbid poison, which has the property, under suitable circumstances, of reproducing its kind, should be capable of being diluted indefinitely in water, like a chemical salt; and therefore it is not to be presumed that the cholera-poison would be equally diffused through every particle of water. The eggs of the tape-worm must undoubtedly pass down the sewers into the Thames, but it by no means follows that everybody who drinks a glass of water should swallow one of the eggs. As regards the morbid matter of cholera, many other circumstances, besides the quantity of it which is present in a river at different periods of the epidemic must influence the chances of it being swallowed, such as its remaining in a butt or other vessel till it is decomposed or devoured by animalcules, or its merely settling to the bottom and remaining there. In the case of the pump-well in Broad Street, Golden Square, if the cholera-poison was contained in the minute whitish flocculi visible on close inspection to the naked eye, some persons might drink of the water without taking any, as they soon settled to the bottom of the vessel.

Duration of Epidemic and Size of Population

There are certain circumstances connected with the history of cholera which admit of a satisfactory explanation according to the principles explained above, and consequently tend to confirm those principles. The first point I shall notice, viz., the period of duration of the epidemic in different places, refers merely to the communicability of the disease, without regard to the mode of communication. The duration of cholera in a place, is usually in direct proportion to the number of the population. The disease remains but two or three weeks in a village, two or three months in a good-sized town, whilst in a great metropolis it often remains a whole year or longer. I find from an analysis which I made in 1849 of the valuable table of Dr. Wm. Merriman, of the cholera in England in 1832, that fifty-two places are enumerated in which the disease continued less than 50 days, and that the average population of these places is 6,624. Forty-three places are likewise down in which the cholera lasted 50 days, but less than 100; the average population of these is 12,624. And there are, without including London, 33 places in which the epidemic continued 100 days and upwards, the average population of which is 38,123; if London be included, 34 places, with an average of 78,832.

There was a similar relation in 1849 between the duration of the cholera and the population of the places which it visited; a relation which points clearly to the propagation of the disease from patient to patient; for if each case were not connected with a previous one, but depended on some unknown atmospheric or telluric condition, there is no reason why the 20 cases which occur in a village should not be distributed over as long a period as twenty hundred cases which occur in a large town.

Effect of Season

Each time when cholera has been introduced into England in the autumn, it has made but little progress, and has lingered rather than flourished during the winter and spring, to increase gradually during the following summer, reach its climax at the latter part of the summer, and decline some what rapidly as the cool days of autumn set in. In most parts of Scotland, on the contrary, cholera has each time run through its course in the winter immediately following its introduction. I have now to offer what I consider an explanation, to a great extent, of the peculiarities in the progress of cholera. The English people, as a general rule, do not drink much unboiled water, except in warm weather. They generally take tea, coffee, malt liquor, or some other artificial beverage at the meals, and do not require to drink between meals except when the weather is warm. In summer, however, a much greater quantity of drink is required, and it is more usual to drink water at that season than in cold weather. Consequently, whilst the cholera is chiefly confined in winter to the crowded families of the poor, and to the mining population, who . . . eat each other's excrement at all times, it gains access as summer advances to the population of the towns, where there is a river which receives the sewers and supplies the drinking water at the same time; and, where pump-wells and other limited supplies of water happen to be contaminated with the contents of the drains and cesspools, there is a greater opportunity for the disease to spread at a time when unboiled water is more freely used.

In Scotland, on the other hand, unboiled water is somewhat freely used at all times to mix with spirits; I am told that when two or three people enter a tavern in Scotland and ask for a gill of whiskey, a jug of water and tumbler-glasses are brought with it. Malt liquors are only consumed to a limited extent in Scotland, and when persons drink spirits without water as they often do, it occasions thirst and obliges them to drink water afterwards.

There may be other causes besides the above which tend to assist the propagation of cholera in warm, more than in cold weather. It is not unlikely that insects, especially the common house-flies, aid in spreading the disease. An ingenious friend of mine has informed me that, when infusion of quassia has been placed in the room for the purpose of poisoning flies, he has more than once perceived the taste of it on his bread and butter.

Alternative Theories

Dr. Farr discovered a remarkable coincidence between the mortality from cholera in the different districts of London in 1849, and the elevation of the ground; the connection being of an inverse kind, the higher districts suffering least, and the lowest suffering most from this malady. Dr. Farr was inclined to think that the level of the soil had some direct influence over the prevalence of cholera, but the fact of the most elevated towns in this kingdom, as Wolverhampton, Dowlais, Merthyr Tydvil, and Newcastle-upon-Tyne, having suffered excessively from this disease on several occasions, is opposed to this view, as is also the circumstance of Bethlehem Hospital, the Queen's Prison, Horsemonger Lane Gaol, and several other large buildings, which are supplied with water from deep wells on the premises, having nearly or altogether escaped cholera, though situated on a very low level, and surrounded by the disease. The fact of Brixton, at an elevation of 56 feet above Trinity high-water mark, having suffered a mortality of 55 in 10,000 whilst many districts on the north of the Thames, at less than half the elevation, did not suffer one-third as much, also points to the same conclusion.

I expressed the opinion in 1849, that the increased prevalence of cholera in the low-lying districts of London depended entirely on the greater contamination of the water in these districts, and the comparative immunity from this disease of the population receiving the improved water from Thames Ditton, during the epidemics of last year and the present, as shown in the previous pages, entirely confirms this view of the subject; for the great bulk of this population live in the lowest districts of the metropolis.

It is not necessary to oppose any other theories in order to establish the principles I am endeavouring to explain, for the field I have entered on was almost unoccupied. The best attempt at explaining the phenomena of cholera, which previously existed, was probably that which supposed that the disease was communicated by effluvia given off from the patient into the surrounding air, and inhaled by others into the lungs; but this view required its advocates to draw very largely on what is called predisposition, in order to account for the numbers who approach near to the patient without being affected, whilst others acquire the disease without any near approach. It also failed entirely to account for the sudden and violent outbreaks of the disease, such as that which occurred in the neighbourhood of Golden Square.

Another view having a certain number of advocates is, that cholera depends on an unknown something in the atmosphere which becomes localized, and has its effects increased by the gases given off from decomposing animal and vegetable matters. This hypothesis is, however, rendered impossible by the motion of the atmosphere, and, even in the absence of wind, by the laws which govern the diffusion of aeriform bodies; moreover, the connection between cholera and offensive effluvia is by no means such as to indicate cause and effect; even in London, as was before mentioned, many places where offensive effluvia are very abundant have been visited very lightly by cholera, whilst the comparatively open and clean districts of Kennington and Clapham have suffered severely. If inquiry were made, a far closer connection would be found to exist between offensive effluvia and the itch, than between these effluvia and cholera; yet as the cause of itch is well known, we are quite aware that this connection is not one of cause and effect.

Mr. John Lea, of Cincinnati, has advanced what he calls a geological theory of cholera. He supposes that the cholera-poison, which he believes to exist in the air about the sick, requires the existence of calcareous or magnesian salts in the drinking water to give it effect. This view is not consistent with what we know of cholera, but there are certain circumstances related by Mr. Lea which deserve attention. He says that, in the western districts of the United States, the cholera passed round the arenacious, and spent its fury on the calcareous regions; and that it attacked with deadly effect those who used the calcareous water, while it passed by those who used sandstone or soft water. He gives many instances of towns suffering severely when river water was used, whilst others, having only soft spring water or rain water, escaped almost entirely; and he states that there has been scarcely a case of cholera in families who used only rain water. The rivers, it is evident, might be contaminated with the evacuations, whilst it is equally evident that the rain water could not be so polluted. As regards sand and all sandstone formations, they are well known to have the effects of oxidizing and thus destroying organic matters; whilst the limestone might not have that effect, although I have no experience on that point. The connection which Mr. Lea has observed between cholera and the water is highly interesting, although it probably admits of a very different explanation from the one he has given.

Case Study Questions

D.1 What are the epidemiologic implications of Snow's observations about sizes of cities and length of epidemics?

D.2 Snow suggested several reasons for the failure of contaminated water to produce disease in all who consume it. Why is it that not everyone gets ill or dies, who consumes cholera pathogens?

D.3 What principles were correct and what were incorrect in Snow's observations about time and seasons and the effects on epidemics? Why?

D.4 Several different theories and hypotheses have been presented. Which of these are consistent with known scientific and biomedical knowledge and common sense? Which of these were not consistent nor supported by scientific and biomedical knowledge and common sense? Why?

C A S E   S T U D Y

II

Working through a Food-borne Illness Epidemic Investigation: Typhoid Fever in Schenectady

Excerpted and adapted from "Typhoid in Schenectady: A Foodborne Outbreak." *Case Studies in Epidemiology,* by El-Ahraf A, and Brin BN, Course Syllabus for Principles of Epidemiology; 1998, California State University, San Bernardino.

Typhoid fever, cholera, and salmonellosis, also referred to as alvine discharge diseases, are infections of the digestive system. Such diseases are often spread because of a lack of such sanitary measures as hand washing before handling food. The lack of food protection and good sanitary measures in food preparation are major contributing causes of food poisoning from these and other diseases.

Typhoid fever was made famous by Typhoid Mary. Mary Mallon, a food service worker, caused many deaths and several typhoid outbreaks in New York in the early 1900s. When finally identified as the source of the typhoid epidemics, bacteriological examination of her feces showed that she was a chronic typhoid carrier. Having made her mark in the pages of history, Mary Mallon, has been taught in history- and social studies-related classes in schools and colleges ever since.

Typhoid fever is one of the multitude of salmonella infections and becomes pathogenic because of the endotoxins it produces. The source of infection is usually the feces of asymptomatic carriers. About 2% to 5% of patients become chronic carriers. Persistent carriers by law must be reported to public health departments and are prohibited from handling food. The stool or urine of ill patients who have an active case of the disease is also a source. The organism enters the gastrointestinal tract and invades the blood stream and lymph system. The incubation period relates to the numbers of organisms taken in (3 to 25 days). Symptoms include a slow onset, chills, malaise, headache, anorexia, muscle aches, fever/elevated temperature, and constipation. As the disease progresses, bradycardia, discrete rounded rose-colored spots in crops, emerge on abdomen and chest, and splenomegaly occurs. Prevention is by purification of drinking water, pasteurization of milk, sanitation and food protection, and control of carriers. Tests include blood and stool cultures, as well as bone marrow cultures, rose spots, and liver tests. Food, water, milk, and seafood are common sources of the typhoid salmonella pathogen (Berkow R, ed. *The Merck Manual.* 14th ed. Rahway, NJ: Merck and Company; 1982).

CASE OF TYPHOID FEVER IN SCHENECTADY, NEW YORK

In 1939, Schenectady was a city of approximately 90,000 people. On June 20th of this same year, the Public Health Department's Health Officer received reports of five cases of typhoid fever within the city. The Health Officer also received a report of one case of typhoid fever in a person who lived about 100 miles away in Massachusetts. The person had visited Schenectady in recent weeks preceding. No cases of typhoid had been reported for the past year up to that date in the city. In the preceding 5 years, the average annual prevalence of typhoid had been two cases per year.

Schenectady's water supply was obtained from surface water. A stream with drainage from relatively uninhabited areas was the main water source. About 8 years before the typhoid outbreak, a modern rapid sand filtration water treatment plant was installed and competently operated by a sanitary engineer. The water supply for the city was chlorinated. Daily bacteriological analyses of water from six points in the water distribution system were conducted and reported to the Health Officer. Schenectady had a modern sewer system. Within the city, 95% to 98% of the houses were connected to the sewer system, which was a good record for 1939.

City ordinances prohibited the sale of unpasteurized milk or the sale of milk other than by certified dairies. Approximately 75% of the city's milk was supplied by two large dairies. One other dairy distributed about 300 quarts of pasteurized milk daily. Consumers, using their own containers, purchased a small but unknown amount of unpasteurized milk from nearby farmers. About 95% of all ice cream was supplied by two large manufacturers. They also supplied ice cream to nearby cities. All shellfish dealers were required to be licensed by the local health department. Shellfish dealers were also required to keep records of the receipt and distribution of all shellfish stock handled.

Typhoid carriers were required to be registered with the public health department. Twenty-one carriers were known and tracked by the health department. A survey of the city's hospitals and all physicians showed a total of 13 known or suspected cases of typhoid, which included the one reported from Massachusetts. From interviewing each case in their homes, epidemiologic data were collected. With the use of a spot map, it was observed that there was no geographical clustering of cases.

From the interviews and epidemiologic investigations with the 13 cases, a table of the information was compiled and tabulated and is presented in Table II.1. The epidemiologic interview gathered usual information from each case as found in almost any survey: name, age, sex, and occupation. For this particular epidemic, as in most food-borne outbreaks, certain specific data must be gathered, and this outbreak included date of onset, sewage, water supply, dairy products eaten, uncooked foods eaten, trips, and foods taken away from home. After studying Table II.1, answer the following questions.

Case Study Questions

1. What key activities and important facts tie each of the individual cases together?
2. Prepare a bar graph chart showing the dates and numbers of cases per day of the outbreak by date of onset for each typhoid case. Is this an epidemic curve? Why? Defend your answer.
3. From the case and epidemiologic data, can you estimate possible date of common exposure (present evidence and facts other than just the date)?

TABLE II.1 Summary of Dates Relevant to Cases of Typhoid Fever in Schenectady Outbreak

					Home Sanitation					
Name	***Age***	***Sex***	***Occupation***	***Onset Date***	***Sewage***	***Water***	***Dairy Products***	***Use of Uncooked Foods***	***Trips***	***Meals Away from Home***
Christiansen, Estelle	15	F	Student	6/7	City	City	Dairylea, Blair's	Clams 6/2	None	Daily at school; Blair's 6/2; M.E. picnic 5/30
Blair, Florence	55	F	Housewife	6/9	Septic tank	Own well	Owns cows, Dairylea	Own garden vegetables	Schenectady	M.E. picnic 5/30; Potters 6/4
Dencher, Mary	65	F	Housewife	6/5	City	City	Borden's, Blair's	Market vegetables	Lebanon 5/1–14	M.E. picnic 5/30
Howard, Flora	64	F	Housewife	6/7	Septic tank	Own well	Own cows	Oysters 5/1; fresh tomatoes	None	M.E. picnic 5/30
Jones, Theda	21	F	Teacher	6/7	City	City	Borden's, Dairylea	Clams 5/21; garden vegetables	Altaville 5/20–21	Altaville 5/20–21; M.E. picnic 5/30
Ostrander, Edith	49	F	Housewife	6/11	City	City	Kingning, Dairylea	Garden vegetables	None	M.E. picnic 5/30
Thurber, Walter	25	M	Mechanic	6/25	City	City	Borden's Good Humor	Garden vegetables	None	Shares lunch daily with fellow workers
Kmiecziak, Robert	14	M	Student	6/18	City	City	Canned	None	None	M.E. picnic 5/30
Wagoner, Dorothy	16	F	Housework	6/16	City	City	Borden's Good Humor	None	None	M.E. picnic 5/30; Pep club 5/3
Wagoner, Grace	44	F	Housewife	6/9	City	City	Borden's	None	None	M.E. picnic 5/30
Wagoner, Robert	40	M	Grocer	6/28	City	City	Borden's	None	None	M.E. picnic 5/30
Woods, Alice	53	F	Housewife	6/7	Septic tank	Own well	Own cows	Garden vegetables	None	M.E. picnic 5/30
Vogel, Ethel	41	F	Mill worker	6/7	Pit privy	Chicope Falls, MA	Canned	None	Schenectady 5/29–6/12	Sister's home—Schenectady; M.E. picnic 5/30

4. Several unrelated cases appeared in the investigation. Explain the exposure to typhoid and implications of the unrelated cases of typhoid and give several examples or possibilities.

5. Briefly outline additional steps that are needed in order to complete this particular investigation.

The Schenectady Methodist Episcopal Church held a Memorial Day celebration at the church, which included a buffet picnic supper. On the afternoon of May 30th, the annual Memorial Service was held at the Methodist cemetery in Schenectady and was followed by a late afternoon picnic supper. A potluck approach was used to furnish the food and was provided by a number of the participants. Supper was served to 33 of the persons who attended the service.

An epidemiologic investigation was held at the Schenectady Methodist Episcopal church. In the investigation, inquiries were made of persons attending the picnic. All persons who attended the supper were interviewed. Interviewers recorded as accurately as possible all the foods consumed by each individual. Information about any previous history of typhoid or any possible symptoms was recorded, as well as information concerning the preparation and serving of foods. Food samples were not available as all food had either been eaten or discarded. An attempt was made to obtain fecal specimens from all individuals who were at the picnic. A series of three specimens was acquired from all persons who prepared and provided food for the picnic.

No previous history of any typhoid illness was confirmed in any case. Laboratory studies, mostly consisting of stool cultures that came out positive, confirmed the clinical diagnosis of typhoid fever in all 13 cases. Additionally, the following laboratory data were obtained for persons who attended the picnic but showed no evidence of the typhoid disease.

- Irene Picket = positive stools on July 4, July 5, and July 6 and negative stools on July 23 and August 2.
- Margaret Bennett = 11 consecutive positive stools, July 2 through October 4.
- Kenneth Rineheardt = positive stools July 4 and July 3 and negative stools at a later date.

6. Of the three persons—Pickett, Bennett, and Rineheardt—who was most likely to have been infected during the church picnic outbreak? Who was most likely to have been infected before the picnic?

7. Which laboratory tests might be administered nowadays that were not generally available in 1939? (Some outside research in medical diagnostic books might be needed to answer this question.) How would these tests help the church picnic investigation?

See Table II.2, which is a checklist of the foods eaten at the Methodist church picnic. Included in the table are the names of the 35 persons/cases involved in the outbreak. The table provides information on whether a person was a case or not a case, and the different foods each consumed, with a key at the bottom about each person's eating of different foodstuffs and the ability to recall the foods each had eaten. See Table II.2 and use the worksheet for food-specific attack rates, Table II.3.

8. Compute the attack rates for those eating and for those not eating each food and the unknowns. Calculate a relative risk for each food. Include data for all 35 individuals (include the use of food-specific attack rates).

TABLE II.2 Checklist of Foods Eaten at the Memorial Day Church Supper

Name	*Case*	*Potato Salad*	*Macaroni Salad*	*Cabbage Salad*	*Summer Sausage*	*Spiced Ham*	*Baked Beans*	*Rolls*	*Cakes*	*Coffee*	*Pickles*
S. Christian	Yes	1	1	2	2	2	2	1	2	1	1
S. Blair	Yes	3	3	2	2	2	2	1	2	1	1
M. Dencher	Yes	1	2	2	2	1	2,4	1,4	1	2	2
F. Howard	Yes	1	1	2	2	2	2	2,4	1,4	2	2
T. Jones	Yes	1	3	2	1	2	1	1	1	2	2,4
E. Ostrander	Yes	2	1	2	2	2	2	1	2	1	2
W. Thurber[5]	Yes	1	2	2	2	2	2	2	2	2	2
R. Kmiecziak	Yes	1	1	2	1	2	1	1	1	1	1
D. Wagner	Yes	1	1	1	2	1	2	1	1	1	2
G. Wagoner	Yes	3	1	3	1	1	2	1	1,4	1	2
R. Wagoner	Yes	1	1	1	2	1	1	1	1	1	1
A. Woods	Yes	1	1	2	1,6	2,6	2,6	1,4	1	1	3
E. Vogel	Yes	1	1	3	1	1	1	1	1	1	2
G. Harmon	No	1	2	2	2	2	1	1	2	1	2
J. Stoddard	No	1	1	1	2	8	8	8	8	1	1
I. Pickett	No	1	1	1	2	2	1	1	1	1	1
J. Bennett	No	1	1	1	1	2	1	1	1	1	1
C. Carrol	No	1	2	1	1	2	1	1	2	1	1
G. Anderson[5]	No	1	2	2	2	2	2	2	2	2	2
N. Brothers	No	1	2	2	2	1	2	1	1	1	2
E. Conrad	No	1	2	1	2	1	2	1	1	1	2
E. Gray	No	1	2	2	2	2	1	1	2	1	2
G. Harrington	No	2	2	2	2	2	1	1	2	1	2
S. McAuliffe	No	1	2	2	2	2	2	2	2	1	2
E. Pickett	No	1,4	2	2	1	2	2	1	1,4	1	1
J. Sailsburgh	No	2	2	2	2	2	1	1	1	1	2
L. Smith	No	1	3	3,4	2	2	1	1	2	1	1
M. Bennett	No	1,4	2,4	2	2	2	2	2	1	2	2
E. Thurber	No	2,4	2	2	2	2	2	1	2	2	2
K. Rhinehardt	No	1	1	1	2	2	1	1	2	1	2
A. Wagoner	No	1	1	1	2	1	1	1	1	2	2
H. Wagoner	No	1	1	2	1	2	1	1	1	1	2
B. Alexander[7]	No	Unavailable for interview									
C. Scofield[7]	No	Unavailable for interview									
M. Harrison	No	1	3	2	2	2	1	1	1	1	2

[1] Recalled having eaten the food
[2] Recalled having not eaten the food
[3] Could not remember
[4] Brought or prepared food indicated
[5] Ate food brought home by Mrs. Thurber
[6] Foods store bought
[7] Not located
[8] Gave contradictory responses regarding the food

TABLE II.3 Worksheet for Food-Specific Attack Rates

Food	*Eating Not eating Unknown*	*Persons Contracting Typhoid*	*Persons Not Contracting Typhoid*	*Total Persons*	*Attack Rate %*	*Relative Risk*
Potato salad:						
Macaroni salad:						
Cabbage salad:						
Summer sausage:						
Spiced ham:						
Baked beans:						
Rolls:						
Cakes:						
Coffee:						
Pickles:						

9. From the array of foods provided, list those which you think would be most susceptible to mass contamination. Identify those foods and conditions that provide a good growth medium for bacteria. Which foods are at high risks for contamination during preparation, serving, and storage, thus making them high possibilities as sources for typhoid transmission?

10. As a result of the worksheet that included food-specific attack rates that you prepared, determine the food or foods most likely to be involved in the typhoid outbreak. Base your determination on the following epidemiologic concepts:

    - A majority of cases should have eaten the food.
    - The relative risk.
    - The ease of mass contamination of the food.
    - List of foods that appear to be of high risk in the transmission of disease but have minimum likelihood because of the scientific basis for not being probable of transmitting the disease. Explain why they are not likely to be suspect.

11. How should an epidemiologist deal with circumstances in which an individual cannot recall a food eaten or who gave contradictory responses about whether or not the food items were eaten?

12. Why is an epidemiologist concerned about attack rates and relative risk among persons not eating particular foods?

13. To incriminate a particular food as a source of disease transmission, what epidemiologic and scientific/biomedical findings are necessary?

14. Are pieces of information missing that leave the investigation incomplete? What are the missing pieces of information or gaps in the investigation?

15. Considering all of the data, information, and evidence, what is the most likely and probable explanation for this epidemic? Be specific about the individual persons and the foodstuffs and other supporting factors; include time, place, and person.

16. As an epidemiologist, how would you prevent and control future typhoid fever epidemics such as this one?

CASE STUDY

III

Common-Source Outbreak of Waterborne Shigellosis at a Public School

Adapted from Bain WB, Herron CA, Bridson K, et al. Waterborne shigellosis at a public school. *Am J Epidemiol.* 1975;101(4): 323–332.

Shigellosis is an intestinal tract infection that is caused by shigella organisms. It has four major subgroups of pathogens. The source of infection is excreta of infected individuals or carriers. Shigellosis is usually spread by ingesting food or water contaminated by fecal matter. In addition, flies are a vehicle/vector of contamination, and fomites have also been implicated in the spread of the disease. Epidemics are often found in crowded populations living with poor sanitation and are a source of bacillary dysentery found in children living in endemic areas.

The incubation period is 1 to 4 days. In younger children, the onset can be sudden. Symptoms include fever, irritability, drowsiness, anorexia, nausea or vomiting, diarrhea, and abdominal cramps. Within 3 days, blood, pus, and mucus appear in the stools. The number of stools increases rapidly to about 20 or more a day—severe diarrhea. In the laboratory findings of sample specimens, the shigella bacteria are found in the stools. The white blood count is often reduced at the onset and goes up to 13,000. Plasma CO_2 is usually low, showing a response from the diarrhea-induced metabolic acidosis. Prevention and control are performed by preventing the spread of contaminated food, water, and flies through sanitation, which may include hand washing before food handling, soaking contaminated clothes in soap and water until boiled, isolating patients and carriers, and stools (Berkow R, ed. *The Merck Manual.* 14th ed. Rahway, NJ: Merck and Company; 1982).

CASE OF COMMON-SOURCE OUTBREAK OF WATERBORNE SHIGELLOSIS AT A PUBLIC SCHOOL

In November 1972, a public school in Stockport, Iowa (population 334), experienced an outbreak of gastrointestinal illness. Of the 269 pupils who attended the public school, 194 (72%) were affected, and 14 of the 23 faculty and staff (61%) were also affected. Laboratory and clinical exams showed that the etiological agent was Shigella sonnei. Of the 698 student contacts with members of infected households, 97 (14%) also developed diarrhea. Secondary cases also occurred in 3 of 32 members of households of the school's staff.

Shigellosis is most often spread from person to person; common-source outbreaks also occur and must be considered in any epidemiologic investigation. Water and food should both be considered as a mode of transmission.

In the second week of November 1972 a physician in Fairfield, Iowa, contacted the Iowa State Department of Health by telephone to report a case of shigellosis infection in a young woman who was from Stockport, Iowa. The young woman/patient lived in an apartment across the street from a county middle school. The young woman shared a common water supply with the school. Several guests who attended a gathering at her apartment on November 4th had experienced gastrointestinal illness.

It was discovered that there were high levels of absenteeism at the school because of gastrointestinal illnesses. Similar illnesses were also reported among members of the local high school boys' basketball team. A high school boys' basketball team from the neighboring town also reported gastrointestinal illnesses. The two teams had played a scrimmage at the middle school's gym on November 15th.

Van Buren County, with a population of 8,643 according to the 1970 census, is a small county located in southeastern Iowa near the Missouri border. This is a rural county, with 37% of the mostly white residents living on farms. Almost 22% of the residents lived below the federal poverty level, and 755, or 22%, of the 3,399 households in the county lacked in some or all standard plumbing facilities. All 6th, 7th, and 8th grade students in the Van Buren School District attend the middle school in Stockport. In November of 1972, the enrollment at the middle school was 289 and 25 teachers and staff.

The layout of the school is an important epidemiologic consideration in this case of a common-source outbreak. The school included a main building; an annex housed the gym and several classrooms. The gym was used for physical education classes, and high school teams in the region used it for practice games. Included in the buildings of the school was an old garage located across the street from the school and east of the main building. The building was used as a shop for industrial arts classes. The easternmost third of the shop building was the private residence/apartment of the young woman mentioned previously here, who also developed shigellosis (see building map in Figure III.1).

The water supplies for the middle school, the gym, the shop, and the private apartment all came from wells on the school grounds (see Figure III.1). Environmental studies were conducted to test the school's water supply. Microbiological testing of the wells was done. The wells' construction was studied. Water flow and cross connection tests were carried out on the water supply and the sewage system of the middle school and nearby buildings with fluorescent dye studies.

The family and guests at the gathering in the young woman's apartment on November 4th were questioned about gastrointestinal illness. The students and faculty and staff of Van Buren on November 30th were interviewed and surveyed. Interviews included customary daily consumption of the water at the school, including the fountain in the gym, illnesses, date of onset, symptoms, school absenteeism, physician visits, or hospitalizations. The two basketball teams also were surveyed plus an estimated amount of water consumption at the scrimmage on November 15th. Most symptomatic and some asymptomatic cases submitted rectal swabs for bacteriological culture using standard laboratory procedures.

To investigate secondary transmission of the disease, questionnaires were distributed to families of students, faculty and staff, and all of the basketball players in order to determine incidence (see Table III.1). A secondary case was defined as diarrhea beginning be-

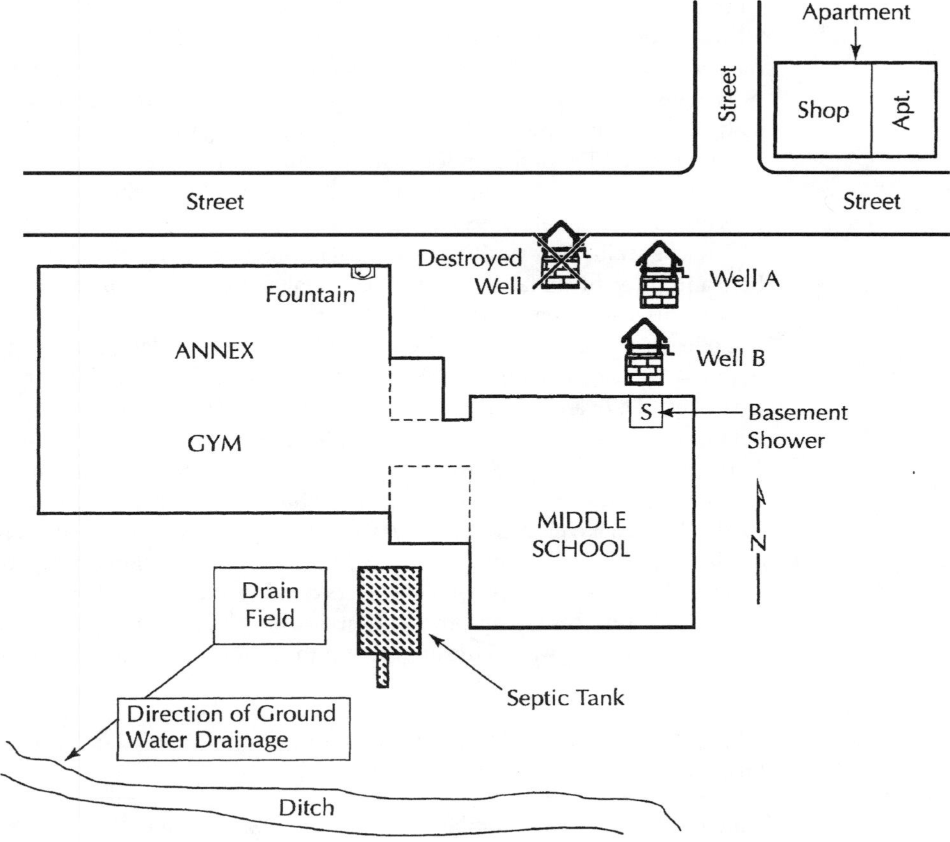

FIGURE III.1 Van Buren County Middle School building map.

tween November 10th and December 4th, among household members (or contacts) of students, faculty and staff, and ball players. Rectal swabs for cultures were obtained from available family members of the groups. Those groups consisted of 10 families chosen at random from the first 40 families to report an apparent secondary infection, three families out of five of the students in which there were apparent secondary cases without illness in the pupil and three families of faculty and staff with apparent secondary infection. Cultures were obtained

TABLE III.1 Shigellosis Secondary Attack Rates

General Secondary Attack Rates			
Questionnaires Returned by	***Total Number***	***Number Returned***	***Attack Rate %***
Families of students	245	169	—
Household contacts	698	97	—
Asymptomatic students	5	37	—

from the index case, an 8th grader and two of the participants in the apartment gathering; all were positive. In the questionnaire, gastrointestinal illness was defined by symptoms: nausea; vomiting; bowel movements that were loose, frequent, or bloody; cramps; or tenesmus. Questionnaires were retrieved from 93% of the students and 92% of the faculty and staff; 194 students and 14 faculty and staff reported gastrointestinal illness in November.

Of the families of the middle school faculty and staff, three returned questionnaires on secondary attacks at 88% or 22 out of 25. Three of 32 household contacts had diarrhea, for a secondary attack rate of 9%.

Rectal swabs were positive for Shigella sonnei for 96 out of 123 symptomatic staff members and three of six faculty and staff. Rectal swabs from 13 of 23 asymptomatic students were positive for Shigella sonnei, as shown by cultures.

Eleven of 12 of those at the apartment gathering developed gastrointestinal illness within 4 days of November 4th. Several students and faculty and staff reported illness in the first week of November (see Tables III.2 and III.3). The first peak in the epidemiology curve occurred on Friday, November 10th, with an average of 12 cases a day for the next 5 days. Forty-five cases occurred on Thursday, November 16th. The outbreak then tapered off rapidly. Male and female attack rates were about the same; grade level showed no difference in attack rates. No clear trends in water consumption and illness attack rates were seen (see Table III.4). From November 16th to 19th, 7 of 18 high school ball players on the visiting team and 10 local high school ball players developed diarrhea. Four of 25 rectal swabs were positive; all four were symptomatic. Diarrhea attack rates among basketball players were directly correlated to water consumption at the school's fountain in the gym.

TABLE III.2 Date of Onset of Gastrointestinal Illness, Van Buren Middle School, Stockport, Iowa, 1972

Date of Illness Onset	*Number of Cases*	*Date of Illness Onset*	*Number of Cases*
November		November	
2	1	16	45
3	1	17	30
4	2	18	7
5	2	19	1
6	1	20	6
7	2	21	3
8	2	22	0
9	3	23	1
10	19	24	3
11	11	25	0
12	12	26	0
13	9	27	2
14	6	28	2
15	14	29	0
		30	1

TABLE III.3 Date of Onset of Secondary Attack Rates of Gastrointestinal Illness in Faculty and Staff, Van Buren Middle School, Stockport, Iowa, 1972

Date of Illness Onset	*Number of Cases*	*Date of Illness Onset*	*Number of Cases*
November		November	
7	1	22	8
8	0	23	2
9	0	24	3
10	1	25	13
11	3	26	4
12	1	27	4
13	4	28	2
14	0	29	9
15	0	30	8
16	5	December	
17	2	1	3
18	5	2	0
19	3	3	5
20	7	4	0
21	3	5	0

The main water sources for the school complex were from the water wells in the schoolyard north of the school house. When the shigellosis outbreak occurred, water well A was in use. Well A supplied water to the shop and to the apartment. Even though shigellosis is rarely transmitted by water, at the time of the outbreak, the water supply for the school became suspected. The suspect well was not chlorinated at the time of the outbreak, and

TABLE III.4 Attack Rates of Gastrointestinal Illness by Usual Amount of Water Consumed Daily at the Middle School

	Students		*Faculty*	
Estimated Amount of Water Drunk	*No. Ill/Total*	*Attack Rate (%)*	*No. Ill/Total*	*Attack Rate (%)*
0 glasses	4/11		3/3	
1 glass	14/19		2/5	
2 glasses	24/36		1/2	
3 glasses	38/57		1/3	
4 glasses	43/56		2/2	
5 glasses	28/38		0/1	
6+ glasses	43/50		3/3	

because it was suspected, it was superchlorinated on November 17th. The Stockport municipal water company had a water system under construction, and special priority was given to connecting the school to the new water supply. The water was connected on November 21st. One of the three wells was destroyed in the process of hooking up the municipal water system. Investigation of the two remaining wells showed that they were shallow bored well cases with ceramic pipe segments, having joints that were not watertight. The outflow pipes of the submersible pump pierced the lining of the well below ground level. The hole allowed seepage of ground water into the well. Well B, which was closer to the school, was not in use at the time of the shigellosis epidemic; however, when the pump in one well was turned on, it lowered the water table in both wells. Well B was located in a slight depression on the surface of the earth and could be contaminated by surface water as well as ground water sources. Indeed, debris was found floating in well B. On the opposite side of the school from the wells was a septic tank that fed a drain field that emptied into a ditch southeast of the school. Attempts with dye were made to show cross-contamination. All efforts failed to reveal any cross contamination by the appearance of the dye in the school well-water supply. Other attempts to show cross-contamination involved using fluorescent dye in the toilet in the apartment located in the shop building, across the street from the school, as well as the school yard storm drains; all failed, with one exception, to show cross-contamination of the well water.

Showers for the students were adjacent to the gym, but visiting teams used the shower located in the utility room on the basement floor of the school. The shower was installed only shortly before the shigellosis outbreak. The shower drained down into a bed of gravel under the basement floor and was known to drain well. Hooking the shower to the sewer system had been considered unnecessary, as it drained well. Dye studies flushed down the drain of the shower, located only a few feet from the wells, showed up in the well water within 3 hours. This same shower was used by three faculty members during the time period of the outbreak. Two of the three faculty members were among those documented with shigellosis on November 13th, and the other was identified with the disease on November 15th and had febrile diarrhea. On November 16th, water samples were taken from the tap in the boy's restroom. They revealed a total coliform count of 125 per 100 ml. A second water sample was obtained from the school on November 17th before the superchlorination of the supply. The second water sample revealed a coliform most probable number of 16+, and Shigella sonnei was recovered from a 1600-ml sample.

Case Study Questions

1. The common-source and first cases of the outbreak were from the well water. Explain how the secondary cases of shigellosis probably occurred; identify the probable mode(s) of transmission in the secondary cases.
2. Was the basketball team from the neighboring community primary transmission cases or secondary? Why? What role did the neighboring basketball team play in secondary cases?
3. In this case, a secondary case was defined as diarrhea beginning between November 10th and December 4th. Why are these dates chosen for this purpose and how do they help determine what a secondary case is in this investigation?
4. Much concern was given to whether a case was symptomatic or asymptomatic. What is the significance of these two states of illness, and why is this important in this particular disease?

5. Calculate the secondary attack rates for Table III.1.
6. What problems or shortcomings did you see in this study? What would be necessary to overcome such shortcomings?
7. What type of sewage system in the school complex was used and how effective was it? What role did it play in disease transmission?
8. What was the attack rate for the students for November?
9. What caused the epidemic to taper off after November 16th?
10. What was the attack rate for the faculty and staff for November?
11. What is the sensitivity for the symptomatic students and faculty and staff using the rectal swab test?
12. What is the specificity for the asymptomatic students and faculty and staff using the rectal swab test?
13. Develop and construct a bar chart of the epidemiologic curve for the shigellosis outbreak using the data in Table III.2. Identify the index case and date, and explain who the index case was. What date was the water chlorinated? What did chlorinating the water do to the epidemic curve?
14. Develop a bar graph of the secondary attack rate for the shigellosis epidemic using the data from Table III.3. Explain why the secondary epidemic curve is different than that of the primary epidemic curve.
15. Calculate the attack rates for the various amount of water consumption as it related to illness onset, found in Table III.4.
16. What are your observations as to the source of the contamination of the well water with Shigella sonnei that caused the outbreak? Give two possible sources for the pathogen getting into the water supply: (1) direct and (2) indirect.
17. What are the control and prevention measures needed for this case and shigellosis?

CASE STUDY

IV

Retrospective Analysis of Occupation and Alcohol-Related Mortality

Adapted from Brooks SD, Harford TC. Occupation and alcohol-related causes of death. *Drug and Alcohol Dependence.* 1992;29(3):245–251.

The liver is the organ that is most often seriously damaged by heavy drinking. Even moderate drinking damages body tissues, which are quickly mended. The more one drinks, the longer, more lasting, and serious the effects on the body. The connection between heavy drinking of alcohol and heart disease has been known for over 100 years. For years, malnutrition was pointed to as the cause of the physiological damage. Malnutrition is still a major factor, but now it is known that alcohol does the damage to the body tissues and organs directly. Areas of the heart affected are the mitochondria (energy-producing cells in the cardiac muscle), which results in alcoholic cardiomyopathy (heart muscle degeneration). Without energy, the heart's pumping action fails over time. Arrhythmia of the heart is also seen in heavy drinkers because alcohol disrupts the natural heart rhythms. High blood pressure and cancer are also caused by heavy drinking. Cancer of the liver, larynx, nasopharynx, and esophagus are seen more frequently in heavy drinkers. Ulcerative lesions are seen in the small intestine. The pancreas is vulnerable to alcohol abuse, resulting in pancreatitis. Alcoholic myopathy or muscle weakness is also seen at serious clinical levels in heavy drinkers (Schlaadt RG. *Wellness: Alcohol Use and Abuse.* Guilford, CT: Dushkin Publishing Group; 1992).

CASE OF OCCUPATION AND ALCOHOL-RELATED CAUSES OF DEATH, CALIFORNIA

Are alcohol-related causes of death associated with similar occupational groups? Is heavy drinking associated with different occupations? Most studies have focused on cirrhosis of the liver deaths related to alcohol drinking. Several research studies found that cirrhosis mortality has been shown to be associated with the following occupations: bartenders, waiters, cooks, longshoremen, seamen, salesmen, wholesale and retail trades, entertainment and recreation workers, truck drivers, garage proprietors, and personal service workers. The studies also found that cirrhosis is highest in lower status jobs—blue collar workers. Also, jobs with high exposure to alcohol use and/or consumption have high drinking levels. Only 8% to 12% of heavy drinkers die from cirrhosis.

Many other alcohol and occupation associated conditions occur but do not get as much focus as cirrhosis of the liver. The more common conditions in which alcohol is implicated as a cause of death include digestive tract cancers, pancreatic disorders, certain cardiovascular diseases, and accidents and injuries.

Which alcohol-related causes of death are associated with which occupations?

The California Occupational Mortality Study (COMS) data set was employed to assess mortality data for the years 1979 to 1981. A 2% sample of employed persons from the 1980 census of California was used. The COMS contains the occupation of each decedent (person who died).

This study, like any occupation-based study, is restricted to the work life span as far as age of subjects is concerned. This study used ages 16 through 64 years. Certain persons, because of their source of work, were excluded as subjects: homemakers, retired persons, students, disabled, military personnel, etc. Only mainstream type employment was used in this study to establish occupations at risk for heavy alcohol drinking. Military/nonworkers/unknowns were also analyzed. Underlying causes of death were used from the ICD-9-CM (see Chapter 2) for cirrhosis, digestive organ cancers, injuries, suicide, and homicide (see Table IV.1).

Thirteen occupational groups were identified, using the Census Bureau's 1980 Alphabetical Index of Industries and Occupations. Age-adjusted mortality rates per 100,000 were calculated for each of the 13 occupational groups (see Table IV.2). The numerator used was the number of occupation-specific deaths in each category of underlying cause of death in California from 1979 to 1981. The denominator for each occupational group was from the 20% sample of the 1980 Census of California used in the COMS, which was 173,438 deaths in California from 1979 to 1981.

Males and whites had the highest percent for each of the causes of death. Older age groups had the largest percentage of deaths for cirrhosis and digestive organ cancers. Younger age groups had higher percentages in injuries, suicide, and homicide. Military/nonworkers/unknowns had a pattern similar to that of workers, except for females, who had higher deaths rates related to alcohol than the female workers. The age-adjusted mortality rate for all other causes of death per 100,000 for the State of California was 238.77.

Research findings show that individuals in certain occupations drink alcohol more heavily than persons in other occupations. Factors that contribute to heavy alcohol consumption include opportunity to drink, time, location, availability of alcohol, work group or social group that has drinking as a custom, job stress, time pressures, and work rotations. Additionally, heavy drinking may occur in jobs that have low job visibility, high turnover, little supervision, and minimal job qualifications. High stress on the job, low accountabil-

TABLE IV.1 Alcohol Related Deaths in California, 1979–1981

Cirrhosis	5.5%
Digestive organ cancers	5.7%
Injuries	13.7%
Suicide and homicide	5.1%
All other causes	64.9%

TABLE IV.2 Age-Adjusted Mortality Rates for Occupational Groups and Cause of Death Per 100,000

Occupational Group	*Digestive Cirrhosis Mortality Rate*	*Cancer Mortality Rate*	*Injury Mortality Rate*	*Suicide Mortality Rate*	*Homicide Mortality Rate*
Executive, administrative, and managerial	13.6	25.1	32.47	13.72	10.02
Professional specialty	15.24	23.76	35.79	20.39	7.97
Technicians and related support areas	19.82	26.47	54.86	22.99	8.83
Sales	16.72	26.17	35.58	17.43	12.62
Administrative support, including clerical	13.5	20.07	23.97	12.15	7.58
Private household service	15.07	22.46	16.79	7.14	17.14
Protective service	36.17	40.46	61.02	33.95	38.13
Other service	29.66	26.46	47.97	18.28	25.6
Farming, forestry, and fishing	41.23	28.56	158.87	23.75	56.68
Precision production, craft and repair	33.98	34.69	91.29	32.78	30.51
Machine operators and assemblers	25.67	27.76	55.66	19.23	26.49
Transportation and material moving	39.58	38.45	112.84	28.41	34.64
Handlers, equipment, cleaners, and laborers	75.97	52.26	129.14	39.33	77.11
State of California	20.07	21.01	50.44	18.71	18.64

ity, and easy access to alcohol are factors that may contribute to heavy and destructive use of alcohol. From an epidemiologic research point of view, all of these factors may serve as confounding variables to occupation and alcohol abuse research.

Certain occupations may allow drinking on the job, as supervisors know little about it. Some people work in the field independently, away from the work site, and other jobs may actually encourage drinking on the job or at lunch. Many studies fail to differentiate between drinking on the job, job-related alcohol consumption, and non–job-related drinking. It is suspected that workplace drinking risks are low as compared with after-hours or lunchtime drinking. Other factors that may contribute to heavy drinking regardless of the work setting are the biological/physiological, familial, social class, religious influences, peer pressure, and other non–work-related factors and variables.

Case Study Questions

1. What occupations are most vulnerable to acquiring cirrhosis of the liver from heavy drinking? List several of the occupations identified by research studies that are more vulnerable to alcohol-induced cirrhosis-related deaths and that have the highest mortality rates.
2. Other than cirrhosis, what major diseases have heavy alcohol use implications as far as causation? List several.
3. Discuss why this study was restricted to ages 16 to 64 years. Discuss the research design implications of the age span restrictions in occupational studies.

4. In this study, which occupations had the highest digestive organ cancer mortality rate?
5. In this study, which occupations had the highest injury mortality rate?
6. In this study, which occupations had the highest suicide mortality rate?
7. In this study, which occupations had the highest homicide mortality rate?
8. Two occupational groups repeatedly exceeded the state average for alcohol-related deaths. Which two were they? Why? Provide an explanation.
9. What figures were used for the numerator of this study? What figures were used for the denominator of this study? Was the use of the numerator and denominator appropriate for age-adjusted rates?
10. Develop and show the formula for the age-adjusted digestive cancer mortality rate for the top four at-risk occupations for this disease found in Table IV.2.
11. What are the possible confounding variables for research in occupations and heavy drinking that lead to fatal diseases? Identify and explain which factors are confounding variables and how they serve as confounding variables.
12. Develop and construct a web of causation along with appropriate decision trees for occupational group-related alcohol deaths.

CASE STUDY

V

Retrospective Cohort Study of the Association of Congenital Malformations and Hazardous Waste

Adapted from Geschwind SA, Stolwijk JAJ, Bracken M, et al. Risk of congenital malformations associated with proximity to hazardous waste sites. *Am J Epidemiol.* 1992;135 (11):1197–1207.

Congenital anomalies or malformations are difficult to pinpoint as to cause. Some congenital malformation causes are understood; many are not. Causes may be single isolated cases, whereas others are multiple and varied. Some malformations at birth are inherited, and some are sporadic in their manifestation. Congenital defects are sometimes apparent and others hidden, taking years to become obvious. About 10% of neonatal deaths are caused by congenital malformations. A major malformation is apparent at birth in 3% to 4% of newborns. By the fifth year, up to 7.5% of all children manifest a congenital malformation. The incidence of certain congenital malformations varies with the defect (cleft lip occurs at the rate of 1 per 1,000 births in the United States) and the geographic area (spina bifida is about 4 per 1,000 births in Ireland and 2 per 1,000 in the United States). Interfamily marriage and culture practices can contribute to congenital malformations, as can perinatal problems and environmental exposures. Genetic factors are responsible for many congenital anomalies and syndromes. On the other hand, multiple factors are often involved in causing congenital malformations. Drugs taken while pregnant, infectious agents, and irradiation are known to cause birth defects. Chemicals in the environment as well as exposure to hazardous materials and waste in the environment and exposure to radiation in the worksite or environment have also been implicated (Berkow R, ed. *The Merck Manual.* 14th ed. Rahway, NJ: Merck and Company; 1982).

CASE ON CONGENITAL MALFORMATIONS ASSOCIATED WITH PROXIMITY TO HAZARDOUS WASTE SITES

Much concern has been expressed by the general public and public health scientists alike over the effects of exposure to environmental pollutants and how they have increased in modern society. It remains unclear whether chronic exposure to toxic chemicals in the environment is present in sufficiently high doses to produce adverse medical effects in humans. Inadvertent exposure to hazardous waste such as Love Canal has increased concern about any adverse effects the exposure might have on reproductive health. It also remains unclear whether individuals who live near toxic chemical waste sites receive doses in sufficient amounts to pose a health hazard, especially to reproductive functions. One concern is that many toxic chemicals present in toxic waste landfills and hazardous waste sites are cytotoxic. That is, they affect cells, tissues, and organs at specific stages of development and inhibit or interfere with normal growth, especially in embryo and fetus growth and developmental stages.

High rates of birth defects have been reported in children exposed to mercury, solvents, and certain toxic chemicals. Community-based studies have been conducted based on reports of clustering of disease around hazardous waste sites. Rarely have congenital defects in infants born to exposed parents been well documented.

This uses a four-tiered hypothesis approach in order to evaluate the relationship between birth defects and the potential exposure to toxic waste sites: (1) Does residential proximity to a waste site when pregnant increase risk of bearing a child with a defect? (2) Do defects of specific organ systems correlate with proximity to a toxic waste site? (3) Were defects associated with off-site migration of chemicals? How does the epidemiologist clarify whether this increased potential health risks? (4) Have chemical types associated with certain organ system defects been evaluated?

Pesticides have been associated with oral cleft (lips or palate) or musculoskeletal defects, heavy metals with nervous system defects, solvents with nervous system defects or digestive system defects, and plastics with chromosomal anomalies. Do the later phases corroborate the initial findings? Finally, this study was to test the association of environmental and health data bases and geographic mapping methods for ascertaining environmental exposures.

Databases of the New York State Department of Health were used: Congenital Malformation Registry (CMR) and the Hazardous Waste Site Inspection Program. The two programs were linked together for analysis of the four tiers of hypotheses. The Congenital Malformation Registry includes reports of all congenital malformations for the state's hospitals, medical facilities, and private physicians diagnosed in children up to 2 years of age. In the state of New York, 917 waste sites in 62 counties were available. New York City sites as well as several other sites were eliminated due to inadequate information. For final study, 590 waste sites in 20 counties were used. Epidemiologic map study approaches included each site being assigned a longitude and latitude using EPA and New York Department of Environmental Conservation records (see Figure V.1, Map of New York State with Waste Sites Identified as Small Black Triangles).

A total of 34,411 cases of malformations were recorded in the CMR for the years 1983 to 1985 and 1984 to 1986 birth cohorts. Any cases that were unusual were eliminated: multiple births, redundant cases, CDC exclusions list to avoid misclassification of malformations, census mapping coordinates missing, addresses incomplete, and locations without a census tract. The study was based on 12,442 congenital malformations and 9,313 cases. One case could have more than one defect.

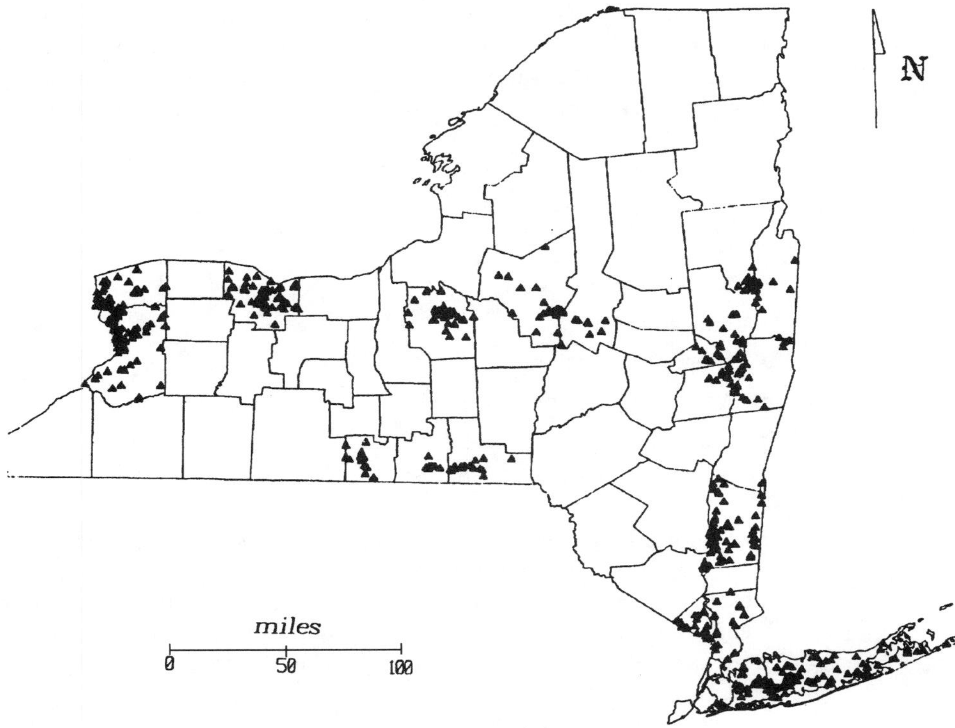

FIGURE V.1 Map of New York state with waste sites identified.

Eight categories of malformations were used from ICD-9-CM (see Chapter 2) that have been reported by research studies in the literature as being associated with exposures to chemicals or toxic substances (see Table V.1). Each individual exposure was unknown, and each probably could have had multiple exposures to a complex mix of chemicals. All cases were put under one general analysis. Each case was then placed in one of the eight categories and analyzed. More than one defect was found present in each case.

TABLE V.1 Eight Categories of Malformations ICD-9-CM

1. Oral cleft defects
2. Musculoskeletal defects
3. Nervous system defects
4. Integument defects
5. Digestive system defects
6. Chromosomal anomalies
7. Syndromes
8. Remaining defects without category

Controls were selected from birth certificate records: 17,802 or 12% of the 506,183 live births for 1983 to 1984 in the State of New York. Cross-checks were made to assure no congenital malformations were included in the control. Confounding variables were excluded from both cases and controls, and the information included the following:

- Maternal age
- Parity
- Race
- Birth weight of the child
- Education
- Length of gestation
- Address and county of residence
- Sex of the child
- Any pregnancy complications

Addresses for cases and controls were each assigned a latitude and longitude. Coordinates were based on census blocks based on Standard Metropolitan Statistical Areas, and Postal Carrier Route centroids were used (a centroid is the center point of the Postal Carrier Route boundary) and zip code centroids. A sample of 500 addresses was taken at random as a test of the mapping methods. The mapping procedure was accurate within 200 feet, 80% of the time.

Hazardous waste sites were assessed using the Hazardous Waste Site Inspection Program (HWSIP), which estimates the likelihood of human exposure. Possible exposure routes into humans include inhalation, ingestion, and dermal contact, which occur by environmental exposure transmission from air, groundwater, surface, water, or soil. This study included all residents within a 1-mile radius of the waste site edge. Still, absolute risk of exposure was uncertain. Assessment was based on a set of scores of a variety of factors: chemical exposure, a probability score chance of contaminant transport from the site, a target factor score that accounts for the population and distance from the waste site, and a weighting factor score giving each exposure a level of relative importance. The assessment excluded the total population portion of the target factor score, to give greater weight to the residents surrounding the waste sites.

Five general categories of chemicals grouped by chemical properties were developed. The five categories were as follows:

1. Pesticides
2. Metals
3. Solvents
4. Plastics
5. Unknown

An exposure risk index was completed for each case. The index accounted for distance and hazard ranking score within a 1-mile radius of the birth residence. Waste sites based on evidence of off-site migration of contaminants were separated from nonmigration sites.

All cases and controls coordinates were matched to hazardous waste sites by a matching program. Distance and direction from the hazardous waste site for the residence of each case or control living within a 1-mile radius of the edge of the site were considered potentially exposed. Risk was determined by association between mothers' (maternal) proximity to waste sites and presence of congenital anomalies (birth defects).

A 12% increased risk for birth defect associated with maternal proximity to toxic waste sites was found. Odds ratios were used to assess the association between proximity to toxic sites and maternal residence. An odds ratio score above 1.01 shows a positive association, and the higher the score the stronger the association. Table V.2 presents the odds ratios for congenital malformation with residential proximity to selected hazardous waste sites. Table V.3 presents odds ratios and exposure risk index for all congenital malformations and for three specific body systems affected by documented chemical leaks at hazardous waste sites. Table V.4 presents odds ratios for congenital malformations for all infants with specific malformations and residential proximity to selected toxic waste sites and chemical groups.

Case Study Questions

1. What are controls in a research study and how are they used? How are controls used in this study?
2. What are confounding variables? How do they affect a research study? What are the problems and limitations of confounding variables in this study?
3. From Table V.2 which malformations had the highest odds ratio? Which malformations had the lowest odds ratio? What is the significance of each?

TABLE V.2 Odds Ratios for All Congenital Malformations and for Specific Malformations in Infants with Residential Proximity to Selected Hazardous Waste Sites, New York State, 1983–1984

Number of Cases[‡]	*Congenital Malformation(s)*	*Odds Ratio*[†§]
9,313	All malformations combined	1.12**
421	Nervous system	1.29*
2,730	Musculoskeletal system	1.16**
1,370	Integument system	1.32**
232	Oral clefts	1.15
429	Digestive system	0.89
245	Chromosomal anomalies	1.18
575	Syndromes[‖]	1.15
4,003	Other (data too limited to infer associations with chemical exposure)	1.01

*$p < 0.05$; **$p < 0.01$.

[†]ICD-9, *International Classification of Diseases*, 9th revision.

[‡]The numbers of cases for the individual organ systems do not add up to the total number of cases for all defects combined because individuals may have had more than one defect.

[§]Adjusted for maternal age, race, education, complications during pregnancy, parity, population density for county of residence, and sex of the child, by logistic regression.

[‖]Syndromes include all defects coded as "syndrome" in the New York State Congenital Malformations Registry, or any child with four or more defects.

TABLE V.3 Odds Ratios and Exposure Risk Index for All Congenital Malformations and for Three Specific Body Systems Affected by Documented Chemical Leaks at Hazardous Waste Sites†‡§

Exposure	*All Malformations Combined (740–759)*	*Nervous System (740–742)*	*Musculoskeletal System (754–756)*	*Integument System (757)*
		Exposure Risk Index		
No exposure risk	1.00	1.00	1.00	1.00
Low exposure risk	1.09**	1.27*	1.09	1.22**
	(1.04–1.15)§	(1.03–1.57)	(1.00–1.18)	(1.08–1.38)
High exposure risk	1.63**	1.48	1.75**	2.63**
	(1.34–1.99)	(0.69–3.16)	(1.31–2.34)	(1.90–3.67)
		Chemical Leaks		
Not exposed	1.00	1.00	1.00	1.00
Exposed, but no leaks found at site	1.08*	1.35*	1.08	1.22*
	(1.02–1.15)	(1.06–1.72)	(0.98–1.20)	(1.06–1.40)
Exposed, and leaks found at site	1.17**	1.16	1.16*	1.38**
	(1.08–1.27)	(0.87–1.55)	(1.03–1.31)	(1.17–1.62)

*$p < 0.05$; ** $p < 0.01$.
†Adjusted for maternal age, race, education, complications during pregnancy, parity, population density for county of residence, and sex of the child, by logistic regression.
‡ICD-9, *International Classification of Diseases*, 9th revision.
§Numbers in parentheses, 95% confidence interval.

TABLE V.4 Odds Ratios for Congenital Malformations for All Infants with Specific Malformation Codes† and Residential Proximity to Selected Toxic Waste Sites Containing Associated Chemical Groups: New York State, 1983–1984

Chemical and Associated Malformation (Reference)	*OR‡§*	*CI‡§*
Pesticides/oral clefts (13–15)	1.27	0.84–1.92
Pesticides/musculoskeletal system (16, 17)	1.20*	1.05–1.38
Metals/nervous system (18–20)	1.34*	1.07–1.67
Solvents/nervous system (21–23)	1.24*	1.01–1.54
Solvents/digestive system (24, 25)	0.91	0.73–1.13
Plastics/chromosomal anomalies (26–29)	1.46*	1.01–2.11

* $p < 0.05$.
† Previously related to chemical exposures in the literature.
‡ ICD-9, *International Classification of Diseases,* 9th revision; OR = odds ratio; CI = confidence interval.
§ Adjusted for maternal age, race, education, complications during pregnancy, parity, population density for county of residence, and sex of the child, by logistic regression.

4. From Table V.3, which body systems were at the most risk of exposure to chemical leaks? What is the significance of such determination?
5. From Table V.4, which three combinations of "chemicals associated with congenital malformation" were the highest? Which chemicals were linked to and associated with malformations according to the odds ratio? Explain the assessment and the meaning of Table V.4.

6. From the three tables and the final assessments, what are the findings of this study with regards to exposure and proximity to hazardous waste sites and congenital malformation? Explain your answer.
7. Pick one form of congenital malformation, develop and construct a web of causation for the disorder, including appropriate decision trees.
8. What prevention and control programs can be implemented to reduce congenital malformations from environmental exposure?

CASE STUDY

VI

History and Epidemiology of Polio Epidemics

Infantile paralysis, as it was first known, was a most difficult disease to understand. For centuries, people became crippled and no one seemed to know why, for the paralysis was not associated with a disease. It was observed that mostly young people were paralyzed, and often the legs or back and also the arms were affected. Historically, this crippling disease was called infantile paralysis or anterior infantile and a variety of other names. The term "infantile paralysis" became popular because this disease was thought to be confined to children, although it had been observed in almost all ages.

Infantile paralysis was studied by physicians/epidemiologists, and the disease was eventually called poliomyelitis. The real breakthrough came when the infection was finally discovered to be a biphasic disease. The first phase of the disease has symptoms that are similar to those of the flu or a bad cold. It was the second phase in which the crippling occurs, as the virus moves from the blood into the central nervous system (CNS), where nerve cells in the spinal cord and/or brain are destroyed and replaced with fatty deposits. The devastating result is the irreversible loss of control of the lungs, limbs, or other musculoskeletal structures. Atrophy of muscles is caused by loss of neuromotor control of the affected muscles. The sensory nerves are mostly unaffected, and feelings remained. The part of the spinal cord affected by the virus is the anterior horn of the gray matter of the spinal cord.

When the two levels of the disease were finally discovered, the door was opened for more effective epidemiologic investigations. The disease, when running its course, did not always progress into the second phase in all people, and those fortunate enough to experience only the first phase usually escaped paralysis.

The virus, when finally discovered, was thought to be harbored only in the upper respiratory tract, but was later found throughout the body, with its highest concentrations in the gastrointestinal tract.

The Salk killed virus vaccine, injected intramuscularly, has a moderate level of effectiveness. Sabin developed a more effective vaccine in the form of a weakened live vaccine taken orally in sugar cubes, thus targeting the higher concentration of the virus in the gastrointestinal tract with the Sabin vaccine being the more effective of the two. From the use of these vaccines, millions of people have escaped the crippling paralysis caused by the poliovirus.

A. BRIEF REVIEW OF POLIOMYELITIS AS IT IS KNOWN TODAY

The virus responsible for polio is very small compared with many other viruses, such as the smallpox and chickenpox viruses. The poliovirus falls in the Enterovirus class of the Picornavirus group. It exists in three immunological virus types: Type I is the most likely to cause paralysis and lead to identifiable epidemics due to the observed paralysis. The infection is highly contagious and is spread via fecal–oral and pharyngeal–oropharyngeal (mouth–throat) routes.

The main source of spread is from the lesser types, labeled as inapparent infections, which occur widely in unimmunized populations. The risk of direct person-to-person transmission comes from the fact that inapparent cases are mistaken for colds or influenza. The apparent/overt (easily seen) outbreak is rare except during epidemics, and even then the ratio of inapparent infections to clinical cases exceeds 100:1. Epidemics are most likely to occur when basic public health measures such as hand washing are neglected, when food sanitation is poor, and through interpersonal transmission by those who think the infection is only the flu. Where sanitation and hygiene are poor, virus circulation can be extensive. When the infection and immunity are acquired in the first few years of life, cases are sporadic and confined largely to children less than 5 years old, and epidemics do not occur. Polio is a seasonal disease occurring in the summer and fall in temperate climates. Tropical climates and underdeveloped countries experience epidemics year round. Unvaccinated populations are at high risk of epidemics.[1]

The virus multiplies in the pharynx and intestinal tract and is present in the blood, throat, and feces during the incubation period. After onset, it can be recovered from the throat for about 1 to 2 weeks and from the feces for 3 to 6 weeks or longer. CNS involvement lasts several days, disappearing as antibodies develop. Factors predisposing patients to serious neurologic involvement include increasing age, recent inoculations (recent DTP is commonly found connected to the onset of poliomyelitis), recent tonsillectomy, pregnancy, and physical exertion concurrent with onset of the CNS phase. In older cases, the first phase might not be accounted for, or the minor illness might go unobserved.[1]

Rotary International has been working toward a goal of eradicating poliomyelitis from the earth by eventually vaccinating every person in all countries, especially underdeveloped countries. There is also much effort being put forth to eliminate the polio vaccination activities in the United States, much as was done with smallpox. The eventuality is that all people are to be protected by vaccination, and the source of the pathogen will be eliminated. Some segments of the public health community are warning that to halt polio immunizations is a bad move and have issued similar warnings about smallpox vaccinations being stopped. In regard to smallpox, the world now has a massive population of susceptibles who could become infected with smallpox—all of those born after 1978. Much media attention has been focused on the few rare cases of children acquiring polio from the immunization process. However, the media fails to point out the millions of persons who could be crippled today from paralytic polio if it were not for the polio vaccine.

Case Study Questions

A.1 Identify the pathogenic agent and the group to which infantile paralysis belongs.

A.2 Identify the locations in the body where this pathogen is harbored.

A.3 Identify the current accepted mode of disease transmission and related epidemiologic implications.

B. FIRST POLIO EPIDEMICS STUDIES AND REPORTED SWEDEN

Some early observations of Dr. Ivar Wickman in several cities in Sweden (Umea, Goteborg, Stockholm, and Tingsryd [population 3,000, 200 miles southwest of Stockholm] in the summer of 1905) follow.

A minor case of the illness, with its outward symptoms (as opposed to the inward progress of the disease as it occurs when it has moved into the CNS) is what Swedish epidemiologist Ivar Wickman observed in the early part of the 20th century. These observations were crucial to detecting and understanding the total picture and scope of the disease and its two-phase process.[2]

Names of Polio

Wickman referred to this child-crippling disease as Heine-Medin Disease in 1907. Jacob Von Heine (1799–1878) was a German orthopedist and Wickman's teacher. Oskar Medin (1847–1927) was a Swedish pediatrician. Wickman named polio after Heine and Medin because they had both conducted the earliest adequate study of the disease.[2]

Other names of polio included "debility of the lower extremities," a term used in the late 1700s; "morning paralysis," used in the mid 1800s, and "Heine-Medin Disease," used in the late 1800s and early 1900s. Most commonly used in the early 1900s, it was called "infantile paralysis." "Anterior poliomyelites" is a term later derived from the work of Dr. John Shaw. With the discovery of the virus, it was called "poliomyelites" and shortened to "polio."[2–5]

The mid 1800s through the early 1900s was an amazing era for advances in microbiology, epidemiology, medicine, and science, all of which in some way contributed to the understanding of polio and the discovery of the poliovirus.[2] Wickman and Medin believed that Bergenholtz deserved credit for observing the first polio epidemic, a minor outbreak of 13 cases in the small village of Umea in northern Sweden in 1881.[2–5]

Age Issues: Not Just a Child's Disease

As early as 1858, Q. Vogt described the first case of poliomyelitis in an adult (Switzerland). Polio was previously thought to occur only in children. In the 1905 epidemic, it was reported by Wickman that 45% of those stricken with the disease were over the age of 10 years, and 21% were over the age of 15 years. Wickman observed that poliomyelitis was not limited to children and that, as epidemics recurred, they included older age groups. The concept of the disease as "infantile paralysis" became obscured.[2]

In 1884, the first accurate account of the encephalitic form or cerebral type of polio was documented by Adolf von Strümpell in Vienna. He suggested that the causative agent could be localized in the brain and the spinal cord.[2]

Epidemiologists struggled for the longest time trying to understand the disease and identify true outbreaks, as the disease goes through a two-phase process before getting to the paralytic phase. At first, only the paralytic phase was clearly recognized and identified as infantile paralysis because the first phase was so easily confused with other diseases such as the flu, common colds, and related conditions. This was the case with an outbreak of polio in Oslo, Norway, which was thought to be spinal meningitis. Epidemics of influenza have also been confused with the first phase of poliomyelitis because the symptoms are quite similar. Such a mistaken occurrence took place in Los Angeles in the mid-1930s, causing a panic among health care professionals. Mild cases of the disease that did not reach the paralytic stage were thought to constitute 5% to 25% of all cases.[2]

Disease investigators of the day were a frustrated lot because of the lack of clear understanding and diagnosis of the disease. Numerous field workers, such as nurses, who were hired to trudge through communities during polio outbreaks in an attempt to trace relationships between multiple paralytic cases often found only dead ends. Countless case questionnaires and forms were completed with the assistance of families in an effort to trace the disease and its transmission. The data from these questionnaires were analyzed in order to trace the spread of the disease.[2–5]

Even though clustering of polio cases was observed in rural communities in Norway and France, it was Sweden's epidemiologists/physicians who further connected polio outbreaks to ruralness and who provided the most advances in poliomyelitis in the years 1890 to 1914.[2]

Karl Oskar Medin Many of the advances in knowledge of polio are attributed to Karl Oskar Medin. Medin is given a great deal of credit for detecting and assembling a comprehensive set of clinical features of the disease—the best effort done to this point in history. The greatest recognition of his work came when he, as a reliable, articulate, and experienced pediatrician, presented his observations to the 10th International Medical Congress in Berlin in 1890. Medin was also concerned about community care (public health aspects) of children. He was chairman of the Stockholm Board of Health from 1906 to 1915. He was also known for his role as an excellent teacher and had many pupils.[2]

Medin was born in 1847 in a small town near Stockholm and attended college at Uppsala, obtaining his medical licentiate at Stockholm in 1875. He was a prominent pediatrician in Sweden, a professor of pediatrics at the Karolinska Institute, and head physician at the General Orphan Sylum in Stockholm, giving him 30 years' experience in pediatric medicine in an all-child setting. Medin clarified the picture of poliomyelitis but gained for Sweden the unfortunate reputation of being the country where the worst outbreaks had occurred at the time.[2]

In 1887, Medin investigated an outbreak of 44 cases. Before that, he had stated that the cases of polio showing up at Polyclinic Hospital in Stockholm were infrequent. Attending to such an epidemic gave Medin considerable experience in dealing with polio in a great number of children.[2]

Medin divided the cases into two groups: (1) the spinal type that consisted of 27 cases of the paralytic type and (2) those with less common signs based on unusual location of the lesions. Medin was able to establish clearly the clinical course of the disease. The site of the pathological lesion had been previously established as being in the spinal cord, but it was Medin who established that there is first a phase that affects the body's total systems and then later a paralytic phase. He established that early minor symptoms and signs, such as fever, headache, and malaise, were symptoms of the early phase and later could (or may not) be followed by serious damage to the CNS. In certain areas of the spinal cord, the lesions could cause paralysis of various muscle groups or organs when the motor neurons were destroyed. Any disease involvement with the CNS always led to complications and some form of paralysis, even if it was minor. Medin followed the patients in the outbreak closely, making astute observations, documenting the early features of the disease, and observing that the disease subsided for a brief interim afebrile period, thus giving the course of the disease a biphasic pattern, with a major bout of fever experienced in both the first and last acute phases of the illness. The minor illness and its accompanying symptoms represented the first phase, and the second phase was more complicated and serious, resulting in paralysis to some parts of the body (see Figure 5.18). These observations were followed and advanced by Kling and his colleagues, including Ivar Wickman.[2]

Why the Scandinavian region experienced the first wave of the extensive polio epidemic is not clear. The epidemic of 1905 was the worst, with over 1,000 cases. It is known that polio seems to occur in rural areas as much as, if not more than, in large cities, and Scandinavia was quite rural at the time. Less exposure to a disease led to the population's having less immunity to the disease. There seemed to be higher immunity in city dwellers and lower immunity in rural populations.[2]

Ivar Wickman Ivar Wickman, Medin's pupil, was thoroughly educated about poliomyelitis by his mentor. Wickman experienced two epidemics while working at the Medical Clinic in Stockholm—one in Stockholm and the other in Goteborg in 1903. Wickman was born in Lund in the southern tip of Sweden in 1872. He studied in Lund and Stockholm and, later in his career, on the European continent. He passed the medical board exams in 1895, at which time he became Medin's assistant in the Stockholm Pediatric Clinic. He wrote a 300-page monograph on polio in 1905, making him one of the leading experts in the field. Wickman, a man with well-known publications and advanced training, including the advanced medical degree of "Doctor of Medicine," applied for the directorship of the now-prestigious Stockholm Pediatric Clinic, feeling sure that he would be accepted for the position. He was not and consequently committed suicide in 1914 at the age of 42.[2]

Epidemiologic Questions

Among the clinical pathological observations made by Wickman was concern with how the agent (of which he was not sure) traveled through the community and how it entered the human host. How did it spread throughout the body, and how was it eliminated? Did it travel within the body along the nerves, in the lymph, or in the blood? From the 1905 epidemic of 1,031 cases, he wanted to know what the nature of the disease was. Was it actually contagious? How did it spread? Was it spread by direct contact with infected sick people? Did healthy people carry the agent? Was it waterborne? Foodborne? Was it spread like typhoid? (We now know the answer is yes—both are feces borne.)[2]

Key Epidemiologic Points

The number of cases was no doubt increased by Wickman's inclusion of cases of both the paralytic type and the abortive/nonparalytic type. Whether to include nonparalytic cases was always a subject of debate among epidemiologists and statisticians. Wickman's astute observation that the nonparalytic cases were as important to the transmission of the disease, if not more so than the paralytic cases, was a major epidemiologic contribution. The abortive type, or nonparalytic cases, and paralytic cases are two ends of a continuum. Nonparalytic or abortive cases were lucky and escaped having a serious outcome from such a crippling disease, with no more than what might seem to be a bad case of the common cold. (The course of the disease ends, either because of a high immune response by the body or because the person gets only a mild dose of the pathogen and/or a mild case of the disease, develops immunity, and is therefore no longer susceptible.) Paralytic cases might die, but most often they were crippled and devastated for life. These advanced cases suffered major or minor deformation of limbs, a total loss of use of limbs, or confinement to an iron lung for the rest of their lives.

Mild cases (abortive/nonparalytic cases) were found to be just as contagious as paralytic cases and could not be ignored. A relationship between main roads and railway routes and the spread of the epidemic of 1905 was established. An association with disease spread was developed based on busy traffic centers, which allowed frequent communication between rural and urban dwellers. Wickman followed many rural outbreaks, pursuing epidemiologic investigations with tireless energy.[2]

It was observed by W. Wernstedt in the 1911 epidemic that, if an outbreak visited a certain locale, in the next few years that area would be spared an epidemic. Wernstedt observed and reported that the areas hardest hit by the 1905 and 1908 epidemics had little activity during the major epidemic of 1911. He attributed this to a natural immunization process caused by past outbreaks. He also observed a reduced incidence of the disease in the following years because of this general natural immunization. Wernstedt is given credit for his observation about acquired immunity to the disease from unapparent infections.[2]

The abortive and nonparalytic cases were of major concern to public health officials and epidemiologists because of their ability to spread the disease and continue to transmit it. The paralytic phase confined a person to bed so that the person was no longer out and about spreading the disease. To the family and more so to the individual, the paralytic form of the disease was of major concern as it changed the lives and structure of families and in many cases ruined lives. Even though to Wickman both forms were equally infectious, the focus of the medical community seemed to be limited to the paralytic form of the disease. Attack rates of paralytic polio in rural areas were about 3.0 to 3.7 per 1,000. Wickman established not only that polio was a disease of the CNS but also that the disease was highly contagious, spread mainly through its subclinical infectious state, and biphasic in its course. All clinical studies done later in monkeys verified not only the clinical but also the public health and epidemiologic observations of Wickman.

In 1911, Kling and his team of virologists proved Wickman's observations to be correct; that is, that the mild or inapparent cases of the infection were indeed very contagious and thus of great concern in the spread of the disease. Kling and his colleagues, by isolating the pathogen in the mucous membranes, were able to show that the agent propagated itself in the mucous membranes and then penetrated them to cause the infection. The infection was spread by both the oral route and the feces route, with the feces/gastrointestinal route being more significant. Kling's virology studies confirmed the two phases of the disease and that the abortive stage was as contagious as the paralytic phase. They also demonstrated that healthy carriers do exist during an epidemic. Studies showed that the virus persists in the throat for about 2 weeks in most cases but that it could be there for as long as 180 days (6 months) and 200 days (7 months). The pathogen's ability to produce inflammation was reduced after the 14-day period, showing that the virus weakens after its acute stage.[2]

Rural Observations

Many investigations observed that rural areas often had more serious epidemics than urban areas. In Sweden, there was a tendency for polio to attack rural areas, especially remote villages in Sweden's sparsely settled countryside. Wickman was able to trace the movements of people during the epidemic. Ruralness seemed to contribute to the disease, due to the fact that lack of travel, remoteness of villages, and infrequent contact with outside people did not allow even a mild form of the disease to be experienced by rural folk, which would have produced immunity. Thus, outbreaks occurred often in rural areas, with the inevitable result of crippled children, partly due to a lack of immunity in infants and youth.[2]

Epidemic Curve

Wickman developed an epidemic curve of the cases. The epidemic curve for this Swedish outbreak was much like other disease outbreaks, a significant epidemiologic point. For epidemic curves to occur, a population of susceptibles must be available, as well as a disease that has an identifiable course and time duration. The disease enters the population with a few cases, and as the pathogen is transmitted through the population, more and more cases occur (see Herd Immunity in Chapter 3, Figures 3.5 and 3.6). Depending on the disease's incubation period and the usual course and duration of a case of the disease, the shorter the incubation and duration, the more pronounced the epidemic curve. What allows an epidemic to continue is the number of susceptibles in the population at risk. In a totally susceptible population, like that in the late 1800s and early 1900s in Sweden, the disease spreads like wildfire, and the epidemic curve is extreme and pronounced. What causes the epidemic to subside and diminish is the number of susceptibles left. Who is left to get the disease? The epidemic curve diminishes when susceptibles have become diseased or have died. The diseased recover and are now immune, or the still-healthy have fled and can no longer be exposed. The epidemic curve diminishes because of the recovery/immunity of the previously ill or the death of the diseased cases. Immunization/vaccination and mild cases of the disease reduce the susceptibles and stop an epidemic by herd immunity. Numbers of nonparalytic cases compared with paralytic cases vary from epidemic to epidemic. The ratio of paralytic to nonparalytic varies because of the circumstances of the outbreaks.[2]

Not only did Wickman recognize that the pathogens often missed the CNS, but he realized that the abortive/nonparalytic cases actually outnumbered the paralytic cases. He learned quickly that paralysis was the dramatic side of the disease, but that if the infected cases were lucky enough to escape paralysis, they were no less contagious. Wickman observed that, in one village in the middle of the epidemic, more than half were of the nonparalytic type. He observed that the infection was spread mostly by the nonparalytic cases.[2]

Observed symptoms in nonparalytic types could be stiff neck, pain, stiffness in the back, or merely a fever. Wickman's colleagues viewed a diagnosis of infantile paralysis in the absence of paralysis as ridiculous. The skepticism would remain for many years to come.[2]

Wickman demanded that poliomyelitis be considered a highly contagious disease. Mild cases (abortive/nonparalytic cases) must also be taken seriously and considered just as contagious as paralytic cases because of their infectious nature. Wickman was as concerned with slightly ill cases and healthy carriers or inapparent cases as he was with full-blown paralytic cases. Clinical and laboratory evidence eventually proved this epidemiologic observation to be true.[2]

In the summer of 1905, Wickman investigated an outbreak in a school near Tingsryd, a village of 3,000, with 18 cases occurring between August and October. The school was the primary site from which the infection spread. Twelve of the 18 attended the school, and the other 6 lived at the school. Six children from only four houses, who had no contact with any of the other 52 attending the school, also came down with the disease, considering both abortive and paralytic cases.[2]

Wickman held that the incubation period was 3 to 4 days to onset of the minor illness phase, with the time period to onset of fever in the paralytic phase being 8 to 10 days. Later, when studies were done with the live attenuated poliovirus vaccine, it was demonstrated that the incubation period to first onset was 3 to 4 days.[2]

Poliovirus Discovered

The poliovirus was discovered in 1908 in Vienna by Karl Landsteiner and E. Popper. In 1911, one of the worst polio epidemics (3,840 cases) of all time hit Sweden. Scandinavia was labeled as the source and breeding ground of the polio disease because much of the reported research occurred there; the 1911 epidemic further emphasized this negative image.[2]

The Swedish medical community, particularly the clinical virologists, tried their best to understand and study the new findings about polio, especially because they now knew the agent was a poliovirus. In the 1911 epidemic, this presented an opportunity for a team from the State Bacteriological Institute in Stockholm to study the clinical and virological aspects of polio. The team was headed by Carl Kling.[2]

Carl Kling went to the Pasteur Institute after the 1911 epidemic subsided and became known as the world's leading authority on poliomyelitis. He was associated with the Pasteur Institute for 25 years and in 1919 was made director of the State Bacteriological Institute in Stockholm. He also made radio broadcasts about polio. He claimed that poliomyelitis was waterborne. He never married and died in 1967 at the age of 80 years, after 50 years of work on poliomyelitis.[2]

Kling and his team obtained tissue samples from victims who had died. Most importantly, they were able to recover poliovirus samples from various anatomical sites throughout the body, showing that the disease invaded more than just the CNS. The team also recovered samples of the poliovirus from living patients, proving that the abortive phase of the disease was just as communicable as the paralytic phase. They also were able to acquire samples of the virus in "healthy carriers."[2]

Kling and his colleagues knew the virus was a filterable virus and therefore could be separated from other material and used experimentally. They also knew that the virus caused lesions in the spinal cord and brain of monkeys and humans. The virus had been shown to be in the mucous membranes of the throat and nasal passages of monkeys as well as lymph nodes next to the small intestine (mesenteric lymph nodes). The agent was also found in the tonsils, pharyngeal mucous membranes, salivary glands of humans and monkeys, oropharynx, trachea, and, especially important, in the blood and the walls and contents of the small intestine. Fourteen fatal human cases of polio confirmed all of the sites. Then 11 acutely ill patients provided specimens, and the poliovirus was recovered from basically all the same body sites in the live acute cases of the disease. Thus, monkey experiments, fatal/dead cases, and live acute cases all produced basically the same findings—that is, the pathogen was found in all the same sites throughout the body.[2]

Doubts by American researchers, physicians, and scientists and some Europeans concerning the presence of the pathogen in the gastrointestinal tract and rectum, as well as doubts concerning the virus's weakening over time, caused delays and setbacks in developing a vaccine well into the 1930s.[2]

Case Study Questions

B.1 Using the data below and a computer spreadsheet, create an epidemic curve bar graph.

Person/Disease: Cases of poliomyelitis recorded in Sweden

Place: Sweden

Time: Monthly reporting for the years of 1905, 1906, 1907; from January 1905 through July 1907

Frequency: For the y-axis of the graph: 50-case increments up to 400 cases

1905 Cases		*1906 Cases*		*1907 Cases*	
Jan. =	1	Jan. =	48	Jan. =	9
Feb. =	5	Feb. =	33	Feb. =	9
Mar. =	4	Mar. =	36	Mar. =	11
Apr. =	4	Apr. =	24	Apr. =	6
May =	8	May =	41	May =	5
Jun. =	20	Jun. =	15	Jun. =	13
Jul. =	138	Jul. =	21	Jul. =	51
Aug. =	367	Aug. =	32		
Sept. =	242	Sept. =	49		
Oct. =	140	Oct. =	22		
Nov. =	69	Nov. =	31		
Dec. =	38	Dec. =	24		

B.2 From the epidemic curve created in Study Question B.1, what have you learned from this case thus far? Discuss the implications and observations of all time aspects of this disease. Discuss seasonal variation, cyclic trends, implication for duration of the disease, and incubation periods.

B.3 List the various names by which polio has been known.

B.4 Discuss and explain the issues of age and its implications for the epidemiology of polio and infantile paralysis.

B.5 Why did physicians and epidemiologists have such a difficult time identifying outbreaks and the spread of polio? Explain and discuss in detail.

B.6 From your reading and study thus far and from studying Figure 5.8, explain and discuss polio as a biphasic (two-phase) disease and the problems this two-phase process posed in investigating polio epidemics.

B.7 List the many epidemiologic observations made by Wickman about infantile paralysis and its spread. Who later confirmed these observations, and how did he verify them?

B.8 What were the epidemiologist observations of Wernstedt?

B.9 Explain and discuss the terms "abortive case" and "anterior case." What are other terms used for each of these two terms? Explain the role of these two terms in polio epidemics. What observations did Kling make about the abortive cases or phase?

B.10 When was the poliovirus discovered? Explain its characteristics and the locations in the body where it was originally discovered.

C. FIRST MAJOR EPIDEMIC OF POLIOMYELITIS IN AMERICA: RUTLAND, VERMONT

It was in the summer of 1894 in Vermont that the first major United States poliomyelitis epidemic occurred. Charles S. Caverly, MD, a practicing doctor, member of the state board of health, and public health officer for the state of Vermont, presented a report on the epidemic. Caverly, though a very successful practicing physician, was excited about public health and epidemiology. He came from a rural area of a rural state, born in Troy, New Hampshire, in 1856. He attended New Hampshire schools and Dartmouth College, graduating in 1878. He received his medical degree from the University of Vermont in 1881. He also did postgraduate work at the College of Physicians and Surgeons in New York City and was professor of hygiene and preventive medicine at the University of Vermont, from which he later received an honorary ScD degree.

Caverly reported that in Rutland County there was an outbreak of an acute nervous disease that invariably was attended with some paralysis. The first cases occurred in Rutland and Wallingford about mid-June. The epidemic progressed through July into surrounding towns.

This first US epidemic was the largest reported in the world thus far, with 132 documented cases. Six of the cases had no paralysis, but all had distinct nervous symptoms. Caverly was one of the first to recognize the abortive nonparalytic cases, even though he probably overlooked hundreds of them. This epidemic was also the first to be studied by a public health officer. From the advantage of his political position, Caverly was able to call meetings and coordinate the exchange of information.

Caverly was most diligent in his effort to identify each case. The previous summer, a small epidemic had occurred 125 miles away in Boston, making the outbreak in some nearby cities somewhat predictable. Public health officials have observed that poliomyelitis epidemics usually terminate when cold weather sets in and show up again in a neighboring city the next summer, much as they did in Scandinavia. (This makes epidemiologic sense, as the new city is where susceptibles are now available. Those in the city of the recent outbreak had naturally acquired immunity yet interacted on a close personal basis for the disease to be communicated.) Caverly was able to show that the age distribution was much greater than previously reported. (Dr. Mary Jacobi in 1886 had suggested that infantile paralysis was limited to children 18 months to 4 years of age.) Caverly reported cases (probably only paralytic cases) of 20 in the 9- to 12-year age range and 12 cases over the age of 15 years. The shift in age to include older age groups, including adults (Franklin D. Roosevelt, the 32nd president of the United States, who served from 1933 to 1945, contracted poliomyelitis at the age of 39), was observed more frequently from this point on. Adults were not excluded from the Rutland epidemic, even though most cases occurred in children. Caverly attempted to classify cases according to sites of paralysis. The death rate from this epidemic was quite high at 13.5%. This figure held with later observations that the older the patient who contracted poliomyelitis, the greater the death rate. Caverly reported a curious observation—that the paralytic disease also affected domestic animals, with horses, dogs, and fowl dying with various types and degrees of paralysis. Dr. Charles Dana, professor of nervous diseases at Cornell University Medical College, verified that one of the fowls with paralysis of its legs had an acute poliomyelitis of the lower portion of the spinal cord, yet Landsteiner in Vienna and Flexner could not produce cases of poliomyelitis in lower animals. Finally, they turned to primates to produce experimental polio, yet this paralytic disease has been reported throughout this era as occurring in domestic animals.

Caverly made some gross mistakes beyond the animal paralysis issue. He suggested that infantile paralysis was not contagious. He seemed to try to define the disease by the old Hippocratic theory of medicine—because heating is mentioned in 24 cases and chilling of the body in only 4 cases, he determined that there was a general absence of infectious disease as a causative factor in the epidemic.

Despite his errors, Caverly made major contributions for his time; he was the first health officer and physician to do a major systematic study of an infantile paralysis epidemic, and he was the first to recognize and confirm the occurrence of nonparalytic cases.

Case Study Questions

C.1 What unique epidemiologic observations and contributions about the epidemic of infantile paralysis were made by Dr. Caverly from his experience in rural Vermont?

C.2 What epidemiologic observations did Dr. Caverly make regarding age of infantile paralysis victims and polio epidemics?

C.3 What were some critical thinking and observational errors regarding epidemiology that were made by Dr. Caverly?

D. SIMON FLEXNER, MD, AND WADE HAMILTON FROST, MD: AMERICAN EPIDEMIOLOGISTS WHO INVESTIGATED POLIOMYELITIS

Flexner

When the news of Landsteiner's discovery of the poliovirus reached the United States, Simon Flexner, MD, the new director of the Rockefeller Institute of Medical Research in New York City, took advantage of the opportunity the new discovery presented. The Rockefeller Institute was well funded, had just had much success in an attack on meningococcal meningitis, and had a well-equipped institute including facilities to handle primates, which was supported by a staff of qualified researchers.

New York had recently suffered through a poliomyelitis epidemic of about 750 to 1,200 cases in 1907. Flexner was appointed as one of 12 members of a committee appointed by the New York Neurological Society to study the polio epidemic. A report was finally produced by the committee in 1910, which included the findings of Landsteiner. Flexner also described in his work, supported by Dr. Martha Wollstein, that they had obtained samples of the pathogen from two fatal cases, one in New Jersey and one in New York in 1909. They inoculated monkeys and were able to pass the 2 strains from monkey to monkey in serial fashion. Most of their work was on monkeys, yet they claimed that what occurred in primates was also true for humans, a statement the medical community questioned. Flexner himself noted that in different species of monkeys the poliovirus behaved differently making animal model research a bit unpredictable and making it hard to develop a protocol applicable to humans.

Simon Flexner, considered a laboratory doctor and one of the foremost experts on poliomyelitis at the time, did not have the answers for many practical questions of practicing doctors: How long was a case of poliomyelitis contagious? Why is poliomyelitis contagious to some and not to others? The key question at the time was this: "How do you best treat poliomyelitis?" The fact that the disease was known to be caused by a virus provided the general practice doctor with no cure or solution to treatment. Viruses are small, difficult to see, and mysterious. Much laboratory work was done by Flexner and his colleagues at the Rockefeller Institute and published in the *Journal of the American Medical Association* from 1909 to 1913 as news updates on poliomyelitis, again establishing Flexner as the expert on the disease.

In 1910, Flexner and his colleagues in the United States and Landsteiner and his colleagues in Vienna were able to demonstrate that the serum of monkeys that had recovered from experimental poliomyelitis contained antibodies (which Flexner called germicidal substances) that, when mixed with a small amount of active poliovirus, would actually neutralize or inactive the poliovirus and render it inert. Later, A. Netter and C. Levaditi, in Paris, found the same antibodies in humans recovering from the disease. This was a landmark discovery that would benefit later vaccine research. For Flexner, this was the last major breakthrough, and his polio research started to subside, as did that of Landsteiner and his colleagues in Europe.

Stubbornly clinging to lines of thinking that are not accurate has plagued medicine from the very beginning—so it was with Flexner. He refused to accept certain clinical facts, which led him away from important discoveries, including virology as a method of clinical investigation. Flexner retired in 1935 from the Rockefeller Institute and died in 1946 before the polio vaccine was discovered and before the discovery that the poliovirus was indeed a family of viruses instead of being a single virus. Flexner was also faced with the separation at that time between practicing physicians and researchers. MDs were to practice medicine and not dabble in anything remotely resembling experimental research. During the 1911 epidemic in New York, Flexner worked at the Rockefeller Hospital instead of at the institute, rigidly clinging to the idea that physicians should practice their art at the bedside in the hospital, not in the laboratory. Thus, as a physician, he was not allowed to do testing in virology. Contention existed between the hospital medical director and Flexner because of the opposition to collaborative work among the physicians and the researchers. Meanwhile, the physicians wished to stretch their efforts beyond mundane medicine into the areas of research. The Rockefeller Hospital study, even though it included 200 cases, offered little insight beyond that provided by the Swedes.

Treatment offered by the Rockefeller groups was similar to that offered elsewhere: mild sedative, bed rest, and medication to control pain. From a public health perspective, cases should be treated like any other communicable disease—they should be made aware of their contagious conditions, be quarantined, and have disinfection carried out. In the wards with poliomyelitis cases, caps and long gowns were worn by those working with patients. Hands were thoroughly scrubbed with soap and a nail brush, and soaked in a corrosive substance.

Two physicians, Rosenau and Brues, in 1912 set forth the theory that poliomyelitis was spread by the stable fly. W. H. Frost and a colleague (J. F. Anderson) were able to show experimentally that this was untrue. Frost relied on a clinical laboratory for his work, much as Flexner did, but also traveled the countryside, much like Wickman in Sweden, going door to door investigating poliomyelitis outbreaks. He gathered serum specimens for laboratory tests, which in turn allowed statistical analysis. The use of statistics in epidemiology was greatly advanced by Frost in this era.[2]

Frost

Frost contributed much to the epidemiology of polio from 1910 to 1930. He quickly grasped the importance of knowing how polio was spread and is credited with establishing a strong foundation of statistics as a basis for epidemiologic study. He was considered one of America's leading epidemiologists in the 1920s and 1930s.

In 1908 Frost was assigned to the Hygienic Laboratory. Two years later, after investigating pellagra, tetanus, typhoid, and water pollution, he was assigned to field investigations of poliomyelitis epidemics, even though he had limited knowledge of the disease. He and J. F. Anderson, the new director of the Hygienic Laboratory, learned quickly, and their involvement with this new disease led to the composition of a 50-page monograph on poliomyelitis, which they called a précis. This document contained subject matter not included in Wickman's 300-page monograph and not covered by the Rockefeller Institute of Medical Science. Frost would eventually become dean of the School of Hygiene and Public Health at Johns Hopkins University.[2]

Frost and Anderson addressed and recorded age of the onset of cases in various epidemics in different environmental conditions. Frost, like Wickman, observed that the disease was more contagious than medical science believed at the time and was quick to point out that direct contact was probably one of the main means of disease transmission. Frost observed in the 1910 epidemic that the disease was transmissible from person to person, probably by direct contact, and appeared to be highly contagious under some circumstances, affecting a considerable proportion of the population of a limited area.[2]

For a short time, the stable fly and other biting insects were implicated as possible vectors of the poliovirus. Anderson and Frost in 1912–1913 tested the stable fly and showed that vectors were not generally involved in the disease's transmission. Frost had worked on poliomyelitis epidemics in Mason City, Iowa, in 1910; Cincinnati, Ohio, in 1911; and Buffalo and Batavia, New York, in 1912. He knew from experience and firsthand observation that vectors were not implicated in disease transmission but that direct person-to-person contact was. Frost was able to observe the disease in different environments and settings, including large cities, small towns, and rural areas. Not since Wickman in Sweden had any other epidemiologist so painstakingly completed statistical studies on epidemics. No other epidemiologist had been afforded the opportunity to make scientific observations and draw learned conclusions on the three dimensions of investigation: close clinical observation, laboratory experiments, and statistical analysis. Frost, like Wickman, had used spot maps to mark the location of the residences of paralytic, abortive, and suspicious cases.[2]

Frost's Epidemiologic Methods

Frost was able to observe increases and decreases in incidence and prevalence in rural versus city settings. He made seasonal and meteorological charts surrounding the times of epidemics. Included in his investigations were other observations of epidemics, such as sanitary conditions of individual cases, milk supply, food supply, observation of paralytic cases in humans and domestic animals, and the presence and absence of flies, mosquitoes, and other insects. His knowledge base was founded on house-to-house surveys, countless clinical observations, statistical analysis of the findings, and years of community-based experience, all confirming that poliomyelitis was spread by direct contact.[2]

Frost came to a most fundamental epidemiologic conclusion: that an accurate diagnosis must be made before an investigation can proceed. In the case of poliomyelitis, the abortive case—those without paralytic symptoms—must be identified, as they are so numerous as to be of great epidemiologic significance. Thus, Frost was able to use the laboratory to achieve a more accurate diagnosis of the poliomyelitis in all types of cases. He was able to collect serum samples from nine cases in the Iowa epidemic and with the help of Anderson analyzed them, thus proving Flexner as well as Netter and Levaditi of France incorrect in their assumptions based on monkey experiments: that the blood of victims recovered from the disease (in monkeys at least) did not contain poliovirus. Frost showed that abortive or unapparent infections of poliomyelitis did indeed contain the antibodies.

Frost and Anderson were always extremely cautious in their claims and reports, which often weakened their position and respect. They were hesitant to make any strong affirmative stance on their discoveries for fear they would not be accepted. The investigators at the hospital of the Rockefeller Institute heard of the findings on Frost's work and themselves went on to show that human sera from recovered adults did have high amounts of polio antibiotics, much as paralytic patients did.

Frost was the first to use such a combination of methods and such a sophisticated arsenal against poliomyelitis, yet he was overly cautious. He observed that during epidemics the incidence of the disease was affected by susceptibility to the infection. Age was one of the key observations about poliomyelitis, with susceptibility being limited to the first half decade of life and the risk diminishing thereafter. (Naturally acquired immunity probably accounted for this factor; either the victim had a mild case and was no longer susceptible, or had a bad case and died, or was paralyzed. After an epidemic had passed through a community, the disease was no longer contagious until a new crop of susceptibles in the form of new children came along.) Early on, the lack of understanding of the role of the abortive, mild, or inapparent cases in a population caused Frost to conclude that widespread immunization of the population against the disease was unjustifiably radical. Frost was able to share his vast experience of poliomyelitis investigation in the 1916 epidemic.

Case Study Questions

D.1 What were the epidemiologic limitations of Flexner's work on polio? List and discuss several of these limitations.

D.2 Who was Dr. Frost, and what were his contributions to epidemiologic investigations of infantile paralysis/polio?

D.3 What did Dr. Frost contribute in the way of understanding modes of disease transmission in poliomyelitis?

D.4 Which specific methods and approaches was Dr. Frost able to use and establish as solid epidemiologic methodology?

E. POLIOMYELITIS EPIDEMIC IN LOS ANGELES, 1934

By the spring of 1934, a great deal was known about poliomyelitis. The mode of transmission was known to be person to person. The two-phase process of the disease was well understood, and mild nonparalytic infections or anterior poliomyelitis as well as paralytic infections were all understood to be major means of contagion. Animals and most insects were eliminated as vectors. It was known that some victims would die in a few days. Some would have crippling paralysis, and others would recover without a sign. The poliovirus had been isolated and identified from most parts of the body—most importantly, the CNS; blood; saliva; gastrointestinal tract, especially the small intestine; mesenteric lymph nodes; and nasopharynx. The damage caused by the poliovirus was known to be done in the spinal cord's anterior horn of the gray matter and in brain tissue.[2]

When the poliomyelitis epidemic hit Los Angeles, many horror stories from past epidemics had been deeply implanted in the minds of medical and nursing professionals. It appears that the medical professionals at the time were well informed about the facts of poliomyelitis, yet most ignored them and, moreover, failed to inform the public. The Contagious Unit of the Los Angeles County General Hospital was responsible for most of the activities of the epidemic, and fear of the disease seemed to dominate its efforts, in spite of evidence that much of the sickness that occurred in June of 1934 was not poliomyelitis.[2]

Physicians and nurses were strained, worried, and terrified of contracting the disease themselves. By June 15, 50 cases a day were being admitted to most hospitals, yet by June 29, only 1 fatal case of poliomyelitis had occurred, producing a sample of the poliovirus. A second case produced another sample on July 4.[2]

When the Poliomyelitis Commission arrived in Los Angeles from Yale University School of Medicine, headed by Dr. Leslie T. Webster of the Rockefeller Institute of Medical Science of New York City, a public meeting was held to review the situation of the epidemic. The meeting digressed to physicians and nurses discussing their risk of getting poliomyelitis and whether they might receive disability pensions if paralyzed by the disease and were disabled in the line of duty.[2]

New interns in training at the Los Angeles County Hospital were deprived of teaching and proper guidance because the attending physicians were afraid of getting the disease and stayed away, consulting by phone instead of going to the hospital. Doctors who worked at the County Hospital in the communicable disease wards were not welcome on house calls because their patients viewed the hospital as a pest house.[2]

No one knew how much of the disease outbreak that year was really polio. Nearly all adults, especially the nurses and doctors, were afraid of getting paralytic polio. In those who got the serious form of the disease, health care providers observed much pain and weakness, but very few deaths occurred. The number of cases of paralysis was much lower than one would expect. The question was this: Could it be another virus or a different strain of the virus? Dr. Webster believed that 90% of the cases were actually not poliomyelitis.[2]

Researchers had little success in searching for the poliovirus in the nasal passages of suspected victims through nasal washings. The disease could not be produced in monkeys or lab animals. Webster believed that the problem was complex and that the infantile part of infantile paralysis was missing because most cases were in adults. The paralysis phase of the disease was also missing, as no paralysis occurred in most cases.[2]

Oral washings with ropy (an adhesive, stringy-type thread that was soaked in a special solution and swirled around in the throat in order to capture samples of mucous tissue) were done routinely. Ropy washes were able to gather even a few flakes of mucus and the debris in it. The ropy washes used a special solution that helped save samplings of potential poliovirus evidence and preserved the specimens for months (101 days) for later study. Even after such a long time, the specimens could be spun in a centrifuge and yield the virus; thus, in future outbreaks, disease investigators would not need to take an army of public health workers along to gather specimens.[2]

Hysteria raged on in the main populace. Not only was the general public afraid of getting the disease, but a major part of the medical and nursing profession was also participating in the fear. Yet officials were not daring enough to tell the public that the disease was not polio. It was disclosed that half of the 1,301 suspected cases were not poliomyelitis. The actual attack rate was estimated to be from 4.4% to 10.7%.[2]

There was no doubt that Los Angeles was visited by an epidemic of poliomyelitis in the summer of 1934, but it was a mild one. Most of the people who were sick that summer were sick either from another disease (encephalitis, meningitis, or influenza) or from a mild form or a different strain of the poliovirus. Patients had atypical symptoms for polio, and the observed symptoms were rheumatoidal or influenzal with striking emotional tones of fear that they might get polio. It was observed by US Public Health Service officer Dr. A. G. Gilliam, of the Los Angeles County Hospital's personnel, "Irrespective of actual mechanisms of spread and identity of the disease, this outbreak has no parallel in the history of poliomyelitis or any other CNS infections."[2]

As an unfortunate outcome of this epidemic and its resulting hysteria, patients who exhibited even a slight degree of weakness were immobilized in plaster casts. This was a common practice in the 1930s, and many were subjected unnecessarily to this treatment.

Case Study Questions

E.1 By 1934, a great deal was known about poliomyelitis. Summarize all that was known about all facets of the epidemiology of polio.

E.2 How serious was the polio epidemic of 1934? What were the social, psychological, and political implications and their effects on the epidemiology of polio surrounding this case?

E.3 What were the final conclusions about the polio epidemic of 1934 in Los Angeles, and what were the implications for the future?

EPILOGUE

Polio epidemics continued across America. The last national poliomyelitis epidemic was in the early 1950s. In 1954, Dr. Jonas E. Salk began immunizing with killed (formalin-inactivated poliomyelitis viruses) vaccine, called the poliovirus vaccine, and later Albert B. Sabin developed the live vaccine, called the oral poliovirus vaccine, usually taken orally in sugar cubes. In the late 1980s, post-polio syndrome was discovered, and investigations of this late phase of poliomyelitis have continued.

REFERENCES

1. Berkow R, ed. *The Merck Manual of Diagnosis and Therapy*. 14th ed. Rahway, NJ: Merck, Sharp and Dohme; 1982.
2. Paul JR. *A History of Poliomyelitis*. New Haven, CT: Yale University Press; 1971.
3. Millard FP. *Poliomyelitis (Infantile Paralysis)*. Kirksville, MO: Journal Printing Company; 1918.
4. Smith JS. *Patenting the Sun*. New York: William Morrow and Company; 1990.
5. Rogers N. *Dirt and Disease*. New Brunswick, NJ: Rutgers University Press; 1990.

APPENDIX

II

Answers to Select Chapter Questions

CHAPTER 1

1. Distribution refers to the relative numbers of people in each of the various categories or populations, such as in different age, sex, or occupational groups. Studying the distribution of disease may involve identifying the number of cases according to age, sex, or occupational groups. When disease occurrence is compared among groups, it is often useful to compare rates rather than counts (i.e., the number of cases divided by the corresponding population).

   Determinant refers to cause. Identifying a causal association requires first evaluating the statistical association between exposure and outcome variables. After a valid statistical association is observed, other factors must be considered (e.g., temporal sequence of events, dose–response relationship, and biologic plausibility) in making a judgment about causality.
2. As many infectious diseases have been controlled in modern times, life expectancy has increased, and noninfectious diseases and conditions have become the primary causes of death in the United States (see Table 1.2). The study of epidemiology includes communicable diseases, noncommunicable diseases, injuries, trauma, mental disorders, birth defects, maternal–child health, occupational health, environmental health, and behaviors related to health (e.g., nutrition, exercise, and seat belt use).
3. The pathogen or disease-causing agent (e.g., bacteria, viruses, worms, chemicals, or any other plant or animal substance or factor that can cause disease, disability, illness, syndrome, or death) thrives, propagates, and multiplies in a medium or habitat called a reservoir (humans, animals, or certain environmental conditions or substances). A pathogen leaves its reservoir by a mode of transmission to a susceptible host. The mode of transmission may be direct transmission (person-to-person contact) or indirect transmission (airborne droplets or dust particles, vectors, fomites, food-borne substances). The final link in the chain of infection is thus the susceptible individual or host—usually a human or an animal.
4. Refer to Table 1.1.

6. Persons aged less than 4 years and more than 80 years are the most vulnerable to falls. Persons who are more than 60 years old accounted for 44% of the total emergency calls caused by nonindustrial falls. Susceptibility to falls is related to development in young children and general health and strength.
7. Age-specific rates indicate that, regardless of socioeconomic status, the risk of falls is initially high in the age group 0 to 9 years; it then decreases, with the lowest levels in the age group 20 to 39 years, and then increases to the high risk in those more than 60 years old. Within each age group, except more than 60 years old, the risk of falls is highest in the low socioeconomic group and lowest in the high socioeconomic group. For those who are more than 60 years old, the risk of falls is highest in the high socioeconomic group and lowest in the medium socioeconomic group. Socioeconomic status likely influences the rates because of its association with general health. In contrast to risk, the burden of falls is greatest in the age group 20 to 39 years because this is where the largest proportion of the population lies. Focusing on the rates is more informative from a risk perspective, whereas focusing on the percentage of total population is more informative from a burden perspective.
9. Six of the top 15 leading causes of death are noncommunicable diseases or events. Risk factors for heart diseases, cancer, cerebrovascular diseases, chronic obstructive pulmonary diseases, and diabetes mellitus are well established. These risk factors are largely related to lifestyle behavior and can be effectively controlled through primary prevention. Primary prevention may lower the risk of most of these diseases or conditions. For example, requiring seat belt use may lower the risk of death in a motor vehicle accident. Stricter criminal penalties may lower the occurrence of homicide. Vaccination may lower the risk of influenza, and not smoking may lower the risk of many of the leading causes of death and conditions. Secondary prevention through screening may help lower the risk of death from many of these diseases and conditions by improving the chance of survival and recovery. For each of the leading causes of death, tertiary prevention can limit disability by providing rehabilitation where disease, injury, or a disorder has already occurred and has caused damage. This type of prevention may help prolong life.
10. By identifying high-risk behaviors, who in a community participates in such behaviors, where these people are located, and whether existing programs are available or need to be developed to reach these people, effective public health prevention and control efforts can be made. Dissemination of risk factor information to the public provides a basis for informed individual decision making.

CHAPTER 2

1. d, h, g, j, b, o, m, a, i, n, p, l, f, k, c, q, e
2. For example, discovery of microscopic organisms, later called microbes, bacteria, and microorganisms; advanced chemistry and histology, which influenced advances in the study and control of diseases in epidemiology.
3. John Graunt and William Farr
4. Experimental
5. Case control and cohort

CHAPTER 3

1. Infectious diseases are generally communicable. A few rare exceptions are shown in Table 3.1. Infectious communicable diseases may be acute or chronic. Noninfectious diseases and conditions are also noncommunicable. These diseases and conditions may be acute or chronic.
2. Congenital and hereditary diseases, allergies and inflammatory diseases, degenerative diseases, metabolic diseases, and cancer. Refer to the section entitled Classification of Diseases.
3. Refer to Table 3.3.
4. Microbe sources (Table 3.4), animal sources (Table 3.5), and inanimate sources (Table 3.6).
5. The time from exposure to the onset of clinical symptoms is the **incubation period**. Incubation period is typically used for infectious diseases. In the context of noncommunicable chronic diseases, the time from exposure to the onset of clinical symptoms is typically referred to as the latency period.
9. As life expectancy increases in the United States, for example, they are becoming more susceptible to diseases that typically affect people of older ages, such as cancer or heart disease. As illustrated in Table 1.2, although heart diseases explained 8% of all deaths in 1900, they explained about 30% in 2000. The percentage of all deaths attributed to cancer also increased dramatically over the century, from 4% to 23%. As life expectancy continues to increase, in part because of decreases in infectious diseases, the noninfectious diseases more common in older ages will explain an increasingly larger percentage of deaths.

CHAPTER 4

1. Nominal
2. The rates are highest in San Francisco and lowest in Atlanta for each of the racial groups. Compared with Atlanta, the rates in San Francisco are 17% higher in whites, 40% higher in blacks, and 106% higher in Asian or Pacific Islanders. Compared with Atlanta, the rates in Detroit are 9% higher in whites, 38% higher in blacks, and 12% higher in Asian or Pacific Islanders.
3. Yes. Some of the difference in rates described in question 2 may be due to differences in the age distribution among racial groups in the different areas.
4. The age-adjusted breast cancer rates are more similar among the geographic areas than the crude rates. Compared with Atlanta, the rates in San Francisco are now only 4% higher in whites, 5% higher in blacks, and 54% higher in Asian or Pacific Islanders. Compared with Atlanta, the rates in Detroit are 6% lower in whites, 10% higher in blacks, and 9% higher in Asian or Pacific Islanders.
5. Breast cancer is more common in older ages. When we adjust for differences in the age distribution, the rates become more similar. Hence, whites have an older age distribution.
6. Compared with Asian or Pacific Islanders, the age-adjusted breast cancer rates are 1.7 times higher in whites and 1.4 times higher in blacks. Hence, race is a risk factor for breast cancer.

7. Identifying differences in lifestyle and characteristics among racial groups would be useful. Some examples include parity, a history of breastfeeding, a history of certain benign breast diseases, the age at menarche, the age at menopause, exposure to ionizing radiation, obesity, first pregnancy at a late age, nodular densities on a mammogram, and socioeconomic status.

8.

	White		***Black***		***Asian or Pacific Islander***	
Age	***Cases***	***Relative Frequency***	***Cases***	***Relative Frequency***	***Cases***	***Relative Frequency***
< 50	3,861	0.2157	1,278	0.3282	463	0.3265
50–54 years	2,161	0.1207	531	0.1364	187	0.1319
55–59 years	2,205	0.1232	406	0.1043	182	0.1283
60–64 years	1,858	0.1038	396	0.1017	168	0.1185
65–69 years	1,828	0.1021	347	0.0891	127	0.0896
70+	5,991	0.3346	936	0.2404	291	0.2052
		1.0000		1.0000		1.0000

The largest percentage of cases is in the more than 70-year-old group for whites but in the less than 50-year-old group for black and Asian or Pacific Islanders. This may be because white women have an older life expectancy such that they are more likely to live to age 70 and older.

9.

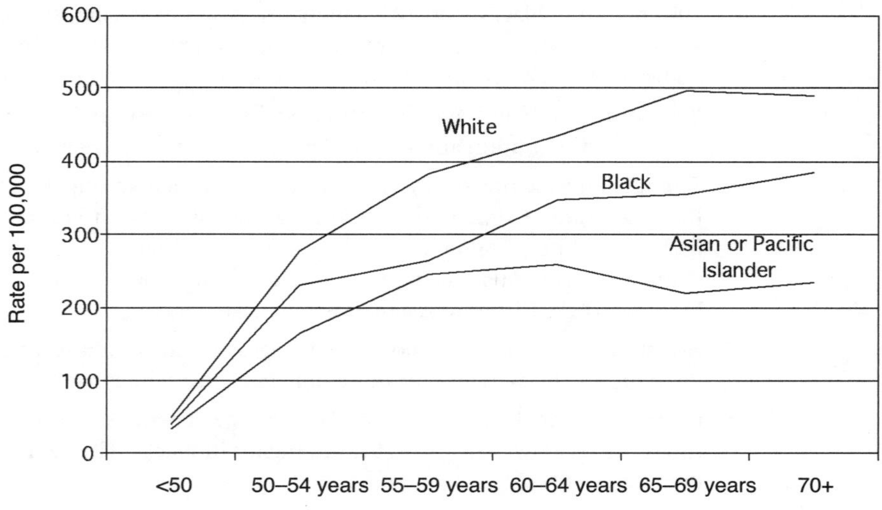

10. 95% CI: 159.1–163.9 for whites, 93.3–99.3 for blacks, and 76.5–84.9 for Asian or Pacific Islanders.
11. The crude rate for whites aged 50 to 69 years is 374.2 per 100,000. The age-adjusted rates (per 100,000) for blacks and Asian or Pacific Islanders, using the white population as the reference, are 284.3 and 215.1, respectively.
12. The *SMR* is 0.76 for blacks and 0.57 for Asians or Pacific Islanders.
13. Whites have an older age distribution than the other two groups; for example, the percentage of the population less than 50 years old is 70% for whites, 79% for blacks, and 75% for Asian or Pacific Islanders. On the other hand, the percentage of the population at least 70 years of age is 11% for whites, 6% for blacks, and 7% for Asian or Pacific Islanders.
16. Disease A has better survival (lower mortality).
17. Attack rate. The numerator is the number of people who become ill; the denominator is the population at risk at the start of the interval. The rate base is 100.
18. $70/390 \times 100 = 17.9$
19. The age distribution is skewed to the left; that is, there are some young outliers, but the participants tend to be older.
20. Nine percent of the variation in pulse (per minute) is explained by exercise (in hours per week).
21. For every additional hour in exercise per week, the pulse goes down an average of 0.05 per minute. This only applies within the range of our data; that is, if hours exercised ranged from 0 to 20 hours per week, it would not be appropriate to extrapolate this result to exercising say 25 or 30 hours per week.
22. Perform the analysis in stratified age groups or simply add age to a multiple regression model or a multiple logistic regression model.
23. 10,000 per 100,000 person-years. 95% CI: 8,614–11,386.

CHAPTER 5

1. For example, diseases of the heart are 1.5 times higher in men. Estrogen in women has been shown to be protective against heart disease. Differences between sexes may also be influenced by differences in risk factors such as smoking, blood cholesterol, blood pressure, and physical activity.
2. For example, HIV/AIDS age-adjusted death rates are noticeably lower in non-Hispanics. Differences between ethnic groups are likely explained by differences in risk factors such as unprotected sex, injection drug use, homosexual behavior, having other sexually transmitted diseases, and mother–infant transmission.
3. Afghanistan is 89.0; the United States is 49.2.
4. The following web site may be useful for constructing the age pyramid plots: http://www.uvm.edu/~agri99/spring2004/Population_Pyramids_in_Excel.html
5. Uterine cervix and corpus mortality decreases over calendar years. Early detection through PAP smear screening likely explains much of this decrease. Breast cancer mortality rates

fell between 1990 and 2001. Early detection through mammography screening and breast-self exams and improvements in treatment likely explains the observed rates.

6. There is a 20- to 25-year latency period.

CHAPTER 6

1. No. The crude death rate considers the number of deaths relative to the population and expresses this rate per 100,000.
2. a. 903 per 100,000
   b. 152 per 100,000
   c. 27 per 1,000
   d. 1 per 1,000
   e. 20 per 1,000
   f. 83 per 1,000
   g. 1,927 per 100,000
   h. 83 per 100,000
   i. 35 per 100,000
   j. 5.2%
3. Desert City is 8%; Sun City is 5%.
6. All causes are 818 per 100,000. All malignant cancers are 182 per 100,000. Accidents are 48 per 100,000. Suicide is 9 per 100,000. Homicide is 39 per 100,000.
7. All causes are 1,603,630. All malignant cancers are 153,470. Accidents are 219,283. Suicide is 45,665. Homicide is 244,305.
8. Accidents are occurring much more frequently than cancer in the younger ages and, therefore, produce a higher number of YPLL.
9. All causes are 9,540 per 100,000. All malignant cancers are 913 per 100,000. Accidents are 1,304 per 100,000. Suicide is 272 per 100,000. Homicide is 1,453 per 100,000.
10. Yes. The rates allow us to make meaningful comparisons because the size of the population is taken into account.

CHAPTER 7

1. Establish the diagnostic criteria and definition of disease, select cases, and controls, and ascertain exposure status while controlling for bias.
2. Selection bias (e.g., prevalence–incidence bias and Berkson's bias) and observation bias (recall and interviewer bias).
3. At the design level, selection bias can be minimized by considering incident rather than prevalent cases, and general population controls can be selected. Observation bias can be controlled by blinding subjects, interviewers, and persons assessing the data. Con-

founding can be minimized by restriction and matching. Also, confounding can be controlled for at the analysis level through stratification or multiple regression analysis.

4. Hospital controls are easily identified, sufficient in number, and relatively low in cost. They are more likely to be aware of antecedent events or exposures. They have similar selection factors to those of the cases and are more likely to cooperate. However, they differ from healthy people such that they do not accurately represent the exposure distribution in the population where cases were obtained.

   General population controls represent the population from which cases were selected. However, they are more costly and involve more time to collect than hospital controls. In addition, population lists may not be available, and it may be difficult for healthy people to participate with their busy schedules. Controls from the general population may also have poorer recall and less motivation to participate than controls from the hospital.

   Special groups are healthier than hospital controls, more likely to cooperate than general population controls, and provide more control of possible confounding factors. However, if the exposure is similar to that experienced by the cases, an underestimation of the true association would result.

5. Case-control studies can be relatively small and inexpensive, require relatively little time, and are useful for studying rare outcomes. They yield an odds ratio, which has nice statistical properties. They may, however, be problematic in establishing a sequence of events. There is also potential for bias in measuring risk factors. They are limited to a single outcome variable. They do not yield prevalence, incidence, or excess risk and are prone to selection and observation bias.
6. Select the cohort representing the population of interest. Exclude those who already have the outcome of interest or who are not at risk of developing the outcome. The cohort is classified as exposed or not exposed. The cohort may come from a single population or from two distinct populations (as in the case of a double cohort study). The unexposed group should look like the exposed group with the exception of the exposure. To minimize loss to follow-up, certain additional exclusion criteria may be necessary. To control for confounding, restriction may be employed. Data should be collected on known confounders in order to control for these factors in the analysis.
7. Selection bias caused by healthy worker effect or loss to follow-up. Confounding.
8. Confounding is evident when a crude measure of association (*OR*, *RR*) differs from stratified measures of association, but the stratified measures are similar. If the stratified measure of association differs across the levels of the stratified variable, then effect modification is present.
9. Prospective cohort study. A retrospective cohort study may also be possible, depending on available hospital records.
10. Prospective cohort study. Identify family members of persons with HIV/AIDS. Identify family members of persons without HIV/AIDS. The family members between the two groups should be similar in age, sex, race/ethnicity, and other factors, with the exception of being associated with someone with HIV/AIDS. Administer a validated questionnaire to both groups at baseline in order to ascertain stress levels, as well as to obtain information on demographics, behaviors, etc. This comparison will allow you to assess the initial similarity or dissimilarity between the two groups. Follow the two groups into the future, periodically assessing stress levels between the two groups. Compare stress levels between the two groups over time.

11.

	Coffee	*No Coffee*
Smoking	120	30
No Smoking	30	120

$$OR = \frac{120 \times 120}{30 \times 30} = 16$$

	MI	*No MI*
Smoking	100	50
No Smoking	50	100

$$OR = \frac{100 \times 100}{50 \times 50} = 4$$

CHAPTER 8

1. Ethical issues, interference with the doctor–patient relationship, administrative complexity.
2. Eliminates conscious bias caused by physician or patient selection, averages out unconscious bias caused by unknown factors, and makes groups alike on average.
3. Confounding
4. Bias
5. A therapeutic trial is an assessment of the efficacy of radiotherapy in prostate cancer patients. A preventive trial is an investigation of the efficacy of a new vaccine (e.g., poliomyelitis vaccine).
6. Factorial design
7. Factorial design
8. Run-in design

CHAPTER 9

1. a—confounding, b—recall bias, c—chance, d—chance, e—selection bias
2. c, b, a
4. Step 1: Academic performance in college is not associated with obesity 10 years after graduation, expressed in statistical terms as $H_0 : RR = 1$.

Step 2: Academic performance in college is associated with obesity 10 years after graduation, expressed in statistical terms as $H_a : RR \neq 1$.

Step 3: For this test, we use an α of 0.05. The sample size is large enough that chance is not likely to explain the results.

Step 4: $\chi^2 = 5.0$ and $df = 1$. The critical value for 1 degree of freedom and α of 0.05 is 3.841.

Step 5: $RR = 1.50$.

Step 6: Reject the null hypothesis because the observed value of χ^2 is greater than the critical value of 3.841. Interpretation: those performing better academically in college are 1.5 times (or 50%) more likely to be obese 10 years after graduation.

5. a. 170/880 = 0.193 or 19.3%

   b. 120/170 = 0.706 or 70.6%

   c. 0.944 or 94.4%

   d. If the prior probability (prevalence proportion) is obtained from the same data from which the test is evaluated, you may use the formulas for *PV*+ and *PV*– presented previously or the following simplified formulas:

$$PV+ = \frac{TP}{TP + TP} = \frac{120}{120 + 40} = 0.75 \text{ or } 75\%$$

e.

$$PV+ = \frac{TP}{TN + FN} = \frac{670}{670 + 50} = 0.931 \text{ or } 93.1\%$$

6. a. Stress Test Alpha

   b. Stress Test Delta

   c. It is desirable to minimize the proportion of false negatives and the proportion of false positives. For example, if you believe it is more important to minimize the proportion of false negatives because you believe it is critical that these people receive treatment, then Stress Test Delta is preferred.

7. For example, fair skin may predispose someone to sunburns and increase his or her risk of melanoma of the skin.

8. Direct involves a causal pathway with no intervening factors (e.g., an automobile accident and paralysis). Indirect involves a causal pathway with intervening factors (e.g., poor diet resulting in high cholesterol and high cholesterol resulting in arteriosclerosis).

CHAPTER 10

1. Attack rate
2. When the epidemic is confined to a localized area
3. Point source epidemic

CHAPTER 11

1. D—see Table 3.1 for examples of infectious communicable and noninfectious noncommunicable chronic diseases.
2. Behavioral, environmental, genetic, and social factors.
3. Chronic diseases tend to have long latency periods and a multifactorial etiology. On the other hand, infectious acute conditions tend to have a single causal pathogen.
4. Breast cancer. Only about 5% of breast cancers are thought to be due to inheritance of a particular form of a breast cancer susceptibility gene (e.g., Li-Fraumeni syndrome). Other risk factors include a history of certain benign breast diseases, early age of menarche, late age of menopause, exposure to ionizing radiation, obesity, first pregnancy at a late age, and not breastfeeding.

APPENDIX

III

Epidemiologic Associations and Societies

American College of Epidemiology (ACE)
Peter Kralka, Executive Director
1500 Sunday Drive, Suite 102
Raleigh, NC 27607
Phone: (919) 861-5573 Fax: (919) 787-4916
E-mail: fkenan@olsonmgmt.com
Founded: 1979

American Public Health Association (APHA)
c/o Sarah L. Patrick, Chairperson
E-mail: Sarah.Patrick@state.sd.us
Founded: 1872

American Society for Microbiology
1752 N Street, N.W.
Washington, D.C. 20036-2904
Phone: (202) 737-3600
Founded: 1883

The Association for Professionals in Infection Control and Epidemiology (APIC)
Phone: (202) 789-1890
E-mail: apicinfo@apic.org

Council of State and Territorial Epidemiologists (CSTE)
C. Mack Sewell—New Mexico, President
2872 Woodcock Blvd., Suite 303
Atlanta, GA 30341
Phone: (770) 458-3811, (770) 458-8516

International Epidemiological Association (IEA)
Dr. Chitr Sitthi-Amorn, President
Chulalongkorn University
4th floor, Institute Building 2
Phyathai Road, Pathumwan
Bangkok 10330, Thailand
Phone: + (66) 2 218-8141
E-mail: schitr@chula.ac.th
Fax: + (66) 2 253-2395

National Foundation for Infectious Diseases (NFID)
Office of Health Communication
National Center for Infectious Diseases
Centers for Disease Control and Prevention
Mailstop C-14
1600 Clifton Road
Atlanta, GA 30333
E-mail: ncid@cdc.gov
Founded: 1950

Society for Epidemiological Research (SER)
PO Box 990
Clearfield, UT 84098
Phone: (801) 525-0231 Fax: (801) 774-9211
E-mail: membership@epiresearch.org
Founded: 1967

Society for Healthcare Epidemiology of America (SHEA)
66 Canal Center Plaza, Suite 600
Alexandria, VA 22314
Phone: (703) 684-1006 Fax: (703) 684-1009
E-mail: INFO@shea-online.org
Founded: 1980

Index

Note: page numbers followed by "t" denote tables